Some reader's comments:

"Just have to say I am feeling great so soon on the reset! I get woken several times at night with our new-born baby but really feeling positive mentally and physically. I have always been a sugar addict and truly I have had no cravings, which is a miracle in itself. During this journey, I have curbed my lifelong habit of horrendous nail-biting and now have beautiful, long and strong nails. This is massive for me as I have never been able to stop this awful habit!!" Hannah Dunn, Rolleston, NZ

'My bowel has become my biggest area of concern in recent years, having been hospitalized in recent months with a bowel blockage and lifelong pain from IBS. At times my abdomen could be so distended and hard to the touch that I was mistaken for being 8 months pregnant! So it is a huge relief to me that this appears to be a thing of the past for me". Michelle Brown, Orari, NZ

It is a great inspirational book that makes so much sense. It inspired me to look at myself and take charge of my health, and I'm doing just that with positive results. I am so pleased I went on this journey, many thanks for sharing your knowledge with me". Ken Billing, Palmerston North, NZ

"The book is very informative, the fast is very hard to achieve, but the results are AMAZING. It really is worth all the effort; it changes your body and your mind". Clara Camargo, Nelson, NZ

"I have misplaced 10 kg since I started reading the book and then the reset. Have no plans to find it. Feeling really good, lots of energy and finding coping with winter mud on farm easier. Sleeping heaps better but still have mind detox to master. The best thing for me is that it is adaptable. It has been interesting that the good choices come easily now. My body is telling me what I need, not my brain. It's a lifestyle for me now and looking forward to the future". Dinah Osborne, RD Ashburton, NZ

TAKE CHARGE OF YOUR HAPPINESS, BELLY FAT & SEXINESS

A WOMAN'S RAPID RESET FOR BODY, MIND AND HORMONES

David Musgrave

Published by Waihi Bush Press, 83 Burdon Rd, Geraldine 7991 NZ

ISBN   978-0-473-45640-5

Contents

CHAPTER 1
A Woman's Rapid Reset for Body, Mind and Hormones

"Do not believe anything I say. Rather take from this book only that which holds the ring of truth for you"

Djwal Khul

Tara was having a wonderful day; all the women from the Moonstone Cave were out picking blueberries. Her lips were blue from the biggest and fattest berries that somehow just didn't want to go into the basket. The clear autumn sunshine was sparkling off the yellows and reds of the leaves of the woodland trees. Tara's happy laugh rang out as young Katyer, who was just budding into her womanhood and attracting the eyes of all the young men of the cave, was telling a funny story about how Kurt had been showing off the night before, trying to attract her attention and ended up flat on his bum.

Tara looked around to find her daughter Ursula, who was getting around so fast now on her chubby little legs, and had a moment of horror when she couldn't see her. Then there was a crash and a scream from around the corner of the blueberry patch, then Mummeeeeee! Tara rushed around the corner and to her horror saw a hole in the leaves where Ursula had fallen into the pit trap, dug by the men to try and catch a bear feeding on the blueberries. She flung herself on the ground and looked down the hole to see Ursula lying in a crumpled heap at the bottom of the pit, with a nasty looking gash in her leg from one of the sharpened sticks planted in the bottom of the hole.

Everyone else was gathered around by then, so she got Melanie and Lucie to hold her legs while she wriggled herself as far as she could get down into the hole, but she was still way short of Ursula's outstretched hand. Young Katyer, who was a renowned climber, often seen perched high on a rock on the cliff behind the cave, ran to grab her deerskin wrap which she had flung on a bush as the afternoon got hotter. "Here you go," she said, "you two hold this end and lower me down, and I will be able to reach her". To Tara's relief, Katyer soon had Ursula in her arms, as she rocked her to soothe her agitated cries for Mummy. Once Ursula had calmed down, they soon had them both out of the hole, and Tara had her baby safe in her arms again. Then all the other woman gathered around, laughing and crying with relief, stroking and touching Tara and Ursula to make sure she was real.

Then Melanie, who was the cave's healer, took charge, sending Katyer to run back to the cave to build up the fire and heat some water. She then ran her hands gently over Ursula's little body to make sure nothing was broken. "She's fine," she said, "let's get her back to the cave so that I can put some salve on that little gash, and we can all have a hot cup of herb tea to calm us all down".

My little story certainly seemed stressful for the women involved, but did the women's reactions sound like 'fight or flight' to you?

Observing these types of behaviors in women, it certainly didn't to a group of women researchers from California, who realized that the classic stress response of 'fight or flight' just didn't describe the way women behave under stress at all. They quickly realized that it was men who described the 'fight or flight' model, and it only applied to men.

They then went on to look deeper into women's hormonal response to stress, and used this information to describe a new model for the way that women respond to stress, which they called 'tend and befriend'.

I will come back to this new idea shortly, because it's important to understand how women respond to stress differently from men, as this has major implications for how you can organize your life to minimize the impact of stress on the way your body feels and on your wellness.

Have you heard of the idea of 'tend and befriend 'before? I would be surprised if the answer isn't NO, yet this important concept is not new science. This unique female stress response was first described seventeen years ago. Interestingly, a 2011 study showed that the time lag from the initial research to routine implementation in medical practice is usually about 17 years, but can be as high as 50 years.

This is why I wrote this book for YOU, because there is a lot of recent ground-breaking research which is not yet being applied by most health professionals, to help you achieve wellness.

Through an intensely patriarchal age, even much of what science, folklore, and food manufacturers got right (and a lot of what they got wrong) was based on either the studies of men or the priorities of men. That is only now beginning to change, with an increasing focus on the distinctive biology and chemistry of women. Women face different challenges from men and require different answers.

When I was in my early 40s, my youngest son had a bad reaction to his MMR immunization at the age of two and ended up with severe eczema and food allergies, and trying to scratch himself bleeding day and night. Two and a half years later somebody gave me a bottle of imported flax seed oil for him, saying, "it's really good for the skin". That turned out to be the understatement of the year, and within a couple of days, his skin was almost magically better (for the full story see www.ITookCharge.nz/Olivers-Story).

The scientist in me wanted to know how and why this had happened, so I started avidly reading the research literature about flax seed oil. What I read very quickly convinced me to start taking it myself, and even though I was pretty fit and healthy and ate reasonably well (I thought), I was amazed at the improvements in my energy levels and skin and just how well I felt all the time.

I was working as a research scientist in agriculture at the time, but I quickly decided to start my own company to bring the benefits of good tasting flax seed oil to New Zealand. So for the past twenty-seven years I have been studying nutrition and, more recently, how a woman's hormone system works so that I can design and manufacture food products that support wellness.

A few years ago, when a woman from a past relationship was in a very menopausal state, she told me "I am going to have to go on to HRT in spite of the risks, otherwise I will probably kill someone, and that's most likely to be you". That worked for me as an incentive to find out a whole lot more about woman's hormones, and within a couple of weeks she was on a supplement of natural progesterone and feeling wonderful and "like she was in the second trimester of pregnancy".

Again, the scientist in me wanted to know how and why this had happened and why so many women really struggle around menopause and their periods, which should be something that just happens naturally. This research led me on a path to where I was able to completely disappear my own quite severe prostate issues (which has similar hormonal origins) and ultimately to this book.

When I first set out on my journey to write this book, I struggled to see how a 72 year old agricultural scientist could credibly write a book for women on how to be well. There were already books on the market written by women doctors, but several factors that they were writing about didn't fit with the current science, as I understood it, so I decided to write it anyway.

When I was researching the chapter on stress hormones, I quickly came across the new 'tend and befriend' model. I hadn't read about this in any book on the subject (and I still haven't), but why not?

I suddenly had a 'light-bulb moment', that my lack of medical training is actually to your advantage in my writing this book, because I don't have any preconceived ideas on how things are, based on my training. This has left me free to bring you the current science as it really is.

The reality is that by modifying your lifestyle in the ways that I recommend in this book, is backed by current research, which supports the idea that your body has an amazing ability to heal itself, but only if you choose to support it to do that. Not many people choose to do the things necessary to achieve these results, but the important idea is, that you can if you choose to. This book is designed to support you through the process of choosing to do that for yourself.

For instance, for over 35 years Dr Dean Ornish has promoted a program scientifically proven to reverse heart disease. Since 2010 this program has been funded by Medicare and other health insurance companies in the USA. His program has now helped thousands of people who have chosen to take back their lives and many now live DRUG FREE. His comprehensive program teaches how to eat real food, reduce stress, exercise regularly and tap into the healing power of community.

"When you make big changes, you get big benefits. And you feel so much better, so quickly, that – for many people – those choices are worth making. Not only to live longer, but live better."
Dean Ornish, M.D

We have also known for some time now that similar approaches can also reverse diabetes, autoimmune conditions and cancer. As of 2014, we also now understand that the amyloid plaque, that we used to think was the cause of Alzheimer's, is actually your brains protective response to multiple assaults, from an inflammatory diet, infections, stress and toxins. So by addressing all these factors, we know we can, in most cases, reverse Alzheimer's and dementia. This is not to say that ongoing research won't improve on what we know now, but we do already know how to reverse the major health conditions of our day, if we choose to.

1.1
The Science of Women

Wellness for women includes some particular challenges.

Women have a more difficult time with their hormones than men, for the simple reason that you have a monthly cycle, which controls the ebb and flow of your sex hormones, driven by the lunar cycle. Everyone has a daily cycle driven by the rising and setting of the sun, called your circadian rhythm, that drives the ebb and flow of your stress, thyroid, and metabolic hormones. The complications that arise from overlaying these daily rhythms on top of a woman's monthly cycle makes a woman a lot more vulnerable to the effects of hormonal upset.

A simple example is that a healthy woman will be producing large amounts of progesterone immediately after ovulation, to prepare your body for if you get pregnant. However, your body uses progesterone to make the stress hormone cortisol, so if you are highly stressed around ovulation, making cortisol becomes the priority for your body. This will leave you low in progesterone, estrogen dominant, likely with PMS and feeling pretty miserable, because progesterone is a prime happy hormone for you.

A woman's path to wellness is littered with such paradoxes and challenges, which I aim to unravel for you.

1.2
The Science of Wellness

At the same time as I have been studying the science of wellness, I have been acquiring some wisdom about how I can be the best possible version of me, free of limiting beliefs and mind talk. As a result of these studies, at 72 years old I can now put my wellness as 99 out of 100. I can challenge myself physically, without my body limiting me in ANY way, and life is very full and wonderful.

I have discovered that not feeling old is not difficult; it just takes lots of knowledge and a little bit of self-love to motivate you to apply that knowledge. This book is my way of sharing all my knowledge and wisdom with you in the hope that your life can become as joyful as mine is.

I have drawn on 27 years of research into food and wellness and put it all together in one place, as a roadmap of a woman's path to wellbeing. You will not find all this information in one place anywhere else. Nor will you get it from your doctor because as an experienced research scientist, I have written this book based on the most recent published science - the way it really is; there have not been constraints to my thinking coming from prior medical training. And I have the benefit of having tested much of the science in satisfying my customers, and in forging my own path to wellness.

1.3
Where it all Begins

Let's see, you're feeling tired, overwhelmed, anxious, overweight, unsexy and often just plain cranky – you 'Feel Like Crap' (Dr Mark Hyman first talked about the FLC Syndrome – wonderful term!).

Add to that; you're totally frustrated with your weight. You've tried everything but failed, so you tried again, and you failed again.

This pattern really starts to do your head in and makes you feel like a failure, and you just want to give up as you start to fall into a downward spiral of low self-worth. Maybe you've even been to your doctor and been told: "I've run a few tests and they are all normal, so maybe you just need an anti-depressant ". If so, you're not alone. In fact, a staggering one in four women in the United States is on some form of anti-depressant medication.

Such a scenario is very common, but is this normal or necessary? Absolutely not!

So how does it happen that we feel like this so frequently in this modern world?

Unfortunately, our bodies evolved at a very different time, so cumulative effects of modern living tend to push your hormones and gut out of balance to the point that you start to Feel Like Crap.

To find the answer to why this happens, we have to go back around ten thousand years to when our species lived as hunter-gatherers as we moved out of Africa to colonize the world. What made us so incredibly successful as a species is our amazing brain that allowed us to develop the capacity for abstract thought and communicate a wide range of emotions.

Underneath that amazing human brain is the primitive core of your limbic system. Its key functions are to keep you alive and to urge you to reproduce. Unfortunately, our food supply in those days was often erratic, so our bodies developed some very powerful hormonal systems to make sure any excess food was stored for emergencies – as fat!

One of the key functions of your brain's limbic system is to continuously and unrelentingly scan your environment to see whether you are 'safe'. If it decides you are 'not safe' then it starts a hormonal cascade called the adrenaline response or very commonly called the 'fight or flight' response.

Now, this is where the confusion begins.

The 'fight or flight response' was first described in the 1930s by Walter Cannon and became the very widely accepted model to describe what happens to your body when you get a fright or come under stress. So the accepted picture has been that all the physiological changes that happen when you get stressed are designed to help you to either fight a lion, or the neighboring tribe, or if things get really sticky, be able to run away to save your life.

But most of the research that was done to develop this 'fight or flight' model was done on men!

In the hunter-gatherer societies we lived in for nearly 2 million years, the key role of men was to go out and kill animals for food or to defend the settlement from attack. This means that in men, the primary response to stress is to fight (confront the stressor with aggression) or flight (flee from it – or in the modern world, social withdrawal or substance abuse).

So for men, the powerful chemical cascade that follows from a surge of adrenaline, to prepare them for extreme physical activity and to minimize the damage to their body if they're wounded, is overlaid by the physical and psychological changes that come with a surge of testosterone.

1.4
Tend and Befriend

A group of researchers in California, led by Dr Shelley Taylor realized that this model doesn't describe the way women behave under stress at all (surprise, surprise). So their new model, which seeks to describe better how women behave under stress, they called 'tend and befriend'.

The inherent way women respond to stressful situations takes them into protective mode for their children and 'tribe' – the 'tend' part; and by seeking out a wider social group, usually women, for mutual defense (or calling your girlfriend or mother for support) – the 'befriend' part.

The major downside of this response, for an individual woman's health, is that whenever they are stressed, women have a very strong inherent urge to look after everyone else, AT THE EXPENSE OF LOOKING AFTER THEMSELVES.

It's clear from the latest research that this 'tend and befriend' response has evolved in the context of women being the primary caregivers for their children, when fleeing too readily at any sign of danger would actually put their children at risk.

All the adrenaline responses in women still happen, with the chemical cascade that prepares you for extreme physical activity and to minimize the damage to your body if you're wounded. The key difference from men is that instead of getting a surge of testosterone, for women their response is overlaid by a surge of the hormones oxytocin (your cuddle and bonding hormone) and estrogen (which reinforces the effect of oxytocin).

It is oxytocin which promotes the psychological behaviors that promote caregiving behavior and underlies the attachment between mothers, their children, their 'sisters' and their partners – the 'tend' part. Some studies also suggest that oxytocin enhances social contact and reduces aggression – the 'befriend' part.

In situations of long-term stress, the main stress hormone at work becomes cortisol, again overlaid with oxytocin, which gives you a hormone-driven way of being able to cope, which can have very subtle but highly undesirable effects on your feelings of self-worth and your feelings around your relationships.

The reality is that you're of reduced use to anyone else if you are not well, so making your own health a priority makes sense. Yet, if you're not dealing with your stress, then your stress hormones are giving your limbic brain a very subtle feeling that you need to look after everyone else first.

The programmed need to tend or look after other people means that you are likely to feel that you need to take on a range of tasks, just because "I'm fine. I can do that for you". In fact, others can probably take on these tasks instead of adding to your already stressful and overloaded day. You might recognize this: as you make lunches for your teenage children and partner, or maybe rushing home from work to prepare a meal for the rest of the family. When what you would really prefer to do is to pop into the gym for a 20-minute workout (Yes, that is all that it needs to take, see Chapter 13 Move Your Body).

Because you are already stressed and overloaded, adding another layer of tasks to be done can add to your feelings of "I'm not good enough" because the reality is, you are not fine. You're overloaded. So you start to feel overwhelmed. You can also set yourself up for feelings of resentment against the people you are tending, which can have a very damaging effect on your relationship with them.

Enter 'light-bulb moment' number two.

I was driving my tractor cultivating a paddock, which is always quality thinking/listening time for me. I was listening to a panel discussion by four women, all specialists in the field of female sexuality, who were discussing why many women struggle to have a healthy libido.

One of them mentioned that her husband often felt to her like "just another child she had to look after". This unleashed a chorus of agreement from all the women on the panel that they often felt the same way, and that feeling like this really messed with their desire to have sex with their partner. None of them had any real explanation as to why this should be so.

It suddenly dawned on me that this was the combined effect of their 'tend and befriend' response to stress, and the resulting lack of 'sexual polarity', yet none of these professionals in the field seemed to know anything about these effects.

You see, one other subtle effect which can happen if you take on doing tasks for your partner, which he or she is quite capable of doing (and maybe didn't ask you to do for them in the first place), is that you are actually treating your partner a bit like a child. If you really want to kill your desire for an intimate sexual relationship with someone, then you treating them like your child (or us behaving like a child) is a really good way to achieve this.

This was when I knew I had to write Chapter 17 Take Charge of Your Sexiness – now there's a challenge for a guy if ever there was one!

1.5
It's Not all Gender and Genes

Although the 'tend and befriend' model does emphasize the differences between the genders, there is no suggestion that your response to stress is written in your genes.

It really comes down to the question 'who am I?' and in any given situation we are very different people, depending on the circumstances.

So for example, the 'who I am' when I'm on the ski field, waiting at the top of a half-pipe, with six meter high snow walls, preparing myself to ski down, is a very different person from the person I am when I am cuddled up with my partner watching a romantic movie and the fire alarm goes off.

In the first situation, my body is in full adrenaline response, overlaid with a surge of testosterone, which puts me fully into my masculine energy. But this is eustress – a beneficial form of stress (because I chose it). I am doing this deliberately for the pure joy of pitting myself against the mountain.

In the second situation, my body goes into distress (I didn't choose it) and a full-on adrenaline response, but this time it is overlaid with oxytocin because we have been cuddled together, which puts me more in my feminine energy. So my first instinct is to make sure my partner is safe before I go to deal with whatever set the alarm off.

We can all think of how some women can behave in the work environment (when they tend to be more testosterone-fueled and in their masculine energy) when they are under stress they can be just as aggressive and in 'fight or flight' mode as any man. Similarly, when a man is looking after his children (when he tends to be more oxytocin fueled and thus more in his feminine mode), and the children are threatened, he will also likely go into his 'tend and befriend' mode to look after them.

It's important to realize that you are more than the primitive responses of your limbic system. You have the potential to modify how you respond to your limbic system's instinctive feelings, by using your higher cortical mind and your intelligence to find an alternative way of responding.

By being aware of these potential reactions to stress that may be happening in your life, then you may find a better way to talk to the others involved to find a solution that works for everyone. You may also be able to use the techniques described later in the book to get your stress hormone levels back in balance.

1.6
The Impact of Stress

It's important to realize that in any given situation, while the symptoms of stress in a man can be quite different from the symptoms displayed by a woman, underneath both behaviors, the entire stress hormone cascade is still going on, AND doing considerable damage to your body, if you do not take active steps to de-stress, ideally on a daily basis.

A lot of this book is about the impact of these stress reactions on how your body burns or stores energy as fat. It focuses particularly on how stress changes the way your brain and your gut work. Also on the way your body responds to changes in your body chemistry – particularly your thyroid hormones, your sex hormones and your metabolic hormones – in other words, 'your happiness, belly fat, and sexiness'.

This book is also about how to be well, and empowering you to choose to live a long and joyful life – the life of your dreams, without limitations imposed by your health and the way your mind works.

I find it sad that when I give a talk and ask my audience to tune into their body and choose a number between 1 and 100 on how well they feel, I have only once had someone put their hand up at 90 and many still haven't put their hand up at 50.

Personally, I will put my hand up for 99 and getting closer to the elusive 100.

At 72 years of age I don't do anything obsessively, but I mostly choose my food with some care (in other words I generally eat dark chocolate), and I do love butter (but saturated fats are NOT bad for you). I don't do exercise for exercise sake, but I am very fortunate that I can easily go out and ground myself in a very beautiful piece of nature and mostly get enough exercise working my 110 Ha organic farm. I do meditate most weekdays and usually do some yoga about once a week.

In other words, I don't stress if I don't do my 'routine' every day – because after all, it's what you do MOST days that determines your health and happiness - it doesn't matter if you miss occasionally. To me, one of the biggest benefits of doing my 'Rapid Reset' is the flexibility it gives me around being able to happily eat whatever food is on offer, without consequences. So, for instance, if I am eating out I will go for what looks the tastiest, or eat takeaways, without a second thought – life is not supposed to be difficult.

To me, it's important that even at my age my body doesn't limit me in any

I read recently, that if you have survived to reach the ripe young age of fifty, statistics show that you are probably about halfway through your life. If you are roughly in this age bracket, I suggest you ask yourself the question:

'Do I want to feel the way I do now for the second half of my life?'

If the answer to this question is NO, then it's time to take charge of your own health and make some changes, probably in several areas of your life.

The reality is that studies have shown that it's much easier to prevent health problems than it is to reverse them. So the longer you leave this decision to seek wellness, the more difficult it's going to be to get to a place where your life is full of juiciness and joy - which is surely where we all really want to be.

way. I will happily point my skis straight downhill for the thrill of speed (and last winter I once nailed three jumps in a row in the terrain park) or spin my partner on the dance floor in a fast milonga until we collapse laughing.

Trust me: getting old does not mean you have to forgo things you enjoy, or have brain fog, or be in pain, or tired, or have low libido, or 'Feel Like Crap'. I believe we were born to be happy here on earth NOW – not in some future realm. But we have to consciously choose to live for happiness and joy and not just let life happen to us, because of the unconscious choices we have made in the past.

That said, the food you eat gives your body very powerful hormonal messages – a calorie is not just a calorie. Food is information to your body, so your body and DNA respond to and metabolizes the four major food groups very differently - carbohydrates, proteins, fats, and dietary fiber.

This means that for most people, a few simple changes in the areas of your life detailed later in the book can make a major change to the way you feel within a few days – your Rapid Reset.

I have written this book around two basic premises.

1.7
How's your Three Legged Stool?

Firstly, that not feeling well in any area of your life is caused by your particular combination of the three following factors. These are what I like to think of as the three legs of the stool of wellness because if you neglect ANY of these three areas, your wellness stool will fall over at some point – probably when you least expect it.

The three legs of wellness are:

1.7.1
The Food You Eat

Do you get optimum amounts of the 40 odd 'essential' nutrients every day – the ones that your body cannot make for itself, so you have to get from your food or supplements?

Please focus on the word 'essential'; because lack of any of them in your diet every day means that the millions of new cells you are growing every day are less than perfect.

There are also a few foods that are no no's, which you do need to avoid actively (most of the time). Note that I deliberately said avoid, not eliminate (except maybe in the short term). Life doesn't have to be difficult to be fun.

1.7.2
Toxicity of the Mind

When we are young, our minds act as a virtual sponge and we believe pretty much everything that is told to us, including negative comments. Your beliefs are acted out in your (usually negative) mind talk – the unpleasant little voice at your shoulder, which I will call your 'ego', which brings a lot of mental and emotional stress into your life.

Every time you say "I can't do ..... because of ....." you are accepting a negative self-belief, which is not actually true, although your ego would like to have you think it is true. Similarly, most of us grow up with some form of the belief: "I am not lovable", which means that until you can let this belief go and love yourself; you are unable to enjoy the wonders of truly loving another person fully.

1.7.3
Toxicity in the Body

"The primary driver of chronic disease in the industrialized world is now environmental toxins" Joe Pizzorno, ND.

Unfortunately, our modern world is rife with chemicals produced in factories. While there are a few natural chemicals that are toxic, nearly every chemical produced in a factory is toxic to some degree, including so-called 'foods'. For instance, I include margarine as a toxic chemical; because there are no enzymes in nature that can digest margarine ('butter is back'

– see Chapter 11 Good Oils Make You Slim and Healthy).

Before the 1970s, the primary drivers of disease were the CHOICES you made, for instance, nutritional deficiencies, nutritional excesses, lack of exercise and smoking. However, over the last 50 years the use of chemicals in industry, farming, medicine and personal care products has increased dramatically. This background toxicity, driven by our widespread use of these chemicals, has led to a strong trend for people to become sick because of the PASSIVE EFFECTS of their exposure to toxins in their food and environment – it's no longer being driven mainly by your choices.

This background environmental toxicity, which is very difficult to avoid, means that unless you are actively supporting your body to detoxify on a regular basis, your liver, bowel, kidneys, and skin detox systems are almost certainly really overloaded and need your active support.

How these three factors manifest in you not feeling well is totally dependent on your unique combination of the fundamental factors outlined below. Nobody else in the world will have your exact combination.

1.8
The Thirteen Most Common Pancakes

My second premise is that ill health is ALWAYS caused by multiple factors, most of them coming from just living in our modern world. For reasons that I will explain later, I have chosen to call these factors: Pancakes. I explain my pancake theory in detail in Chapter 12 Detoxing Your Body and in Chapter 15 Heal Deeper.

For most of you, unless you are specifically working to minimize them, to a greater or lesser extent ALL these Pancakes will be impacting on your health. The rest of the book is devoted to explaining these Pancakes and how you can minimize or eliminate them, to restore the legs of your stool of wellness.

1. Ongoing issues with self-destructive mind talk from your ego, which seeks to keep you in the past or worrying about the future, rather than living in the NOW. Chapter 2 How Your Brain Works

2. Sufficient distress in your life to be causing your body some health issues from the elevated stress hormone levels. Chapter 4 The Effects of Stress on your Body

3. Issues with a stuttering thyroid, which comes from the impacts of toxins, stress and mineral deficiencies. Chapter 5 Your Energy Hormone - Thyroid

4. Less than optimum amounts of all the essential minerals you need to be well. Chapter 6 Thyroid – the Canary in Your Coalmine

5. Some degree of estrogen-dominance, which comes from our ongoing, widespread exposure to the toxic xenoestrogens in our environment and food, that disrupt your hormone balance. Chapter 7 Why Your Sex Hormones Are Out Of Balance

6. Some degree of insulin and/or leptin resistance and metabolic syndrome, because of your intake of sugar and refined carbs. Chapter 8 The Hormonal Reasons Why Diets Don't Work

7. Some degree of imbalance of your gut and skin microbiome and the leaky gut that goes with it, because of our overuse of antibiotics, sanitizers and prescription drugs. Chapter 9 Bugs Are Important

8. Some degree of gluten intolerance and damage to your body from eating too many refined carbs. Your genes for burning glucose for fuel are fully up-regulated, so you struggle to burn fat for fuel – you are 'glucose- adapted'. Chapter 10 Bad Carbohydrates Make You Fat and Sick

9. The EFA (Essential Fatty Acid) balance in your body is heavily laden towards Omega-6 dominance, and you are not eating enough undamaged fats. Your genes for burning fat for energy are down-regulated, so you are not able to efficiently burn fat for fuel, i. e. not 'fat-adapted'. Chapter 11 Good Oils Make You Slim and Healthy

10. Some degree of chemical toxicity, which is underlying some of your health issues. Chapter 12 Detoxing Your Body

11. A need to move your body a bit more (or maybe even a bit less) to achieve the wonderful benefits that accrue from exercise. Chapter 13 Move Your Body

12. Some degree of sleep deprivation and negative mind talk coming from your ego. Chapter 14 Detoxing Your Mind

13. Less than optimum amounts of all the essential vitamins, proteins and phytonutrients you need to be well. Chapter 16 Your 'Rapid Reset' Plan

The widespread occurrence in people's lives of all the thirteen Pancakes listed above can lead to extreme frustration in your search to alleviate your symptoms and achieve greater wellness.

Unfortunately, the majority of medical doctors are highly trained in 20th Century medicine, which focuses on 'what' you have, so they can fit your particular set of symptoms into a box called a 'diagnosis', which leads to a 'treatment' - usually a pill. (In fact, the better doctors are at finding a 'diagnosis', the more highly they are regarded by their peers).

When your body is telling you that things are just not right, it can be extremely comforting to get a diagnosis from your doctor. You finally know what's wrong with you. "Oh, the relief!"

The problem with a 'diagnosis' is that it tells you little about how your particular combination of diet and toxicity of the mind and body brought you to that place. So having a diagnosis can actually get in the way of you finding what changes you as an individual need to make to get you to a state of wellness.

1.9
The Big Three

We have known for some time how to prevent and even reverse conditions such as heart disease, obesity, and diabetes. Not many people choose to do that, but we know how they could achieve this if they wanted to. More recently we have learned how to prevent and even reverse cancer and Alzheimer's – this science is very new.

At the same time, as a population, we are getting fatter and sicker and the 'Feel Like Crap Syndrome' is increasingly common. Why is this? A big part of the problem is that there is an awful lot of money to be made from the existing system.

Big Food - produces abundant, cheap 'food', rich in available energy, but often almost devoid of available nutrients because it is processed at high temperatures, denaturing many of the essential proteins and vitamins. Many such foods contain lots of damaged oils and preservatives; both added to give them a long shelf life. Some also employ teams of scientists equipped with sophisticated brain scanners, to make sure that their products are very tasty, have exactly the right 'crunch' and light up the addictive centers of your brain as much as possible (See Chapter 10 Bad Carbohydrates Make You Fat and Sick).

Big Pharma - produces a wide range of drugs designed to suppress your symptoms, but which usually do not do anything to treat the underlying cause. They all come with side effects that affect some people, often necessitating another drug to suppress the side effects.

They all deplete your body of essential nutrients - which ones depend on the drug. For instance, statins seriously deplete your body of enzyme CoQ10, which is vital for your mitochondria (the little energy factories in your cells) functioning, which can leave you feeling low in energy.

Some drugs are little or no more effective than a placebo. For instance,

SSRI's widely used to treat depression are no better than placebo for mild to-moderate depression. Again, in spite of billions of dollars being spent on developing and testing drugs for Alzheimer's, the currently available drugs Aricept and Namenda, which are commonly prescribed for Alzheimer's patients to help to manage behavioral symptoms and to sometimes slow the development of more serious symptoms. The latest review of ten studies involving 2714 people has now shown that these two drugs actually increase the rate of mental decline and there are no drugs available yet to halt or reverse the progression of this scary disease.

Big Media – are highly paid by the first two to promote the status quo and to keep you confused about what to do best for your health. Dangerous myths, such as the old food pyramid from the USDA (1992), which promotes the high-carb-low-fat mantra, or that eating saturated fat is bad for your heart, are still widespread in the media.

In some cases, this disinformation campaign even extends to the scientific literature. In 2016 it emerged that in the 1960s, the sugar industry paid Harvard scientists to publish research in a prestigious, peer-reviewed Journal, which downplayed the role of sugar in causing heart disease, at the same time highlighting the hazards of eating fat.

"Given these three extremely well-funded forces working against you feeling well, is it surprising that you may struggle with your life and have some degree of FLC syndrome?" Me.

1.10
Functional Medicine

The 20th Century medicine model does an amazing job of helping with acute, or short-term conditions like broken bones, or a chopped off finger or a lung infection, or a baby born with a malformed heart. It is not well equipped to reverse complex, long-term chronic conditions like diabetes, thyroid malfunction, autoimmune conditions, heart disease, Alzheimer's, and cancer.

On the other hand, the rapidly evolving 21st Century medicine model now focuses on 'why' you have a particular set of symptoms, so that practitioners can use evidence-based medicine to understand the whole-body implications of your unique set of symptoms. They are also using technology to crunch the numbers as part of the process of learning to understand how our microbiome and other factors interact. So science and technology are disrupting the way we will practice medicine in the future, in the same way they are disrupting so many other fields.

Once they understand the 'why', a 21st Century medicine practitioner will work with you towards achieving a life free of symptoms. Such an approach is often called Functional Medicine or Integrative Medicine. To illustrate the importance of finding the 'why' for you - if your 'diagnosis' is that you have low thyroid function, presenting as low energy levels, and you are struggling with your weight, then this could have come from any of the legs of your stool of wellness.

1. The food you eat is lacking in the building blocks of iodine, selenium, and iron, and low in Omega-3. To deal with these issues, you would need to start eating and supplementing differently, in a comprehensive program, including some high-quality sea vegetables and an Omega-3 supplement, such as flax seed oil and move to a diet rich in healthy fats.

2. Your mind is not dealing with long-term stress coming from negative personal relationships, a job you really hate, or feelings of overwhelm about your life as a whole. Such stress leads to high levels of cortisol, which majorly interferes with your thyroid hormone function. I share some ideas on how to deal with such issues around stress in Chapter 14 Detoxing Your Mind

3. Toxicity in your body and/or leaky gut, often leading to Hashimoto's thyroiditis, which is an autoimmune condition, where your immune system starts to attack your thyroid gland. To deal with these issues you would need to undertake a comprehensive whole body detox program, with particular emphasis on your liver and gut and, in the short term, go onto a low carb, gluten-free diet as part of a strategy to allow your gut to heal.

As you can see from these examples above, what you need to do to correct the underlying low thyroid function, completely depends on 'why' it's malfunctioning in the first place. Taking a synthetic thyroid drug is unlikely to lead to you having a long and healthy life.

If you are fortunate enough to be under the care of a skilled Functional Medicine practitioner, you are likely to find that all your symptoms are reversed, by addressing some of the causes of your ill-health. Wonderful.

1.11
Heal Deeper

"Mainstream medicine ... in the Western World is focused on treating the smoke but ignoring the fire ... of inflammation"

David Perlmutter, MD, FACN, ABIHM

I personally believe we should aim higher than this, by addressing all thirteen Pancakes, which are almost certainly impacting on your health. In different ways, all these Pancakes cause inflammation, and there is a rapidly growing consensus among health scientists that uncontrolled inflammation is the major underlying factor in ALL disease.

The science around longevity is expanding rapidly, and there is some evidence that humans should be able to live a healthy and productive life for about 120 years. Can we really do this?

Up to now, there have been five so-called 'Blue Zones' identified, where people routinely live to be over 100 years. These hotspots of old age range from Sardinia in Italy, to Okinawa, Japan, to Loma Linda, California. There have been some things in common identified between these five zones. I address them all in this book.

In this book, I outline the factors that are causing inflammation in your body and my recommendations for a comprehensive set of lifestyle changes. These are all aimed at dampening down the fires of inflammation, to set you on the road to wellness.

This book is designed to empower you to make the choices you may need to make to modify your three fundamental factors, with the objective of helping you along your own journey to wellness.

I have had it said to me, "That sounds like a lot of hard work." I don't see it that way at all.

It has only taken KNOWLEDGE for me to feel wonderful at 72 and not feel limited by my mind and body. I don't see it as hard work to do any of the things I do. I see that my life is full of fun things to do, wonderful food to eat and wonderful, often challenging, but very satisfying, relationships.

"You can spend a lifetime learning from your own mistakes,
or you can spend lunch learning from someone else's."
Tony Robbins

The wonderful thing is, that once you start the process of becoming 'fat-adapted', your body mostly runs on ketones (little water-soluble packs of energy made from fat from your body or your food, that supercharge your brain and your body – see Chapter 11 Good Oils Make You Slim and Healthy) and fat, so it rapidly turns into a virtuous cycle.

So you have stable and abundant energy and a clear brain, which makes you more productive, so you feel good about yourself, so you can easily make time to exercise, or play with your partner, children or pets, which improves your relationships, which boosts your libido, and so you can easily make time to de-stress, which helps you to sleep better, which means you wake up in the morning full of energy, which makes it easy to make good choices about what you eat for breakfast and the rest of the day. It can often be as easy as that.

Only YOU can know the state of your 'stool of wellness' and its impact on your body and your life. This book is my gift to you, to give you the knowledge of the potential harm any shakiness in your stool's legs, or the size of your Pancakes, could be doing to you - 'the What'. I then give you the knowledge of what you can do to change things and so empower you to choose what you want to do about it – 'the How.

"Live as if you were to die tomorrow. Learn as if you were to live forever." Mahatma Gandhi

I hope you enjoy the journey to wellness. I am personally aiming for 169 years – my magic number.

"Fear is good because it tells us what we have to do, and the more scared we are of something, the more sure we can be that we have to do it."
Robert Kiyosaki

CHAPTER 2

How Your Brain Works

"Life is either a daring adventure, or nothing"

Helen Keller

I like to think of the brain as the conductor of the symphony, controlling the detail of what is going on at any one time. More importantly, it also controls the mood and tone of your body's behavior.

Like a great symphony, your body's health is all about balance, because it's when things get out of balance, for any reason, that you start to feel unwell.

Your brain conducts the symphony mainly by controlling when and how endocrine hormones are released in response to outside stimuli. In doing this, it responds to feedback loops between your brain and your body (particularly from your gut and your heart) that work to help keep things in balance.

2.1
Brain Structure

At an elementary level, when you look at a human brain the most obvious thing is that it consists of two hemispheres: the left and right hemispheres. Each hemisphere is unique in the specific types of information it processes, which I will talk about later. Normally, the two hemispheres are connected to each other through a broad band of nerve fibers deep in the brain (the corpus callosum) – and work together to generate a seamless perception of the world, with integrated input from both hemispheres.

If you could look at a live brain, the other very noticeable aspect is how soft it is (about the consistency of soft butter) compared to the very hard, ridged skull that surrounds it.

This is why you need to take care of your head, and playing sports like soccer, where you can be repetitively hitting your head against a hard ball doesn't make a lot of sense. (This is particularly so for young girls, whose higher functions are more concentrated at the front of their brain).

Modern technology has allowed huge advances in our understanding of how our brains work and has demonstrated that many of our previous ideas are just NOT CORRECT. It's not helpful to think of your brain as just a machine or computer that rusts or deteriorates with age. It's only in the last fifteen years or so that we have understood that your brain is always regenerating itself right through your life (which a machine cannot do), by growing new brain cells and new neural connections. We also know that how you live your life has a profound impact on how effective this process is.

We now know that it is NOT true that once you pass childhood, you don't grow any new brain cells, or that for every drink of alcohol you consume, you kill many brain cells, and they don't regrow (that myth was probably created by a parent of teenagers). By growing new neural connections and new brain cells, your brain can restore close to normal function, even from major trauma, stroke or dementia, and even allow someone on the autistic spectrum to normalize their behavior.

We now know that the way your brain grows and functions remains hugely plastic into old age – you should not accept that you cannot change your brain at any point in your life. However, to restore your brain function you will need to accept responsibility for pushing yourself to learn, eating the right building blocks (particularly Omega-3 and turmeric) and engaging in exercise most days to achieve this – there is no magic pill which will do this for you.

The great news is that there are newly developed simple steps that you can take to help support your brain during this process. Of course no two brains are alike, but therapies involving quality brain games (for example BrainHQ see www.ITookCharge.nz/Brain), light stimulation with a cold laser and modified musical soundtracks have all been shown to be effective in some cases. Such research has huge implications for a very wide range of conditions involving your brain, such as having a stroke or being diagnosed with autism or Alzheimer's.

Another idea that has been turned upside down is that specific areas of the brain are totally responsible for specific functions. We now understand that there is much more interconnectedness between areas of the brain than was thought, and much more overlapping of function.

For instance, there is an area right at the back of the bottom of the brain called the cerebellum which we used to think was purely about balance and fine motor control. Older tests for drunken driving, like walking in a straight line or touching your finger to your nose, were all about cerebellum function. We now understand that as well as fine motor control, the cerebellum is also involved in fine-tuning our intellect and personality, and our emotional processing.

We used to think there was an 'older' specific area buried deep in the brain, called the reptilian brain, which controlled all of our basic survival instincts, including our reaction to fear and fighting, our need to eat and have sex to reproduce. Surrounding that was a 'more recent' area called the limbic brain that we used to think was the seat of all our emotions.

Both these sections of our brain are more about survival, and perceive a world as a potentially frightening place filled with rivals competing for the same scarce resources. We now know that they process the information coming from all our senses and it either initiates our stress reaction or attaches an emotion to it. It's important to realize that any feelings of lack and scarcity come from our more primitive brain and that you can use the more recently evolved cerebral cortex part of your brain to choose not to dwell on these feelings.

While we now know that these basic survival instincts don't all happen in a specific primitive part of your brain, for the sake of simplicity and to allow you to relate what you might have read elsewhere, I am going to refer to the brain functions around these more basic survival instincts as the Limbic System and our higher brain functions as the cerebral cortex.

We will talk more about your limbic system and how it controls the production of hormones that control the way your body responds to stress, food and sex.

2.2
Limbic System

When you are new-born, the cells of your limbic system grow new connections in response to stimulation from your senses. Although your limbic system functions throughout your lifetime, it doesn't mature over time and is not aware of time in the same way your cerebral cortex is.

These factors mean that, even when you are an adult, when your emotional buttons get pushed you can have flashbacks and retain the ability to react like a two-year-old, which has profound implications for the way you respond to stress.

Recent research has shown that a child's brain operates mainly in what is known as a theta state, where the brainwaves only vary in frequency between 4 – 8 cycles per second. This state is where you learn most efficiently; you are at your most creative and tuned in to your intuition. However, this also means that until you were about six or seven years old, your brain was a bit like a sponge with no real judgment, so you tended to believe everything that was said to you.

This plays out in various ways, so for instance, if an adult says to you as a child, when you are happily singing away to yourself -"stop that horrible noise, you can't sing" you are likely to go through life with the belief you can't sing. (The reality is: if you can talk you can sing! – did your ego have a response to that statement? See if you can remember why).

Unfortunately, such reactions can go much deeper than this and affect your whole view of your self-worth. For instance, if an adult says something along the lines of "Aghh - you've done .... again, you're hopeless" that is likely to become ingrained in your mind as a belief that 'I'm not good enough' or 'I'm not enough'.

Or maybe as a baby, you didn't form a close attachment to your mother because of some lack of touch, eye contact, emotional unavailability, neglect or abuse. Such early-life trauma has been shown to powerfully affect your future self-esteem, social awareness, ability to learn and even physical health.

Such an event can then become wired into your ego's negative self-talk that 'I'm not enough' and which your ego then uses to beat you up. This can then become a major stressor throughout your adult life, affecting both your brain and your physical health, particularly your ability to maintain a healthy size.

Getting to understand which of your beliefs are real and which are not real, particularly if they came from your childhood, is an important part of the process of detoxing your mind.

2.3
Cerebral Cortex

The portion of the brain that separates humans from all other animals is the very deeply convoluted outer level, the cerebral cortex. Although other mammals do have a cerebral cortex, the human brain has one that is nearly twice the thickness and is believed to have at least doubled the functionality of the brains of any other mammals.

The cerebral cortex contains fields of neurons – cells that transmit nerve impulses – which we now believe are what make us uniquely human. These are the most recently developed neurons and they create circuits that give us the ability to talk, to think linearly as in complex language, to make music, and the ability to think in abstract symbolic systems like mathematics.

The wonderful thing is that this part of our brain is hardwired for joy, creativity and innovation, and asking the big questions like 'who am I'? It is the part of your brain that asks the question 'how can I live a long and healthy life without being affected by FLC, a debilitating illness or dementia?' (which is presumably one of the reasons why you are reading this book).

As you get older and your cortical cells mature, they become increasingly integrated into complex networks with other neurons throughout the brain. This creates the ability to choose to form a new picture of the present moment, rather than just reacting to the emotional response from the limbic system. The new information from your cerebral cortex allows you to re- evaluate responses triggered by your limbic or immature part of your brain, and purposely choose the more mature response.

2.4
The Feminine Life Force

The sages speak of "the feminine life force", which we now understand is associated with the role of the mitochondria in our cells. Almost all of your cells contain mitochondria, tiny structures which convert the energy from our food into energy that our bodies can utilize to sustain life and growth. Your mitochondria do contain DNA, but unlike the DNA from your cell nucleus which comes from both parents, your mitochondrial DNA only comes from your mother's egg cell, and so carries your matriarchal lineage – your feminine life force. (Because your mitochondrial DNA only mutates very slowly, a simple saliva test can show you what part of the world your mother's female ancestors come from).

Your mitochondria are much more than energy factories; they also regulate how every cell ages, divides and dies. In the normal course of events, damaged cells, such as cancer cells (which your body is forming all the time), are programmed by their mitochondria to die rather than to reproduce out-of - control to form a cancer tumor.

Given the role of mitochondria in energy metabolism, it is not surprising that your individual brain cells can each contain thousands of mitochondria. Although your brain only represents about 2% of the weight of your body, when your body is at rest your brain consumes about 20% of your body's energy needs. In the process of converting food into usable energy, your mitochondria also produce free radicals. Research has shown that fat burns cleaner and produces less free radicals in your cells, than when they are burning glucose (from carbs). It's like the difference between burning wood to cook your meal or natural gas – a lot less 'smoke' from the gas.

Free radicals can cause a chain reaction of oxidative damage if they are not mopped up by antioxidants. Because your brain uses such a lot of energy, it's very vulnerable to not getting sufficient antioxidants from your diet to mop up the free radicals produced in converting this energy, particularly if you are in a glucose-adapted state (see Chapter 11 Good Oils Make You Slim and Healthy).

If free radicals, sugar-damaged proteins, trans fats or toxins damage your brain's mitochondria, causing inflammation, then this sets in motion the destruction of some of your brain cells. Recent research has shown that these factors are the mechanism behind all degenerative brain conditions, including brain fog, Alzheimer's, Parkinson's, Multiple Sclerosis and Fibromyalgia.

Other organs in your body that consume a lot of energy, such as your heart, liver, kidneys and muscles also contain large numbers of mitochondria, even up to 40% of their weight.

2.5
Am I 'Safe'

Buried right at the bottom of the limbic system is the amygdala, which is the part of the brain that is constantly scanning your environment, your emails, and your marriage to see whether you are 'safe' – perhaps filling in the details with imaginary stuff when the threat is vague or unclear. i.e. "I'm sure he must be having an affair, he seems to be working late a lot". The amygdala also governs your fear and rage response.

As soon as your amygdala gets triggered by an unfamiliar or perhaps threatening situation, which may mean you are 'not safe", it almost instantaneously raises the brain's level of anxiety, focuses your attention on the immediate situation and changes the way your body works in a very dramatic way. You breathe faster. Your blood flow increases, as it is shunted away from your digestive tract and directed into your muscles and limbs, which might require extra energy and fuel for running and fighting. Your pupils dilate. Your awareness intensifies. Your sight sharpens. Your perception of pain diminishes. Your immune system mobilizes into high alert. Your liver releases a surge of glucose into your bloodstream.

Many of your body's responses get communicated via chemical messengers in the blood - hormones. However, there is a direct nerve connection between the limbic system and the adrenal glands, which are responsible for initiating your adrenaline response, so that this happens in milliseconds to potentially save your life. (We now know that there is also some energetic communication happening between parts of the body and even with other people – that 'magnetic' attraction is real and comes from your heart).

This is great if someone has just thrown a plate at your head, as it allows you to duck out of the way. Under these circumstances your attention is shifted completely away from the higher-reasoning activities to focus solely towards life preserving behaviors because of the needs of the present moment.

My Big Adrenaline Rush

In an evolutionary sense, the adrenaline response is designed to allow your body to move very fast and for you to have all the strength possible to allow you to cope with emergency situations.

While many of us have heard of the 'fight or flight' response, very few in this modern world have actually experienced situations where the 'fight or flight' response saves our life.

I want to share a wee story with you which illustrates a couple of really important things about the adrenaline response.

One day I was walking down into the farmyard with my wife, two young women and my young son. When we got into the yard, around the corner came a young bull that had been hand raised, so had no real fear of humans, but he had just had his first taste of a heifer in heat, and he was on a testosterone hangover.

When he saw us he just put his head down and charged, quite fast. Nobody had any weapons, but I was wearing steel-capped boots, so I went out towards him and kicked him in the nose as hard as I possibly could. That didn't do anything at all to stop him and the next

few seconds are a bit blurred, but I ended up standing pinned against a shipping container, with the bull's horns on either side of my pelvis and my hands on his horns.

That lasted a very short time before he flung his head sideways and just threw me into the air. I was flying through the air horizontally and tumbling, and when I was about half a meter off the ground, I happened to be in a position to look under my arm and saw the bull coming very close to me with a very nasty look in his eye. This made me realize "F... he's serious".

In the time it took me to drop from my body being horizontal and straight half a meter above the ground, I was able to twist my body, curl and land on my shoulder and roll in such way that I landed on my feet out of the bull's path.

So let's fast-forward the 20 minutes or so it took to get him under control and back in his paddock. I was due to leave to go to speak to a farmers' field day at that point, and while I was feeling a little bit roughed up, I felt not too bad. So I decided to get in the car and head off to the field day, which was about 40 minutes away. Half an hour later, when I was just going

through a small town and driving around a roundabout – I remember very clearly exactly when it happened – the adrenaline response just stopped, and suddenly my body hurt – a lot.

In fact, I had two broken ribs and pretty severe bruising, but up until that point when the adrenaline stopped, I really wasn't aware of that.

I guess there are two messages I would like you to take from this little story.

Firstly, just how amazing your body can be when you are in the adrenaline response. I still find it hard to believe that I was able to react so quickly to save my life from that bull. I have heard of people who have lifted a car off a loved one who's been pinned in a car accident.

The second moral of this wee story is that I really didn't know that I was living on adrenaline at the time that I decided to go to that field day. My body wasn't feeling the pain, and while I guess in hindsight, I was feeling a bit 'amped up', I had no idea that I was as badly injured as I was.

How much of your life do you spend running on adrenaline and not realize it?

2.6
'Fight or Flight' vs 'Tend and Befriend'

These self-preserving behaviors happen in response to a surge of adrenaline, which prepares your body for instant action.

The initial research that tried to explain the body's response to an emergency focused on the physiological and psychological changes that happened to men under stress. These were described as the 'fight or flight' response, which describes accurately the way that males tend to respond in an emergency.

While the limbic system controls instinctive behaviors, such as aggression and dominance, it now emerges that, for men, the functional changes that come from the adrenaline response (that prepares their body for extreme physical activity and to minimize damage from a wound), are overlaid by the emotional changes that come with a surge of testosterone.

Recent research has focused on the reality that the way women tend to respond to an emergency is more likely to be quite different from the masculine 'fight or flight' response. The more common feminine response has been called the 'tend and befriend' response. This better describes the instinctive nurturing response, which happens when a woman or her family come under any threat.

Both types of response have strong biological reasons for their development, which are based on the way that our society was operating up until about 10,000 years ago and how we managed brain activity at that time.

When humans were hunter-gatherers, men tended to be out hunting often dangerous animals for food and had to make instant decisions to fight or run away in dangerous situations. Their strength and hunting skills also made them the first line of defense when their settlement was threatened.

On the other hand, women tended to stay grouped in or around the settlement, gathering and preparing food, and looking after children. While the adrenaline response in women still happens, we now know it is overlaid by the release of the hormone, oxytocin.

Oxytocin is produced in all of us when we hug and kiss, or have skin contact, and is an important part of an orgasm. Women produce oxytocin more readily than men and also have lots of estrogens that enhance the bonding effects of oxytocin. Oxytocin is also an important component of what happens when women give birth or breastfeed. It is this powerful combination of oxytocin and estrogen that promotes caregiving behavior and underlies the close attachment between mothers and their children - 'tend'.

So in stressful situations, women are more likely to make physical contact or hug and kiss. Some studies also suggest that oxytocin enhances social contact and reduces aggression – 'befriend'.

In stressful situations women instinctively tend to look to other women for support as a mother puts the needs of children and others around them first – EVEN AT THE EXPENSE OF THEIR OWN HEALTH. Unfortunately, this tends to play out as a stressed woman looking after everyone else around her, rather than looking after herself. In this modern world the tendency for a woman to reach out to other women in her 'tribe' can be long phone calls to mum or a girlfriend, or the need to meet 'for a coffee'.

This hormonal difference means that fleeing or fighting are much less likely to be the first or primary instinct for women under stress as they tend to be for men. This is not to suggest that in some circumstances women can't be as aggressive as any man, or that your genes determine the way you behave – far from it. Nor do I want to suggest that men can't slip into a nurturing role in a stressful situation, if that's what their families need at the time.

It's just that the fight or flight model really doesn't describe the way most women respond to stress most of the time. More importantly, it doesn't describe the strong tendency of women not to put their own health first. How YOU respond to stress and deal with stress has major implications for your health.

2.7
Your Emotional Brain

"The human mind is not a terribly logical or consistent place."
Jim Butcher

When any of your senses are stimulated the messages are immediately processed first through the limbic system, so that by the time the message reaches your cerebral cortex or higher thinking center, you've already placed a feeling on how you view the situation. Is this pain or is this pleasure? Then you have the potential to modify the way that you respond to that information.

While many of us think of ourselves as 'thinking creatures that feel', because 'thinking' comes from our huge cerebral cortex, we actually feel with our limbic brain first. So we are really 'feeling creatures that think' – that's why we buy things because of the emotional response we get from them and then justify the purchase to ourselves (and our partners).

To put it another way, the feelings you experience – the emotional experiences of sadness, joy, anger, frustration or excitement – are the emotions that are actually generated by the cells of the limbic system.

But it's important to realize that the biochemistry of any emotional response by your limbic system only persists for about 90 seconds. You then have the ability to modify your response to your emotions through your higher thinking centers.

What this means in practice is that when you have an angry response   to something, if that angry feeling in your body lasts for longer than 90 seconds, then your higher thinking centers have actually made a choice, whether conscious or unconscious, to continue to feel and probably express your anger.

I find it a huge help in being able to let go of anger to ask myself the question "why am I choosing to stay angry with this person I love". It's not the easiest question to ask in the moment, but I find I am getting much better at asking it over time.

"It's important to realize that the biochemistry of any emotional response by your limbic system only persists for about 90 seconds. You then have the ability to modify your response to your emotions through your higher thinking centers."

2.8
Right Brain

The right brain deals primarily with the global picture and right here, right now.

It is more concerned with the richness of the present moment, and when you are governed more by your right brain, then you are likely to be enthusiastic, carefree and friendly.

You may notice that one person is taller than another, but there is unlikely to be a judgment made, so to your right brain you are all equal members of the human family.

Your right brain is more open to new possibilities and more likely to think outside the box, so tends to be highly creative and willing to try something new with enthusiasm.

The language areas of the right brain seem to supply a wider sense of context and more global meaning.

More importantly, your right brain seems to be more open to the eternal flow, where you exist at one with the universe, right now. It is less likely to be bogged down by your past or fearful about the future and what that may or may not bring.

2.9
Left Brain

In contrast, the left brain is more about the detail of the local picture and organization. It has an amazing ability to process huge amounts of information, and from that identifies patterns. It specializes in being able to categorize, organize, describe, judge and critically analyze absolutely everything – including all the energy and information about the present and intuitive possibilities created by your right brain.

It is also an amazing multi-tasker and partly measures its value by how many things that it crosses off your to-do list.

Your left brain thinks in language, particularly the precise meanings of words and sequences. The language center of your left brain works to make sense of the world based on minimal amounts of information, by taking whatever details it has to work with and weaving them together into a story.

Unfortunately, this means that sometimes it will fill in the blanks with stuff that it makes up in the form of alternative scenarios or 'what if' possibilities, as it tries to fill the gaps between what you really know and what seems likely to fit. This can seem like the stirring up of drama and trauma that may play out as thoughts such as "what did that look between .... and his secretary mean at the party tonight? What if they are having an affair", and similar scenarios.

Your left brain seems to be the primary seat of your ego - the unconscious mind talk in your head that speaks to you almost constantly about the past or the future, unless you are fully present. Your ego can spend a lot of time and energy degrading, insulting and criticizing yourself (and others) for having made wrong or bad decisions, as your left brain runs rampant on automatic.

It is your ego or unconscious mind that has the capacity to allow you to be a sore loser, hold a grudge, tell lies and even seek revenge.

2.10
Your Unified Brain

For most people, the two hemispheres of the brain complement each other and give you a seamless perception of the way the world is. So most people are really good at utilizing the different skills and different characteristics of the two sides of the brain, allowing them to support and complement each other.

Some of us can be a bit more unilateral in the way we think and can either:

- Exhibit rigid thinking patterns that are analytical and critical (extreme left-brained).

- Seldom connect to a common reality and live with 'our head in the clouds' (extreme right brain).

Creating a healthy balance between your two characters gives you the ability to remain flexible enough to welcome change (right brain) yet remain connected enough to follow through with a plan (left brain).

2.11
How to Combine the Best of Both Sides

The exciting thing about understanding the differences between your right and left brain is that you realize you have a choice in how you react. For instance, if you approach me with anger, then I can either choose to reflect your anger (left brain) or approach you with a loving heart (right brain) and diffuse your anger.

The limbic system automatically triggers the angry response, lasting about 90 seconds (as mentioned above), as it attaches a feeling to the outside stimulus. While it's certainly easier to stay with the preprogramed reaction of the limbic system and your left brain, (which tends to be what your ego wants you to do). The path to a more joyful and productive life is to recognize the power your cerebral cortex gives you to make a choice, and respond in a more positive way in any given situation.

Being proactive in this way means starting to take responsibility for your choices and hence the direction your life moves in.

"The reality is that whatever your life is now, is absolutely the result of the choices you have made in the past. Maybe many of those choices were not conscious, but you still allowed things to happen, which is an unconscious choice." – Me.

If you don't like the way your life is now, then it would be great if you could accept that you have created your life, no one else did it for you, which is the beginning of you starting to get better at making choices. The beginning of change starts with you accepting that you are more than your life now, so that you want to change.

The personal development coach Brian Tracy, suggests that if something feels like it has gone wrong for you, if you get triggered, and you feel out of control, tell yourself "I am responsible." You might be upset and pissed off, but keep saying it to yourself, and keep looking at it from the angle of how you are responsible - only then will you discover the way in which you are responsible. Only then will you see ways of changing your situation and giving yourself more power in the process.

I will talk much more about how you can retrain your brain to make better conscious choices later in the book. For now, I want to talk about how what you eat can impact on how your brain functions.

2.12
Inflammation and Your Brain

Inflammation is part of the healing response as a kind of spot treatment. The swelling and redness and pain that occurs around a healing cut or an insect bite or an overextended joint, is all part of your body's mobilizing of resources to heal the damage.

If however, the body is under constant attack from an irritant like gluten, or in fact any other toxin, then the immune system turns the inflammation response on and it can stay on. This leads to the immune system pumping out chemicals like inflammatory cytokines, which are carried throughout the body by the bloodstream and across the blood-brain barrier into the brain.

This shows up as the presence of antibodies to the irritant, created by your immune system or increase in systemic inflammation in your blood and your body. This uncontrolled inflammation is widespread in western cultures. There is now a lot of research linking such inflammation to being the fundamental cause of ill-health and early death associated with heart disease, diabetes, Alzheimer's, cancer and virtually every other chronic disease you can imagine.

It's easy to think of arthritis as an inflammatory condition because we can see the redness and swelling and feel the pain, so we see the connection between the arthritis and (if we choose to use them) your doctor prescribing drugs such as ibuprofen and aspirin, which are marketed as anti-inflammatory drugs.

It's probably not quite so easy to see the connection between inflammation and heart disease, because we can't see the redness, swelling or feel any pain, but the research is showing that unchecked inflammation is a major contributing factor to heart disease. (Of course, we have been conditioned to think that high cholesterol has this role). But you can probably accept that your doctor prescribing a low-dose aspirin is a useful tool in reducing the risk of heart disease and strokes, which it does by reducing inflammation and thinning the blood.

It can be even harder to see the connection between brain inflammation and everything from multiple sclerosis and epilepsy to autism, depression, and Alzheimer's. Like the heart, we can't see the redness and swelling or feel any pain (because the brain has no pain receptors) but recent research is clearly showing that an inflamed brain is the primary cause of these conditions. While the use of anti-inflammatories to treat such conditions is not common, their use has reduced the risk of Alzheimer's and Parkinson's in a couple of studies, so that some doctors may prescribe them for this purpose.

2.13
Eating for Your Brain

2.13.1
Omega-3

Your body is very good at creating what it needs, where it needs it, because it is encoded in your genes.

You are probably aware of the need to get adequate amounts of the Omega-3 long-chain polyunsaturated fatty acids, DHA (Docosahexaenoic acid) and EPA (eicosapentaenoic acid) in your diet. These are commonly found in fish oils. These are both important building blocks for your brain, particularly DHA. Your brain is around 60% fat, and about 20% of that should be these Omega-3's.

If you are a mother, you are likely aware that your baby's growing brain needs a lot of Omega-3. For most women, the first pregnancy is not usually a problem as the baby can usually extract enough Omega-3 from your body without you having any noticeable symptoms. However, if you do not consciously rebuild your Omega-3 stores before any subsequent pregnancies, then your baby will be at much higher risk for learning disabilities, and you will also be at higher risk for postnatal depression.

It seems your brain is also particularly efficient at converting the shorter chain Omega-3 ALA (alpha-linolenic acid), found in vegetable oils like flax seed or chia seed oil, into the DHA it needs. When people were supplemented with flax seed oil, the amount of ALA and EPA measured in their blood went up, but the amount of DHA in the blood didn't change. However, when they measured the changes in Omega-3's in the brain, the amount of DHA had also gone up. This is not entirely surprising given that our species evolved on the plains of central Africa where there was not a lot of access to high DHA oil from seafood.

To have a vibrant, healthy brain requires you to consciously make sure you get adequate Omega-3 in your diet.

2.13.2
Gluten Sensitivity

I am sure you are asking at this stage "why is he talking about gluten in a chapter on the brain". It's likely that the first thing you think about in relation to gluten sensitivity is gut problems and coeliac disease. Until recently you would have been considered completely correct, but we are also starting to understand that gluten can also contribute to a leaky brain.

We now know that gluten sensitivity is a major causative factor in developing the leaky gut syndrome that drives a lot of inflammation in the body. Similarly, gluten can cause the gaps between the cells in the blood-brain barrier to open up to allow foreign particles into your brain, which contributes to brain inflammation and brain shrinkage. Yes, size really does matter when it comes to your brain.

While the science on this subject is very new, some researchers working in this field are finding some degree of allergic reaction in over 90% of the people they are testing.

I explore this issue in greater detail in Chapter 10 Bad Carbohydrates Make You Fat and Sick

2.13.3
A High Carb (Carbohydrate) Diet

The latest research is showing that, as a population, to a very large extent the high levels of fast carbs we consume on a regular basis, are driving the rapid rise in obesity, diabetes, dementia and Alzheimer's. Science now understands that the high levels of blood sugar, which go with insulin resistance and diabetes, are also negatively affecting the brain.

If you have chosen to go with a 'low fat' diet, you might not have thought of your diet as being 'high carb.' However, the reality is if you are not using fat for fuel (being 'fat-adapted') you are either eating lots of carbs to provide your energy or your body is having to make carbs from your protein intake.

When blood sugar levels are high, glucose can damage proteins by attaching to the protein to form what is called a glycated protein. It is these damaged proteins which are one of the key factors driving the physical damage seen in brains with Alzheimer's, for instance.

We have known for a long time that brain disorders and dementia are associated with brain shrinkage, but the research which is showing that such brain shrinkage can happen as a result of blood sugar spikes is very recent. Research is also showing that the blood sugar levels linked to these results are not unusually high. This is why dementia is starting to be referred to as Type III diabetes, because it shares the common origin of uncontrolled blood sugar levels.

2.14
Busting the Myths

Just to be clear, what I'm saying probably challenges some long-cherished beliefs. It's true that many years ago these beliefs were formulated as scientific theories, which is a legitimate part of how science works.

Unfortunately, many of these theories have been comprehensively shown to be not correct. They have since been shown to be myths, which do nothing to help you along the path of wellness. Unfortunately, these same myths help to ensure that some very large industries make an awful lot of money, which means they can afford to spend a lot of money to maintain the myth and stop us learning the truth.

The three most dangerous myths are the following:

*   A low-fat, high carb diet is good

- All cholesterol is bad
- Saturated fat is bad

I repeat, these three statements have no current scientific backing so please, for your health's sake, accept that these three statements are simply not true. More on this later!

CHAPTER 3

It's Not You; It's Your Hormones

"Hormones can either make you feel like crap, or like a rock star, ready to take on your mission"

Sara Gottfried, MD

Your body produces hormones in amounts that are constantly varying dynamically, in response to what is happening in your body, what's happening in your environment, and what's happening in your mind. Your body makes them on a moment-by-moment basis. Your hormones are your control messengers in a vast, interrelated body-wide network. These hormones are chemical messengers, which essentially control who you are - your behavior, emotions, sexiness, immune system, and how you burn food as fuel.

Yes, you can attempt to use willpower to change your behavior, but that's incredibly hard to sustain in the long term when, for instance, your hormones are telling you loud and continuously that you need to store more fat!

Similarly, it can be very difficult to respond positively to your partner's suggestion to make love if your levels of estrogen, progesterone, and testosterone are out of balance and you have zero libido.

So, to a very large extent, it is your hormones and biochemistry that drive your behavior.

Your endocrine glands, which include your adrenal glands, thyroid, ovaries, pancreas, and adipose tissue (fat cells), produce an incredibly complex range of hormones. They release these hormones into the bloodstream, enabling them to travel throughout the body carrying messages to every cell and controlling many important functions of the body.

This also means that they must be removed from your body when they are no longer needed. It is one of the key roles for your liver to break down such hormones ready for excretion out of your body, to maintain your hormonal balance and wellness. This means that if your liver/gut detoxification system is overloaded, your body is not clearing your excess hormones efficiently, making it hard for your body to maintain hormonal balance. There is a continuous cross-talk between your brain and your gut and every other part of your body, so what is happening in one part of your hormonal system will ALWAYS influence all your other hormones. Nothing ever goes on in isolation in your body.

For instance, the building block for many of your hormones is cholesterol, but your body is all about survival, so its priority is to use cholesterol to produce cortisol, for without cortisol you would die. Unfortunately, your sex hormones are also made from cholesterol, so if your body is low in cholesterol and you're very stressed and producing lots of cortisol, then you don't make many sex hormones, and life isn't much fun.

One of the reasons that women are more susceptible to the impact of stress than men is that having high cortisol levels can not only reduce your production of progesterone, but it can also block your progesterone receptors and getting the progesterone signals into your cells is key to you being a happy woman.

Your hormonal system is incredibly complicated, and the brief description that follows is only to highlight some of the more important hormones and some of the interactions that I think are important for you to understand for your journey to wellness.

3.1
Your Three Musketeers

This very powerful quartet, are the guys you really want on your side in taking charge of your happiness, belly fat and sexiness, and they are the key ones I will be talking about in the rest of this book. They are your Stress Hormones, your Thyroid Hormones, your Sex Hormones, and your Metabolic Hormones.

3.2
Stress Hormones

The main hormones that control how your body responds to stress and life-threatening situations are adrenaline and cortisol. Both of these are mainly produced by your adrenal glands, which sit on top of your kidneys. However, recent research has shown that your gut is also a significant producer of cortisol, which is perhaps why your gut is often where you first feel 'stressed'.

Your adrenal glands also produce aldosterone, which helps to regulate your blood pressure and the mineral balance in your body. Your aldosterone levels are closely related to cortisol levels, so if you are stressed, and your cortisol level is high, then your aldosterone levels are almost certainly high as well. This can lead to high blood pressure, low potassium levels, and muscle cramps.

If you get to the point of adrenal exhaustion, which goes with long-term stress, then your cortisol levels plummet, as do your aldosterone levels. This leads to low blood pressure, a high pulse or palpitations, and a craving for salt. Big clue: if your dog loves licking your legs this is a good indication that you are losing salt and may be low in aldosterone.

As I said, it's complicated.

The importance of your stress hormones is explained more fully in Chapter 4 The Effects of Stress on your Body.

3.3
Thyroid Hormones

Your thyroid gland in your throat produces two key hormones, T4 (thyroxine – relatively inactive) and T3 (triiodothyronine – the active one) and small amounts of T2 and T1, which appear to be only active within the thyroid.

The amount of T3 that your body produces is key to you feeling energized, and comfortably warm, and is a big part of managing your weight. If you're not making enough of this hormone you are likely to have problems with brain fog, ongoing tiredness, weight gain and constipation, and in the long term, you are at greater risk of Alzheimer's.

Unlike your stress and sex hormones (made from cholesterol), the key building blocks for your thyroid hormones are the amino acid, tyrosine, and iodine – T4 is 65% by weight of iodine. Adrenaline and dopamine are also made from tyrosine.

Your body can make tyrosine from other amino acids but under prolonged stress, needing lots of adrenaline, your body might not be able to make enough tyrosine. However, there are many good food sources of tyrosine. All animal and fish proteins, eggs, beans, peanuts, and almonds all contain useful levels of tyrosine, so getting enough in your diet is not difficult.

The importance of your thyroid hormones is explained more fully in Chapter 5 - Your Energy Hormone - Thyroid

3.4
Sex Hormones

The key sex hormones are estrogen, progesterone, and testosterone (Yes, women also produce some testosterone). These guys are responsible for your menstrual cycle, keeping your joints and vagina lubricated and maintaining your libido, and they help regulate your mood and emotions, sleep, vitality, fluid retention and body shape.

In women the main source of your sex hormones is your ovaries, but your adrenal glands and fat cells also produce sex hormones. A significant amount of your progesterone is made in your adrenal glands, so this production tends to get shut down when you are stressed and your adrenal glands are prioritizing making stress hormones.

Fat cells are quite active producers of estrogen so, particularly after menopause, the amount of fat you carry can have a significant effect on the total estrogen loading in your body, which can lead to estrogen dominance.

How your sex hormones interact is described more fully in Chapter 7 Why Your Sex Hormones Are Out Of Balance

3.5
Metabolic Hormones

Your key metabolic hormones are Leptin, Ghrelin, and Insulin.

The full description of the role of your metabolic hormones in your journey to wellness is described in Chapter 7 The Hormonal Reasons Why Diets Don't Work

3.6
Other Important Members of the Team

3.6.1
Oxytocin

Oxytocin is a brain hormone, which is often called the 'love hormone' because your levels of oxytocin tend to be higher during intimate experiences. However, your oxytocin levels are also raised during stressful experiences, particularly in women as part of their 'tend and befriend' response to stress.

Psychologically, higher levels of oxytocin create feelings of calm and closeness. This calming effect can be very useful in a stressful situation because losing your cool in a dangerous situation can very quickly make things go pear-shaped if your children pick up on your panic.

Oxytocin plays a very important role in bonding with people, but has other roles, particularly

Oxytocin is also often also called the "cuddle hormone" because physical contact is a powerful way of raising your oxytocin levels. When I first discovered this, I initiated what I call an "oxytocin hug" in my family, lasting about 20 seconds.

Try one of these with someone important in your life and notice how, during an extended hug like this, you will start to feel calmer and closer to the person you're hugging – a delicious experience.

The effect is multiplied many fold if you have direct skin-to-skin contact in the hug, which is a very powerful argument for sleeping naked with your partner to enhance your feelings of closeness, intimacy and bonding with them.

during pregnancy, birthing, and breastfeeding, in regulating the birthing process, and in creating the amazing bond that happens between mother and child. If the contractions are not strong enough for delivery in the third stage of labor the mother will often be given some synthetic oxytocin to help move things along.

Normally, the levels of oxytocin continue to rise after a birth to help contract the uterus and stop bleeding. This whole process can be aided by the mother being given the naked new-born baby to hold on her chest, as skin-to-skin contact is a powerful way to raise your oxytocin levels. If, for some reason, this bonding process doesn't really happen – often the case with nervous first-time mums – this can be another situation where oral oxytocin may be used.

Of course, skin-to-skin contact is also part of the sexual act and encourages the desire to be kissed and cuddled by your lover. Just being touched raises your oxytocin levels; this creates increased sensitivity to touch, especially in your erogenous zones around your neck and genitals. It also creates feelings of intimacy and desire, which enhances the desire to be touched further.

This all works in a delicious spiral eventually leading to orgasm. Oxytocin and dopamine are the two hormones released in large quantities during orgasm, to generate the intense feelings of happiness and pleasure.

Women actually need more oxytocin to reach orgasm than men, which is a key reason why a 'quickie' seldom does it for a woman. During peak sexual arousal a woman's level of oxytocin can reach levels much higher than a man's during orgasm, which is one of the reasons why she is capable of enjoying multiple orgasms more easily than a man (See Chapter 17 Take Charge of Your Sexiness and the sequel to this book for men).

We know that oxytocin can also promote good health by boosting our immune system. For instance, oxytocin plays a role in why pet owners heal more quickly from an illness; why those in relationships live longer than singles; and why support groups can help for people with chronic diseases or addictions.

Oxytocin seems to do this by its calming effect and by helping to achieve restful sleep. While we don't completely understand how this works, it seems that the key reason is oxytocin's powerful ability to counteract the effects of your stress hormone cortisol.

3.6.2
Serotonin

Serotonin is your happiness or contentment hormone, but it is also involved in regulation of your appetite, digestion, sleep, mood, memory, pride and self-esteem, and sexual desire.

Most people think of serotonin as being a brain hormone, but actually around 90% of the serotonin in your body is made and used in your gut. Your gut is increasingly being called your second brain (ever had a gut feeling?) and there is a fascinating new field of research showing that the composition of the microbiome you have in your gut, really matters for your brain health. There are even strains of probiotics being developed which can enhance serotonin production (See Chapter 8 Bugs Are Important).

A highly refined or high GI (Glycemic Index) carb intake increases your blood sugars, which immediately depletes the feel-good brain hormones serotonin, dopamine and GABA (gamma-aminobutyric acid – see 3.9 GABA), which can severely affect mood and feelings of well-being. It gets worse if the refined carbs include gluten, because for many people gluten causes a degree of inflammation, which also blocks the production of your feel-good brain hormones (See Chapter - 9 Bad Carbohydrates Make You Fat and Sick).

Serotonin is one of the main brain hormones you need to feel happy, and one of the ways to get a very short-term increase in the amount of serotonin your body makes is to eat lots of sugar. This happens because the protein precursor to serotonin is the amino acid, tryptophan, and when you get a surge in blood sugar, the insulin spike to get the sugar out of your bloodstream also removes all the amino acids, except tryptophan. So you get a brief burst of disproportionately high tryptophan levels into the brain, which gives you a short-term increase in serotonin and feeling good, followed by a crash when your blood sugar plummets because the insulin spike has driven all the sugar into your cells.

So if you're low in serotonin and feeling unhappy, then you are very vulnerable to bingeing on comfort food. Over time this see-saw effect can lead to sugar cravings, but your brain eventually becomes desensitized, and using sugar in this way often ends up as mood disorders.

Sugar also works to generate the pleasure response from a dopamine release, (see below) which makes you doubly vulnerable to craving high-sugar foods on a bad day. For instance, a good friend of mine wrote a very funny song called "When you're feeling down the best way up is chocolate" – so true!

The other way to get the same happy effect that you get from sugar, but without the nasty crash afterwards, is to work out. This is because exercise works in a very similar way to insulin to move all the other amino acids from your bloodstream into your muscles, except for tryptophan, which enhances your serotonin levels. Studies are showing that moderate exercise works better to lift your mood than any antidepressant drug (See Chapter 13 Move Your Body).

Your natural rate of serotonin production is partly dependent on your exposure to sunlight, which is why some people get the winter blues when they are not getting enough sunlight exposure.

A very powerful way of enhancing your natural serotonin production is to combine the above two effects: go out and exercise in nature and come home feeling really good about yourself. It works way better than an expensive gym membership!

"The other way to get the same happy effect that you get from sugar, but without the nasty crash afterwards, is to work out..."

The fact that serotonin is involved in your feelings of happiness has led to the theory that if you could reduce the rate at which serotonin is removed from around the neurons, you would have a cure for depression. This has led to the production of huge quantities of a range of drugs called SSRI (serotonin reuptake inhibitors – e.g. Prozac, Wellbutrin etc.), which are designed to maintain high levels of serotonin in your brain, and in theory, stop you being depressed.

Do they work? – Unfortunately, for mild-to-moderate depression they are little or no better than placebo, so no they usually don't. They are, however, very widely prescribed by doctors because of very effective advertising by the drug companies. While they can level out your mood to some extent, so they may help to relieve the lows, they also prevent the highs, making life feel flat, and many women feel like they have a "chemical brain".

Unfortunately the high level of serotonin lingering around your neurons from the use of such drugs inhibits your own natural production of serotonin and leads to your own serotonin having a reduced effect on your mood in the long term.

It gets worse. The lack of highs also relates to sex as well and sexual side effects of SSRI's are relatively common (somewhere between 36% and 98%), so the feelings of arousal during sex and the intensity of the orgasm can be greatly reduced.

Moreover, worse yet, these side-effects don't necessarily stop when you stop taking the drugs, so you are vulnerable to increased feelings of suicidality, and a very large study of post-menopausal women on antidepressants showed a 45% increased risk of stroke and over 30% increased the risk of death from all causes. There is even an internet community called 'persistent SSRI sexual side effects'.

My recommendations in Chapter 16 Your 'Rapid Reset' Plan will do a lot to improve your serotonin levels, and this may be sufficient for many women, but I will give you some alternatives if you feel you need additional support.

3.6.3

Dopamine

Dopamine is the 'reward' brain hormone, which has many complicated effects on the body. This is the biochemistry that drives your feelings of pleasure and satisfaction, but it also has to do with lust and love and milk production and addiction and movement and motivation and attention and psychoses.

Dopamine works with leptin, cortisol, and melatonin to regulate your daily body rhythms, which are vital for balanced hormone production.

Dopamine is also involved in learning. If something feels really good, then it's dopamine that leads you to want to repeat the experience. So dopamine is the driving force behind the cravings in your life, for things both good and bad.

> *"If something feels really good, then it's dopamine that leads you to want to repeat the experience... dopamine is the driving force behind the cravings in your life, for things both good and bad."*

As such, a dopamine hit is highly addictive so it is a key driver of addictive behaviors around foods such as sugar, but also around alcohol and drugs and smartphones. Addiction can happen because you become reliant on the stimulation of your dopamine receptors by a particular substance or the ping that tells you that you have a new message on your phone.

Even worse, when you frequently stimulate your dopamine receptors by seeking pleasure from a substance, the receptors can become desensitized so that it requires a larger dose of whatever feels good to you, before you get the same level of pleasure.

Conversely, if some experience feels really bad then dopamine will help you to avoid it in the future.

In the context of this book, a high level of cortisol from long-term stress severely depletes your brain of dopamine, but part of dopamine's ability to promote good health and lift your mood also comes from its ability to counteract the effects of cortisol.

Happily, dopamine and oxytocin are both released in large amounts during your orgasm, so I've seen it claimed that the combined surge of dopamine and oxytocin from about three orgasms in a lovemaking session, is enough to give you pretty much a full hormonal reset.

3.6.4
GABA

The primary functions of your brain hormone GABA are to reduce anxiety and promote a deep, restful sleep. These are both important for a healthy immune system and the production of HGH (Human Growth Hormone), which enhances muscle growth and body repair. GABA also has a role in enhancing learning and memory formation.

As usual for your body, it's the balance that is important, so too much GABA will usually make you drowsy, which is how drugs like Valium and alcohol work to make you drowsy. However, sometimes excess GABA can have the opposite effect, making you feel anxious or panicky and bring on physical symptoms such as tingling, feeling flushed and increased heart rate. Excess GABA may also bring on unpleasant sleep disorders, which can also happen with Valium and alcohol.

On the other hand, too little GABA can bring on a range of mood and brain disorders, such as feelings of stress, anxiety or depression. There is also increasing evidence linking low GABA with conditions such as autism, schizophrenia and Parkinson's disease.

Taking GABA supplements can work for some people to enhance their mood and sleep, but many people do not seem to respond at all. This may be because in some people the tight junctions of the blood-brain barrier are not allowing the GABA to enter the brain, while for some others the GABA can get into the brain or it may be affecting the GABA receptors in the gut. This may also mean that what you are eating at the time you take the GABA, and the condition of your gut microbiome can influence whether you have a desirable response to GABA or not – treat it with care.

CHAPTER 4

The Effect of Stress on your Body

"In Chinese medicine, stress is the root cause of all disease and is just as important as, if not more important than, diet"
Dr Josh Axe, DNM, DC, CNS

It's important to realize that your body's 'stress response' to a stressful event has evolved over millions of years and was designed to ensure your survival in crisis situations, like a sabre tooth tiger attacking your cave or a drought causing a famine. It's equally important that you recognize that it co-evolved with our 'relaxation response', which is designed to reverse all the potentially negative effects of stress on our body (See Chapter 14 Detoxing Your Mind).

While stress has always been a part of our lives, it's only in relatively recent times when the Industrial Revolution started the large-scale movement of people away from farms and villages and into cities, where life is more impersonal, that distress has become part of everyday living for many people. We now know that chronic distress is impacting negatively on our health and is a prime causal factor in the recent explosion of chronic conditions like heart disease, diabetes, infertility and dementia.

What is the scale of the problem now? The American Psychological Association has been surveying stress levels in the USA for eleven years now, and this year's results showed that women are reporting stress levels 16% higher than males, with the gender gap widening.

Around 80% of Americans reported experiencing at least one health symptom as a result of stress over January 2017. The symptoms were both physical and emotional and included headaches (34 per cent), feeling overwhelmed (33 per cent), feeling nervous or anxious (33 per cent), or feeling depressed or sad (32 per cent). Over one-quarter of the women surveyed reported using eating as one of their methods of dealing with their stress. Hmmm.

Unfortunately, in this modern world, we tend to use the term 'stress' to describe the negative impact of situations in our daily life that can lead to feelings of being overwhelmed. This can lead many people to believe that ALL stress is bad for you, which is not necessarily the case.

4.1
Eustress

Not many people are familiar with this word, which has the same root as euphoria. If you choose to put yourself in a situation, which you instinctively know will trigger an adrenaline response, then this can be an example of 'Eustress ', or positive stress.

This is usually a short-term situation where you choose to deliberately put yourself under pressure to achieve something positive in your life.

A key aspect of eustress is that it feels exciting. It motivates you to do something challenging, focuses your energy, and actually improves your mental and physical performance.

Of course, the impact of different situations varies for everyone, but some examples of eustress or positive stress could include situations as diverse as getting married, or having a baby, or having to perform in public, or bungee jumping, or skiing a very steep slope.

4.2
Distress

Distress is the type of stress that you probably become more familiar with as you get a bit older. It is the stress that has a negative impact on your life and is usually perceived as something a bit (or even a lot) outside your control and that you didn't consciously choose.

So distress feels completely different from eustress, in that it usually feels unpleasant, causing anxiety or concern for your ability to cope with the situation – you may even feel you are running out of 'cope'. Distress can be both short- or long-term and usually leads to decreased performance and can lead to quite severe mental and physical problems.

The distress can come from situations as diverse as the breakup of a relationship, negative self-talk about how you are not enough, conflicts with colleagues at work, money problems, feelings of inadequacy, having issues with sleep, or an injury or illness.

I hope you are starting to notice something really important: that stress, either eustress or distress, can come from either emotional, mental, or physical sources.

A key aspect of stress is the wide variety of situations that can be seen as stressful, so this can include the routine hassles like getting the family out the door each morning or dealing with a difficult colleague at work. We can also have one-time events that can have a profound effect on our lives, such as moving house, getting married, and having a baby. And then we can have the ongoing long-term demands, such as dealing with a chronic health condition, caring for a child or an ailing parent, or negative self-talk about how we're 'not loveable'.

Another important aspect of stress is that we don't generally enjoy the extremes of stress, either high or low. Most people do not enjoy the feeling of living an ongoing high-stress lifestyle, where you are constantly living on the edge or past the edge and then running out of capacity to cope. However, neither do we enjoy the complete absence of challenges provoking stress – that's called boredom. So what most people seek is a comfortable middle ground between too much stress and lack of stress.

Of course, everyone is different, so there are some people, more often in their twenties and early thirties, who choose to go into a high-powered, high-stress job, such as being the editor of a high fashion magazine. For them, this type of job is long-term eustress, in that it feels exciting and challenging and gives a sense of living on the edge.

At some point such a lifestyle tends to move into distress, as your stress hormone (adrenal) system starts to get overloaded. So you start to find that the early morning coffee you needed to get you going requires another one mid-morning to keep you going and another one at lunchtime, or perhaps a glass of wine over lunch, and another coffee mid-afternoon when you suddenly run out of energy. By the end of the day you are feeling tired, but wired, and you really, really need that glass of wine (or two) before dinner to 'relax' at the end of the day.

So what used to be fun and exciting can start to move into being plain hard work, and getting out of bed seems to take more and more effort. Add into this mix a long-term relationship and maybe the demands of a young family and you start to feel like you're running out of cope and your waist size is steadily increasing (See Chapter 8 The Hormonal Reasons Why Diets Don't Work).

What's happening here is that the constant living on bursts of adrenaline and the high levels of cortisol that go with this lifestyle, gradually depletes your adrenal gland's ability to respond to stress and you are likely to be on a slippery slope, potentially heading towards adrenal exhaustion – you do not want to go there.

4.3
The Hidden Effects of Stress

The instinctive response from a woman's limbic system to stress is the 'tend and befriend' response, which is the combination of the effects of adrenaline and oxytocin on your body.

In long-term stress, the main hormones at work become cortisol and oxytocin, which gives you a hormone-driven way of being which can have very subtle, but highly undesirable effects on your feelings of self-worth and your feelings around your relationships.

Your stress hormones are giving your limbic system very subtle feelings that you need to look after everyone else first. The sense of the need to tend or look after other people means that you are likely to feel that you need to take on a range of tasks for others, even though you feel overloaded already.

Because you are already stressed and overloaded, adding another layer of tasks to be done can add to your feelings of 'I'm not good enough' because the reality is you are not fine, you're overloaded, and so you start to feel overwhelmed. You can also set yourself up for feelings of resentment against the people you are tending, which can have a very damaging effect on your relationship with them.

The other subtle effect which can happen if you take on doing tasks for your partner, which he or she is quite capable of doing (and probably didn't ask you to do in the first place); then you are actually treating your partner like a child. If you really want to kill your desire for an intimate sexual relationship with your partner, then treating your partner like a child is a very effective way to achieve this.

Your reality needs to become, that you're no use to anyone else if you are not well, so you have to put your own health first.

It's important also to realize that you are not the primitive response of your limbic system; you are so much more than that. You have the potential to modify how you respond to those subtle feelings by using your higher cortical mind and your wonderful intelligence to find a better way.

The techniques described later in the book will assist you in getting your stress hormone levels back in balance.

"Your reality needs to become, that you're no use to anyone else if you are not well, so you have to put your own health first."

4.4
What Causes the Stress Response?

The stressors in the modern world tend to be very different from those that we were exposed to when we were living in small tribes on the plains of Africa.

We used to live in an environment where the adrenaline response was something that most often happened in cases of emergency (distress) when urgent action was needed. This is not to say that we didn't experience eustress, with the hunters likely coming home on an adrenaline and testosterone high, flushed with success after a challenging or difficult hunt.

However, we now live in a world where, for many people, eustress has become an accepted part of modern living, with people expecting to have some thrills all the time.

Indeed, for some people, the constant thirsting for the next buzz, the next challenge, the excitement, the stimulation of life on the edge is the only way they can cope with the boredom of their mundane lives.

Choosing to live like this is not a bad thing; it's just that our adrenal system is not designed to cope with this sort of level of stimulation, particularly when your body's hormonal systems are already challenged by toxins in the body and mind and are not properly supported by a healthy diet. This means you need to actively destress at the end of your day to stop your adrenal system from falling apart under the strain.

4.5
Coffee

One of the most common stressors in this modern world is coffee or caffeine drinks. Me

I know you don't want to hear this, but that little buzz you get when you have your coffee is because of the adrenaline that your body produces in response to the caffeine.

I will go into the details shortly, but one of the key things that happens when you drink coffee is that you get a surge of blood sugar released into your system. This spike in blood sugar is not needed in most modern situations because you're likely to be sitting still, so your body's response is to produce insulin to mop up the excess sugar floating around in your bloodstream by diverting it into your cells. However, your muscle cells don't need it when

When I decided that I wanted to cut down on the amount of coffee I was drinking, I decided to switch to hot chocolate when I went out to a cafe for a little treat. Somehow a cup of tea just doesn't feel special enough to do it for me at a cafe, although a chai latte or turmeric latte came close.

My coffee of choice is an unsweetened long black, so the milk and the sugar in the hot chocolate and the chai latte really didn't feel that great to my body and just didn't have the right taste.

I used to think, "why would you bother" about decaffeinated coffee, but because I love the bitterness and the taste and smell of a good coffee, I decided to give it a go.

I was actually pleasantly surprised. The flavor was a little less full, but the smell was there and without the side effects of the adrenaline buzz it was a pretty nice alternative, and I still get all the antioxidants. Most of the time I will go for a decaf long black when I'm out at a café, but on the right occasion I will go for a regular long black.

you're at rest so, by default, it gets pushed into the fat cells around your belly where your body can access it again quickly if it needs to.

Before you slam this book shut in horror and don't read any further, I am not saying you have to eliminate coffee from your life. However, you do need to realize that there can be a world of difference in the way your body responds to coffee depending on how and when and why you drink it.

If you have your coffee as part of your morning ritual with your loved one, or that coffee you have when you go out for brunch on Sunday with a friend, your body is in a relaxed state and can usually cope with the downstream effects of the adrenaline surge caused by the coffee, with no ill effects.

If, on the other hand, you are using coffee to help you cope with the distress in your life, to help you to get into your day and get through your day, then you are simply adding more adrenaline into your already wired body and adding to the problem. Your body is unlikely to be able to cope with this in the long term.

It's really important that you get real about what coffee is for you – because, of course, everyone's response to coffee is different.

For some people it makes the heart race and gives the shakes, but it also loosens the bowels, so it may be a way to keep yourself regular and stop the bloated belly and the discomfort that goes with constipation.

For others it dulls your appetite so you unconsciously grab another coffee instead of eating a proper lunch, which can lead to a blood sugar crash in the afternoon, which means you need a sweet treat and another coffee to get you through the afternoon.

Is the amount of coffee you are drinking

contributing to your restless, poor quality sleep so your body is not able to completely restore overnight, so you wake up tired and needing coffee to get you going in the morning?

Do you feel like you need coffee as part of your coping mechanism when things get crazy and hectic and stressful at work?

Is it just an excuse to take some time out from your crazy day?

Or is it just a gentle lift to your mood when you meet a friend for lunch, and you love the taste, and you don't feel any ill effects at all?

Yes, coffee does contain 164 different antioxidants and a study published about ten years ago showed that the average American got more antioxidants from coffee than from any other source. In spite of all the hype about this at the time, what this study really showed us is just how bad the SAD (Standard American Diet) is. The reality is that caffeine is the major active ingredient in coffee and the major impact of coffee is the negative impact on the stress hormones in your body.

The other negative effect of caffeine is that within minutes of consuming caffeine the blood flow to your brain decreases by around 30%, so while you might feel that caffeine helps your brain to function better, the reality is quite the opposite.

Only you can know the real impact of coffee on your body and your life. I can only give you the knowledge of the potential harm it could be doing to you, which then empowers you to choose what you want to do about it. Me

If you are having more than a few coffees a week, you might want to look at stopping coffee for a month and take close note of any changes. You may even be shocked by how much more energy you have without caffeine in your life.

4.6

Physical Stress

In this modern world we tend to do everything in a rush, partly because of the economic pressure we put ourselves under to achieve the goals we set, which means that both members of a partnership are going out to work, or being a solo parent, is becoming increasingly common.

So your distress can look like - you push the snooze button on the alarm because you are just so tired and then it goes again and you know you are going to have to rush to get the family out the door. You don't have time to do more than inhale a plateful of sugary breakfast cereal before you bundle everyone out the door and into the car and you're late, so the traffic is going to be a nightmare. Then you get a call on your mobile from someone at work wondering why you're late for a meeting and you eventually get there and your boss yells at you for messing up his meeting and it's all downhill from there.

You have started your day running on adrenaline, and you're already way behind on your carefully planned day and your to-do list, so you set yourself up for the real killer, which is:

4.7
Hidden Stress

This comes from the mental and emotional stress that you create for yourself from things your ego says to you. Things like – "Why did I hit that snooze button so I was late, I've let my boss down again, now I'm never going to get that promotion, how are we going to cope financially, God I really need a holiday, but how are we going to afford it, I'm so hopeless and … is going to be mad at me and I couldn't go on holiday anyway because I'm getting so fat I couldn't put on a bathing costume, I'm so hungry I could eat my arm off, maybe if I just have a coffee. "

Whatever the story you're telling yourself, or rather your ego is telling you, it is not true; it's just the story your left brain is making up to keep you stuck where you are because your ego doesn't like change.

This is where the critical part of this book comes in with how to detox your mind, because you can never be truly well and live the life you deserve with this sort of crap going on in your head most of the time (See Chapter 14 Detoxing your Mind).

4.8
Your Bodies Automatic Response to Stress

Now I want to go back to the basics about why the adrenaline response evolved and what it's designed to do; more importantly, what it does to your body whether you want it to or not.

It's important to realize that the hormonal changes that happen in your body under either eustress or distress are under the control of your automatic (autonomic) nervous system, so they are not under the control of your conscious mind. It's the job of the limbic system in your brain to constantly scan your environment for potential danger. Most of your hormonal system communicates via chemical messengers in the blood. However, there is a direct nerve connection between the limbic brain and the adrenal glands which initiate your adrenaline response so that it happens in milliseconds.

So in the first instance, the adrenaline response is designed to save you or your family's life in emergency situations.

The physiological changes that happen when you get the adrenaline rush are a very ancient response to an emergency. The changes are designed to increase your speed and strength and to minimize the effect of damage if you are wounded. They are all changes that are designed to improve your body's chances of surviving in a crisis situation, where there is potential for you to be wounded, or have to protect your children from danger, or to have to run for your life.

The changes are very widespread and look like this:

- Your heart starts to beat harder and faster, and your body constricts the blood vessels to your kidneys and digestive system, and your blood pressure rises. These changes are designed to help move the blood around your body faster, so that you can react quickly and your muscles have all the oxygen they need to carry out whatever needs to happen. These changes mean the blood flow to your muscles increases around three-fold.

- The restriction of the blood supply to the kidneys and digestive system means that your kidneys and gut pretty much shut down.

- The muscles need extra oxygen for tending, fighting or fleeing. To supply this extra oxygen you start to breathe faster, your breathing becomes shallow, and the airways in the lungs widen. This is because you are trying to get the maximum amount of oxygen into your lungs and get rid of the carbon dioxide, so that your body gets a lot of oxygen going to all tissues to enable it to respond quickly.

- The muscles also need extra fuel in a hurry so your pancreas, which regulates your blood sugar, is stimulated by adrenaline to produce glucagon to stimulate the release of fast burning glucose as fuel for your muscles. In this modern world, an adrenaline response seldom requires lots of physical activity; the resulting blood sugar spike then stimulates the release of insulin to store the surplus as belly fat so that it can be readily accessed the for next emergency or stress event. More on this in Chapter 7 The Hormonal Reasons Why Diets Don't Work.

- The blood supply going to your skin increases, which promotes sweating.

- This is designed to help keep your body cool in the event of extreme physical exertion. I am sure you all know the feeling when you are in a stressful situation, such as when you are going to perform in front of a crowd, and your body starts dripping with sweat. Those embarrassing wet patches under your arms are a key example of what happens automatically in your body when you get into a stressful situation.

- The production of your happy sex hormones - progesterone and testosterone, gets shut down so your libido takes a nose dive.

- The detox and repair systems of your body pretty much shut down.

- Blood clotting factors increase so your blood can clot more quickly to help reduce the risk of blood loss if you are injured in an emergency, but this gives you increased risk of a heart attack or stroke.

- The spleen, which stores oxygen-carrying red blood cells, releases them into the bloodstream to help get more oxygen to your muscles.

- To give access to extra speed and strength, the muscles of your body tense. This is why we commonly suffer tension headaches in times of crisis or need a shoulder massage.

- To help you see more clearly, your pupils widen to let in more light.

- Your hearing becomes sharper.

- Adrenaline primes the area of the brain called the Amygdala to feel increased anxiety and fear, and your thoughts race - this takes you out of the present and your ability to feel joy.

- You are way less sensitive to pain.

When you look at the previous list of the changes that happen automatically in your body in

Because cortisol regulates your blood sugar levels, if your evening meal is a high fast-carb, low-fat combination – which tends to get burnt very quickly by your body – then you are likely to run short of blood sugar during the night.

This will prompt your body to release cortisol, to prompt your pancreas to produce glucagon to restore your blood sugar levels.

Unfortunately, this surge in cortisol is also highly likely to wake you up and make it difficult for you to go back to sleep.

response to stress, it's hardly surprising that various estimates suggest that around 70 to 90% of all doctor visits are due to stress-related disorders. The list pretty much mirrors the major health issues we confront, which is why it is important to find ways to de-stress at the end of your day.

So written another way, the previous list can look a bit like this:

- Raised blood pressure and clotting factors – Heart disease or stroke
- Kidney and digestive system shut down – Digestive tract disorders like constipation, heartburn, acid reflux and bloating.
- Kidney disorders and bladder infections
- Raised blood sugar – Diabetes or belly fat
- Reduced progesterone and testosterone – Low libido, impotence, or infertility

4.9
Cortisol

"Cortisol is magical. It has this incredible ability to, within seven minutes, to halve your IQ. It makes you fat. It makes you old. It makes you stupid."
Kerwin Rae

Adrenaline is your emergency response stress hormone, but you also have another stress hormone called cortisol, which is produced by the adrenal glands and is responsible for several key functions in your body.

The normal role of cortisol is to control your blood sugar and blood pressure, and it also modulates the inflammatory response in your body. Without adequate levels of cortisol, we would die.

In situations where your body becomes exposed to more long-term stress (either eustress or distress), your cortisol levels will become elevated and distorted, which has many unwanted consequences. In an evolutionary sense, long-term stress and elevated cortisol only happened in extreme events like famine or war, when life was continuously perilous, and the food was scarce, which means your body is not well adapted to cope with sustained high levels of stress. Because of your increased cortisol levels, your body now believes your survival is threatened, which is the signal for your body to conserve resources to ensure long-term survival by slowing your metabolic rate (hello tiredness and belly fat).

When life is running smoothly and all is wonderful, then cortisol follows a diurnal pattern where it peaks in the early morning as part of your wake up to make you feel like bouncing out of bed and rearing to get into your day. Following this peak, cortisol levels normally drop steadily over the day to reach around 60% of wake-up levels by noon, dropping a further 40% by early evening.

Ideally, they would then drop to around 10% of your wake-up levels by 10 p.m. so that when you do fall into bed you go into a deep, restorative sleep to allow your body and brain to rebuild after your day. Your cortisol levels will then remain low until around 2 a.m. when they start to rise steadily towards wake up levels again.

This, of course, explains why it's really important for your wellness to get to bed around 10 p.m. ready to sleep (not to go on Facebook on your phone). This will allow you to drop into a deep, restful, restorative sleep and your body and brain have time to repair before cortisol starts to rise again at 2 a.m. It also explains why an hour of sleep before midnight really is worth about two hours of sleep after midnight.

4.10
Cortisol and Stress

If your adrenaline response has been active during the day, then the fall in cortisol levels doesn't happen so gracefully.

If you do not take active steps to de-stress during the evening, then it's highly likely that you will get a cortisol spike during the evening which can make getting off to sleep a challenge and seriously disrupt your sleeping patterns.

If, after an adrenaline-filled day, you then spend the evening sorting out your children's homework and dirty clothes, catching up on all those emails you didn't have a chance to get to during the day and checking what your tribe is up to on Facebook, evenings like this will likely result in you feeling like you have got your second wind and you couldn't possibly go to bed now. In reality, what you have got is a surge of cortisol in response to the ongoing stress, which will make it really really difficult for you to drop off into the deep restful sleep your body and brain needs to repair itself.

It's really important for your wellness to make sure you have about an hour of relaxing, screen-free, you-time before you are ready for sleep.

So if elevated cortisol is telling your body that food is scarce, or you create an artificial famine by going on a diet, then two nasty things happen. Your metabolic rate slows down so that you burn fat more slowly, but cortisol is also catabolic, which means that it breaks down protein from your muscles into the constituent amino acids. In a real stress situation these extra amino acids would be used to repair damaged tissues. However, in the modern world, these are simply converted back to glucose and burnt as fuel or stored as belly fat.

So, over time, you get reduced muscle mass which limits the ability of the muscles to store glycogen, so even more of any glucose spike has to be stored in fat cells. This sets you up for the dreaded cellulite, because instead of building muscles, the extra glucose in the blood is deposited as fat.

4.11
The Sugar-Fat-Stress Connection

In response to the stress hormones released in an emergency, your body tries to burn only glucose (which it can mobilize very quickly) to provide the energy it needs, rather than fat (which provides a steady, more slow-release form of energy). There is a very close relationship between the adrenaline response and what your body burns as fuel.

The pancreas produces two counteracting sorts of hormones; glucagon, and insulin. If your limbic brain is stimulating adrenaline production to tell your body you need to react quickly, then your pancreas will release glucagon which acts to break down the glycogen (many glucose molecules bound together) stored in the liver and muscle tissues, into glucose. This produces a surge of fast burning glucose in the blood to fuel the action your brain thinks is needed. Insulin regulates your blood sugar by triggering your cell membranes to let glucose into your cells.

The problem with this scenario is that in this modern world the stress response seldom requires a burst of physical activity. The release of glucose from the liver and muscles translates into a spike in your blood sugar, which is not actually needed by your muscles so does not get burnt to provide quick energy.

Your body then recognizes that because high blood sugar levels are dangerous in the long term, so it instructs your pancreas to produce insulin to remove the excess glucose from your blood, and the spare glucose gets pushed into your fat cells. In particular, the visceral fat cells around your belly.

So the characteristic body shape which forms in response to stress is the belly fat around your middle, sometimes called a muffin top.

There is another interesting twist to the sugar and stress response because cortisol regulates your blood sugar. It's highly likely that one of the biggest causes of stress in your body is unstable blood sugar, which can make you feel the same as you would feel if something makes you angry, frustrated, or frightened. Whenever your blood sugar levels change too fast or get too high your body releases cortisol to stabilize them.

You function at your best when your blood glucose levels are kept within the range of 75 to 95 ng/dl, (or 4-6 nmol/l) and the more time you spend outside this range or, the more often it spikes within this range, the more your body feels stressed.

Once you have gone through my 'Rapid Reset' and become 'fat-adapted', your attitude to breakfast will need to change, as you are unlikely to feel like eating at all in the morning and, in fact, the later you eat, the better it is for your brain health. I now find that I don't need my first meal of the day until late morning or even early afternoon because I am running on fat most of the time – 'fat-adapted'. When I am going out before late morning I will have a high-fat breakfast, but I don't have to - it takes away the need to run your life around meals.

The characteristic fat storage pattern of long-term stress is the development of adipose fat around the midline – our belly fat, sometimes called a muffin top.

4.12
Why Breakfast is the Most Important Meal of the Day

As I have mentioned before, if your blood sugar falls too low your body will interpret this as the beginning of a famine.

When your alarm goes do you leap out of bed, dash into the shower, throw some clothes on and then grab a cup of coffee as you race out the door?

Now stop - and think about what's wrong with

this scenario. You are already running on adrenaline, then adding in some caffeine, which both do a wonderful job of spiking your blood sugar and storing belly fat. On top of this you have taken no food so your body thinks you're going into a famine and starts to pump out cortisol, which really adds to the fat storage scenario.

The other reason that what you do first thing in the morning is so important, is that your body sets up your blood sugar regulation for the whole day, based on the first events after you wake up. If you have had a normal restful sleep your body will have transitioned into a mild fat-burning mode (See Chapter 11 Good Oils Make You Slim and Healthy), and your body will stay in this state if you make the right food choices.

All you have to do to break the fat storage cycle is to slow down a little and have some real, low carb food to eat for breakfast. To stay in the fat burning mode you want a moderate protein, high fat, low carb breakfast, and some gentle exercise – maybe a short walk, but any exercise is good. It also enhances the effect of spending a few minutes to visualize your day, thinking about how you would like to feel and what you'd like to have happen.

Such a routine actually sets your body up to preferentially burn fat for energy for the rest of the day, rather than burning glucose. Yeah - a fat burning scenario for a change.

If you really are in a hurry, please don't inhale some sugary breakfast cereal, which will just give you a blood sugar spike and add to the fat storage. The idea that breakfast should be some sort of dessert, to give you energy, has only come from high-pressure advertising and is not based on any science.

A much much better alternative is to take a couple of minutes to mix up a high fiber, green smoothie, made with full-fat yoghurt or coconut cream. Or, as a last resort, as you rush out the door, grab a handful of nuts, like almonds. Either of these will give you some high-quality protein and fats, but few carbs, so your blood sugar stays stable and your body stays in mild fat burning mode, which is perfect for your brain function and your waistline.

All you have to do to break the fat storage cycle is to slow down a little and have some real, low carb food to eat for breakfast.

Your brain has a very high requirement for energy and many people mistakenly think that this means it needs lots of glucose or sugar to function well. There is a growing body of evidence that your brain actually functions around 70% better on ketones, which are water-soluble molecules your liver makes from fat to allow the transport of fat from your blood into your cells, ready to be burnt as energy.

This is why eating some coconut oil works much better as a pick-me-up mid-afternoon than a sugary snack (See Chapter 11 Good Oils Make You Slim and Healthy). And also, why having plenty of coconut oil in your diet helps to prevent the development of dementia or Alzheimer's.

4.13
Stress and Diabetes

When you subject your body to long-term stress you become a prime candidate for metabolic syndrome (sometimes called syndrome X), where you will end up with elevated blood pressure, increased belly fat, elevated cholesterol, and you can start to develop insulin resistance.

The insulin resistance happens because of spikes in blood sugar which go with your stress hormone responses, start to desensitize the insulin receptors on your cell walls, which should trigger the cells to take in more glucose. When your insulin receptors become desensitized and your cells are not removing the excess glucose from your blood, then your body tells your pancreas to release more insulin. This further stresses the insulin receptors. You are then on a slippery slope, likely heading towards Type II diabetes and dementia (increasingly called Type III diabetes), if you don't make some drastic changes in your lifestyle.

4.14
Stress and Cholesterol

The elevated cholesterol that is part of the metabolic syndrome discussed above is actually a response from your body to stress.

Cholesterol is the building block for cortisol, so in response to long-term stress, your body starts making more cholesterol, so that it can make more cortisol, which is essential to control your blood sugar and blood pressure. Without adequate cortisol to control these functions, you die.

Yet how many doctors, when you present with higher cholesterol levels, discuss with you the stress levels in your life or order a cortisol test, rather than reaching for the prescription pad to write you out the script for a statin drug to lower your cholesterol levels.

The reality is your body needs cholesterol because:

- It is the key component of the cell walls that provides the stiffness necessary for correct functioning of your tissues.

- Your brain requires high levels to be healthy; in fact, your brain contains 25% of the cholesterol in your body.

- Cholesterol is also the precursor to the other steroid hormones in your body, most notably your sex hormones and Vitamin D.

So what are some of the more common side effects of statins?

- Loss of muscle function, often with muscle and joint pain.

- Memory loss.

- Loss of libido and sexual dysfunction.

Now wait a minute: don't those two lists look a bit like cause-and-effect to you? They sure do to me.

So is there any evidence of a beneficial effect from taking statin drugs for women? When you look in the research literature you will not find a large-scale study shows that use of statins leads to any increased life expectancy at all in women – even those already diagnosed with cardiovascular disease. The same applies to women in lower risk categories for cardiovascular disease, nor have statins been shown to prevent heart attacks or strokes in women.

Statins are in fact classified as a 'pregnancy Category X medication', meaning that they are known to cause serious birth defects and should never be used by a woman who is pregnant or planning a pregnancy.

4.15
Stress and Alcohol

After a long and stressful day, many people succumb to the temptation to pour a glass of wine (or two) to help you unwind. While it might feel like this is what is happening to your body when you drink some alcohol, unfortunately the reality is not so nice.

Alcohol is not like caffeine in its effect on the body in that there is no short-term effect on your stress hormone levels. However, a recent large-scale study has shown that alcohol consumption raises cortisol levels and slows the rate of decline in your cortisol levels during the day. The authors also suggested that a woman's cortisol levels were more affected by alcohol than men's.

It is thought that the effect of alcohol on cortisol levels is probably happening because alcohol damages liver function, which may reduce the liver's ability to detoxify excess cortisol.

Any increase in your evening cortisol levels is going to have an impact on your ability to drop into a deep, restful, restorative sleep. The alcohol may help you to go to sleep initially, but the elevated cortisol levels will mean that your sleep is not as restorative and that you are likely to be wakeful later in the night.

Given that alcohol converts to acetaldehyde in the body, which is a known carcinogen, it's not surprising that even moderate alcohol consumption greatly increases your risk of breast cancer. Alcohol also increases estrogen levels, particularly in pre-menopausal women, so a combination of these two factors means that for each daily standard drink you have, your risk of breast cancer increases by 11%.

I will discuss this issue further in the estrogen section, but the evidence is so compelling that I invite you to look hard at the choices you make around alcohol.

4.16
Stress and Marijuana

As changes are happening in many parts of the world around the legality of using marijuana, potentially making people more curious about using it, it is worth considering how it may fit into counteracting your stressful day.

A bit like alcohol, the research is starting to suggest that what you think is happening by way of relaxation is not the reality of how marijuana is affecting your body.

For women, the effects of marijuana on your stress hormones are quite similar to alcohol, in that you get an overall increase in the amount of cortisol produced, although it doesn't seem to affect the daily rhythm so badly. The raised cortisol may mean that you don't feel as relaxed as you might expect to and may even feel a little paranoid.

Given the ability of marijuana to increase your cortisol levels you might want to reconsider whether potentially using it to help you unwind would really help you. Since nothing really stands still, if it's not helping you then it must be harming you! Other alternatives are discussed in Chapter 14 - Detoxing your Mind.

4.17
Stress and Depression

Everyone's route into depression is going to be different, but there is no doubt that there is a strong linkage between distress and depression.

The feelings of sadness, hopelessness, helplessness, or worthlessness that go with the feelings that you are gaining weight and 'running out of cope' often go with not dealing with the impact of long-term stress.

The relationship between stress and depression is complicated and can be circular, in that stress can lead to behaviors like drinking more than normal, which can actually raise cortisol and add to a chronic stress burden, and increase the risk of major depression because alcohol is a known mood suppressor.

One close connection is, that if you have chronically elevated cortisol levels, you seldom sleep well, which can be a trigger to a bout of depression. There is also a negative effect of cortisol on serotonin levels (the powerful feel- good hormone needed for restful sleep), and cortisol actually damages serotonin receptor sites. Most antidepressants work by trying to increase the availability of serotonin in the brain.

The fact that women are twice as likely to have depression as men suggests that there is also a strong involvement of the sex hormones in depression as well, especially progesterone which is the happy hormone for women.

The strategies advocated later in the book to detox your body, move your body and detox your mind are designed to bring all your hormones into balance and will have a powerful effect on your mood.

CHAPTER 5

Your Energy Hormone - Thyroid

"Hypothyroidism—a 'Silent Epidemic' of Misdiagnosis"

Steven Hotze, MD

Understanding thyroid function is crucial to improving your health, your body shape, and how you feel, because EVERY cell in your body has a thyroid hormone receptor, which means that how your thyroid is functioning affects EVERYTHING.

Your thyroid gland is a little butterfly-shaped gland that wraps around the breathing tube in your throat area. The thyroid gland makes hormones that play an enormous part in regulating your metabolic rate, as well as temperature regulation, immune function, mental health, and energy levels.

I like to think of the thyroid as your body's accelerator pedal. If your thyroid is optimal, then your body hums along feeling wonderful and nothing is a problem. This is because it is the regulator of energy production at the cellular level and so determines your metabolic rate. So, if your thyroid is sluggish, then you commonly feel cold and suffer from mental slowness, weight gain, depression and fatigue.

Adult humans with low thyroid hormone levels are considered to have hypothyroidism.

Unfortunately, thyroid issues affect many women – somewhere around 30-40% of the population in the USA.

5.1
How your Thyroid Works

Your thyroid is an important part of the very complex adrenal system, which regulates the minute-to-minute control of your bodily functions.

The coordination of all your various body systems starts with the nervous system, which works through nerve impulses to maintain your body in a stable equilibrium (homoeostasis). The endocrine system performs a similar function by the use of hormones delivered throughout the blood and lymphatic circulation systems.

There is a high degree of inter-dependence between the two systems, with certain parts of the nervous system both stimulating and suppressing the release of hormones from the glands of the endocrine system. Similarly, your mind may either inhibit or promote the generation of nerve impulses.

Nerve impulses tend to produce their effects very rapidly, but the effects of stimulating the nervous system tend to be short-lived. Some hormones can also react very quickly, while others have their effect over much longer time periods.

Coordinating these two systems to maintain a stable equilibrium throughout the body is a small portion of the brain buried deep in your limbic system, called the hypothalamus, working in conjunction with your thyroid gland.

Among other things, your hypothalamus responds to the presence in your blood of leptin (your master metabolic rate hormone – See Chapter 8 The Hormonal Reasons Why Diets Don't Work) to control the production of TSH (thyroid-stimulating hormone). It is the TSH that then stimulates the thyroid to make the thyroid hormone, called T4 (thyroxine) because it contains four atoms of iodine.

T4 is essentially a storage hormone that is continually circulating in your blood or is stored within your tissues, but it's not able to actively enter your cells so doesn't really affect your metabolic rate or your symptoms. There is an intricately balanced signaling system that, depending on local demand, controls the conversion of the inactive T4 into the active thyroid hormone, known as T3, because it contains only three atoms of iodine.

With the help of the minerals selenium, zinc and iron, the conversion to T3 happens mainly in the gut, liver, muscles, brain and your thyroid. The other factor that's important for getting the active T3 into your cells is the presence of healthy fats in your cell membranes (See Chapter 11 Good Oils Make You Slim and Healthy).

Only then is the thyroid hormone, in the form of T3, able to get into your cells, with the help of cortisol, to do its job of controlling the activity of the mitochondria. Your mitochondria are the little powerhouses within your cells that take molecules of food energy and convert them into the form of chemical energy that your body uses to fuel all its functions.

It is T3 that controls your metabolic rate and your capacity to burn fat, as well as many other bodily functions. The actions of T3 in your body, are what I like to think makes your thyroid your body's accelerator pedal. This is because it is actually the active T3 that is the regulator of energy production at the mitochondrial level in your cells and so determines your metabolic rate and your energy levels. It controls the conversion of energy embedded in your food into energy usable by the body.

Hence, if your thyroid is sluggish and T3 levels are low, then you feel tired, even depressed; everything is hard work, and you have a strong tendency to gain weight.

Similarly, the inactive T4 governs the 'potential' for your body to make the active T3. As a result, the measuring the levels of the T4 precursor hormone and TSH are 'potentially' useful measures of thyroid activity in the body. These are the tests most often ordered by your doctor if you go to them with a potential thyroid issue.

If your TSH level is high, your brain wants to see more thyroid hormone made – you have an under-active thyroid (hypothyroidism), and conversely, if your TSH is low, your brain is acting as if you are making too much thyroid hormone – that you have an overactive thyroid (hyperthyroidism)

As well as the things already mentioned, your thyroid also affects your:

- body temperature
- heart rate and blood pressure
- muscle strength
- skin condition
- vision
- menstrual regularity
- PMS
- bleeding tendency
- cholesterol levels and risk of heart attack

As you can see, having a healthy thyroid is also crucial to normal immune and brain function.

5.2
Thyroid and your Brain

Compared to the rest of your body, your brain uses a lot of energy to function well, so your brain cells have the highest numbers of mitochondria in them. Of course, this also means that your brain needs a lot of T3 to function well. Consequently, an underactive thyroid (hypothyroidism) can lead to a slowing of mental processes, progressive loss of interest, poor memory for recent events, fading of your personality, and even depression (with a paranoid flavor), or dementia.

An overactive thyroid (hyperthyroidism) can lead to marked anxiety, impatience, over activity, sensitivity to noise, problems with sleep and appetite, and even depression (with sadness), and potentially schizophrenia.

Unfortunately, the effects of thyroid malfunction can easily be mistaken for mild, or even quite severe mental disorders.

It is not uncommon for frontline doctors to miss this connection between the thyroid and mental state, and some people end up being wrongly diagnosed, treated with drugs and even hospitalized for months. One review of some of the co-factors involved in depression found that over half of the people diagnosed with treatment-resistant depression showed evidence of low thyroid function.

Normal brain development and growth in the fetus and in children is also closely interlinked with thyroid function. Developmental brain disorders like ADHD and autism can be the result of disrupted thyroid function.

5.3
How do I Know if I Have a Thyroid Problem?

Unfortunately, thyroid malfunction is very common in modern life, with estimates suggesting that up to 10% of the population have some form of thyroid malfunction and women are around eight times more likely to have a stuttering thyroid than men. Even worse, estimates suggest that up to 60% of those with thyroid malfunction don't even know it, so they struggle on with below par energy levels, perhaps thinking "I'm not as young as I used to be". It doesn't have to be that way.

In a healthy body the amount of inactive T4 produced depends on the level of TSH produced by your pituitary, and there is a powerful feedback loop between the amount of T4 in the blood and the levels of TSH produced. If you are hypothyroid and your thyroid is not making sufficient thyroid hormones to meet your body's needs, then the pituitary increases the amount of TSH produced to try to stimulate the thyroid into making more T4 thyroid hormone.

You would logically think that this means you only have to measure the amount of TSH in your blood, and maybe the amount of T4 and you would get an accurate picture of how the thyroid is functioning – in fact many doctors think this way. Unfortunately, the whole relationship between your thyroid gland, your pituitary gland, and your other hormones, such as cortisol and sex hormones, can get very complicated. In fact, one estimate suggested that there are over 20 ways in which your thyroid hormone system can malfunction.

5.3.1
Blood Tests

So if your doctor suspects you have a thyroid problem, they will look for evidence around the feedback loop described above. Typically this means a blood test for levels of TSH and the storage thyroid hormone T4. If your T4 levels are low and TSH levels are high, this suggests that your thyroid is not able to function correctly and you are likely to get a prescription for some form of supplemental 'T4' - Synthroid (a synthetic approximation of T4) is the MOST WIDELY PRESCRIBED DRUG IN THE USA.

One of the controversial issues is: what constitutes a high level of TSH and a low level of inactive T4?

Many doctors rely on reference ranges supplied by the testing laboratories. Unfortunately, the blood samples sent to a laboratory mostly come from people who are not that well, which often includes people with some degree of thyroid malfunction. This skews the data towards the lower end of the range of levels in the overall population.

Next, the data is statistically analyzed and a reference range calculated, based on the variability of the data, using an arbitrary rule that defines 95% of the tested population as "normal", which gives an answer which is in no way based on how much thyroid hormone your body needs to function optimally.

It is relatively common for doctors to decide on whether to treat your thyroid symptoms, based on a reference range that is skewed toward including many with impaired thyroid function, (so it really is what is 'normal for sick people') and often with little regards for your symptoms.

Not surprisingly, there is debate around what normal TSH levels really are. A normal reference range for TSH from laboratories is often given as 0.4 to 4.0 (in the past, it could be as wide as 0.5 to 5.0). With HYPERthyroid (i.e. your brain is wanting your thyroid to slow down because your T4 levels are too high) defined as TSH being below 0.4 and HYPOthyroid (i.e. your brain is wanting your thyroid to speed up production of T4 because of your T4 levels not being high enough) as TSH being above 4.0. While this might seem a relatively narrow range, somebody with a TSH of 0.4 looks and feels completely different from someone with a TSH of 4.0.

In 2002, the American Association of Clinical Endocrinologists recommended that the range for acceptable thyroid function shift to a TSH of 0.3 to 3.0, which they estimated would probably double the number of people who were diagnosed with abnormal thyroid function.

About the same time, the National Academy of Clinical Biochemistry suggested that, in future, the upper level of TSH is likely to be reduced to 2.5. This was because a very detailed Turkish study found that 95% of healthy volunteers with no thyroid problems had a TSH value between 0.4 and 2.5. The authors recommended that the therapeutic target for TSH should be between 0.5 and 2.0. However some Functional Medicine doctors report abnormal metabolic function at levels of TSH between 1.5 and 2, so you can see that relying on TSH test alone, as many doctors do, could easily result in you not getting the treatment your body requires to be well.

This is where YOU understanding your blood test numbers become really important because, unfortunately, it is relatively common for doctors to work to older standards.

If you are symptom-free, well and good. However, you presumably had some symptoms of thyroid malfunction to prompt your doctor to authorize the blood tests in the first place. Thus, if your doctor bases their decision on whether to treat purely on older standards for blood results, rather than the newer standards and how your body is behaving, then you are likely to be left with a set of symptoms, of varying severity perhaps, but obviously not feeling totally well.

That is not the state you probably want to aim for, which is presumably why you are reading this book.

Another key problem with relying solely on blood tests is that the tests only show how much thyroid hormone is circulating in the blood, and tell nothing of how well the hormones are functioning on a cellular level. The active T3 can only work INSIDE the cell, not on external receptors.

	Hyperthyroidism	Optimal	Probable Hypothyroidism	Overt Hypothyroidism
TSH – uIU/mL	< 0.4	0.5 – 1.5	> 2.0	> 3
fT4 – ng/dL	high > 1.8	1.1 – 1.3	low/normal < 1.0	low < 0.8
fT3 - pg/mL	high > 3.5	2.8 – 3.3	low/normal < 2.5	low < 2.0
Basal temperature °C	> 36.8 (or fever)	36.6 – 36.8	36.5 – 36.4	< 36.4
Basal temperature °F	> 98.2 (or fever)	97.9 – 98.2	97.8 – 97.6	< 97.6
Pulse	70 - 100	60 - 70		40 - 60
Patch Test		> 13 hours	7 - 12 hours	2 – 6 hours

This is where YOU understanding your blood test numbers becomes really important, because, unfortunately, it is relatively common for doctors to work to older standards.

All that said, your T3 levels fluctuate rapidly in response to your immediate stress levels and what's going on in your day. Because of the buffering effect of your storage T4 levels, then your TSH levels respond more slowly, but even they vary within the day, so your low is typically around half of your peak. These factors mean that any blood test is only a snapshot in time and could potentially give quite a false picture of your thyroid hormone levels.

Getting caught in traffic on your way to the doctors and getting stressed about being late, or getting an angry message from someone while you're sitting in the waiting room could be enough to distort your TSH test results enough to give an inaccurate picture of how your thyroid system is performing in your life.

5.3.2
The Whole Picture

If you have decided you likely have a thyroid function problem, then I recommend you check several other factors. My approach to this is based on the work of Dr Broda Barnes.

Firstly, the very first thing after waking, check your morning temperature with a clinical or accurate mercury thermometer and record the numbers. This is best done after the 2nd and 3rd day of your period, and definitely not during ovulation. This test should be performed by placing your thermometer under the armpit for 10 minutes immediately upon waking and before you start moving around. This is slightly more accurate than taking your oral temperature. Repeat the test three days in a row.

Secondly, at the same time, take your pulse for 60 seconds and record.

Thirdly, use our Iodine swab (or get a bottle of Lugol's Iodine or Iodine Tincture from your pharmacy) and do a Patch Test, which gives a guide to your body's stores of iodine. This simply involves spreading a couple of drops onto a small area of your inner wrist and noting how long it takes for the yellow color to disappear. The lower the level of iodine in your body, the faster it will be absorbed into your body. It's not totally accurate, but it does give a good indication of your body's relative level of iodine. If it takes less than half a day to disappear, you are very likely to be low in iodine – it doesn't rub off or wash off.

How you feel has to be the ultimate indicator of whether you have a thyroid issue or not. No tests are completely definitive, but if you and your doctor measure the seven factors in the table above, they will give you a pretty good indication.

5.4

Thyroid Resistance

The other issue around blood tests is that hormone resistance has been documented for several hormones, including insulin, adrenaline, cortisol, progesterone, and thyroid hormones. Hormone resistance can happen when endocrine disruptors from pollution in your environment, or long periods with excessive levels of hormones, effectively jam your hormone receptors.

In stress situations, your body can make a disruptive thyroid hormone called Reverse T3, which is inactive (like T4), but it can get inside your cells and block your thyroid hormone receptors, which can quickly lead to thyroid resistance, so measuring Reverse T3 levels can sometimes be helpful.

Your thyroid receptors are inside your cells, so measuring hormone levels outside the cell in your blood, saliva, or urine doesn't really tell you much if the receptors inside your cells are jammed. Your cells can still not be getting enough T3 to make you feel well.

5.5
Stress and your Thyroid

A normal level of cortisol – not too high and not too low – is very important for normal thyroid function. One of the important functions of cortisol is to work synergistically with T3 at the cellular level, to make them both work more effectively.

In situations of ongoing stress your body believes your survival is threatened, so responds by increasing your cortisol levels to signal your body to conserve resources to ensure long-term survival by slowing your metabolic rate. It does this in multiple ways by telling your pituitary to make less TSH, which means your thyroid makes less T4. It gets worse, because cortisol also tells your cells to make less of the active T3 which gives you your get up and go and, at the same time, to make more of the blocking Reverse T3.

Thus many people who have an imbalance in their cortisol levels commonly have thyroid-like symptoms, even though they can have apparently normal thyroid hormone levels from their blood tests. Conversely, adrenal problems can also masquerade as thyroid problems and not be treated properly.

5.6
Sex Hormones and your Thyroid

One of the key functions of your thyroid hormones is to control the conversion of the energy from your food into usable energy, by fueling the mitochondria in your cells. One of the key functions of estrogen in your body is to work with insulin to store fat so that you have the necessary energy reserves to maintain a pregnancy and raise a child (your body is all about the survival of your genes).

As you can see, estrogen and thyroid hormones have somewhat opposing actions, so if you have excessive levels of estrogen, the high estrogen stimulates the production of the protein that binds to T4, and so reduces the amount of T4 available in your blood to be converted into the active T3. This can effectively block the action of your thyroid hormones and cause hypothyroidism. Excessive estrogen is called Estrogen Dominance (See Chapter 7 Why Your Sex Hormones Are Out Of Balance).

The interaction between estrogen dominance and your thyroid can also do nasty things to your libido by messing with your sex hormone balance. There is probably also a direct effect of low T3 on your libido, as Functional Medicine practitioners have reported that their women clients' libido can improve following thyroid treatment.

5.7
Autoimmune Conditions and your Thyroid

Conventional medical training is a lot about diagnostic training in reading peoples' list of symptoms and putting them in a box called X disease or Y disease. Conventional medicine typically then treats the symptoms, using drugs or surgery, often with scant regard for what might have been the cause. This approach has been spectacularly successful in dealing with acute medical conditions such as an infected wound, accident trauma, a stroke or heart attack.

Such an approach has not coped well with the recent explosive growth in chronic inflammatory lifestyle conditions such as irritable bowel, diabetes, obesity, arthritis, or autoimmune conditions like Hashimoto thyroiditis Rheumatoid arthritis, and mental conditions such as depression, dementia or Alzheimer's.

There is a rapidly growing movement of medical doctors taking a radically different approach (often called Functional Medicine or Integrated

Medicine), where they recognize that the same set of symptoms can come from radically different causes in different people. Functional Medicine practitioners focus on tracking down the cause or causes in the individual and then trying to eliminate or treat those causes.

Not surprisingly, the Functional Medicine approach is highly successful with treating chronic conditions and even includes complete reversal of conditions like diabetes and dementia and even autoimmune conditions – conditions in which your immune system produces antibodies against its own healthy cells and normal components of your body. The conventional medical view is that 'most autoimmune diseases are a chronic condition, which can be controlled with treatment, but not reversed'.

Most articles on thyroid conditions will tell you that Hashimoto's thyroiditis is the most common 'cause' of thyroid malfunction. In reality, it's just a list of symptoms of low thyroid function; sometimes with structural changes in the thyroid detected by ultrasound and accompanied by raised thyroid antibodies. This syndrome was first described by a Japanese doctor. Similarly, Grave's disease in which antibodies mimic the action of TSH and continually stimulate thyroid cells to produce more T4 is described as the most common 'cause' of hyperthyroidism.

Both of these conditions are described as autoimmune diseases because both of these syndromes are characterized by increased levels of thyroid antibodies in the blood. Commonly this has been described as the body making a mistake and developing antibodies that damage its own healthy tissues. Because family history is a strong predictor of the occurrence of an autoimmune disease, you are also likely to be told that you have faulty genes.

Recently some researchers decided that the idea of the body attacking itself did not really make sense and delved deeper into what these auto-antibodies (self-antibodies) really are and what they do. Such research has offered a potentially more rational explanation of what happens in an autoimmune condition.

It indicates that your body's immune system detects one of the body's normal proteins, which has been damaged by a 'toxin' – often mercury or another environmental toxin, or high levels of glucose in the blood. In this scenario the damaged normal protein appears to the body's immune system as 'non-self' and as such stimulates the production of antibodies to the 'alien' or 'non-self' protein.

The wonderful thing about this potential explanation is that it does not describe your body as making a mistake from which there is no recovery. Rather, it points the way to correcting the autoimmune condition, by removing the toxins which damaged the cells in the first place, and supplying the nutritional factors required to build healthy new cells and move towards a full recovery. Such an approach is how Functional Medicine practitioners are achieving the wonderful results they do.

Your thyroid is particularly vulnerable to autoimmune conditions because it has such a high requirement for iodine that it has a special 'pump' mechanism to scavenge iodine out of the blood supply. Unfortunately, this same 'pump' mechanism can also pick up thyroid disruptors, such as phthalates from soft plastics, soy isoflavones, flame retardants and many pesticides, from out of the blood supply and concentrate them in the thyroid. These can then become the toxins that stimulate the development of an autoimmune state, which goes on to damage your thyroid hormone production system.

5.8
Other Autoimmune Conditions

The latest thinking on autoimmune conditions and how they develop, described above, suggests that if your body has sufficient toxicity to cause one autoimmune condition, then the chances of you developing another autoimmune condition are much higher.

Basically, any symptoms of an autoimmune condition are thought to be reflecting the effects of toxicity in the body. Thus, if you have ANY form of autoimmune condition, then you are likely to have some form of thyroid malfunction, because the thyroid is so vulnerable to toxin damage because of the thyroid 'pump'.

Because of the prevalence of, and under-diagnosis of thyroid conditions, the American Thyroid Association recommends that everyone over 35 should have their thyroid function tested every five years and, if you have coeliac disease or gluten intolerance, you should have the full range of thyroid tests. This is because gluten intolerance is such a common autoimmune condition.

The latest thinking on gluten intolerance is that it is hugely underdiagnosed, such that nearly everyone has some degree of intolerance to the gluten protein. This can manifest as anything from low-level inflammation to full-blown digestive issues such as IBS (Irritable Bowel Syndrome), bloating and pain, diarrhea, and/or constipation. Unfortunately, at the lower end of the spectrum, you may not experience any digestive symptoms at all, but it can manifest in other parts of the body making it really tricky to diagnose.

I discuss gluten intolerance in more detail in Chapter 10 Bad Carbohydrates Make You Fat and Sick.

5.9
Symptoms Matter

It's absolutely crucial that you understand that how you feel, and what your symptoms are, matters more than any other factor or test result. Symptoms are your body trying to tell you that something is not right.

From here, if you do not have access to a Functional Medicine doctor, you have two choices:

- You can go the route of trying to sort out what your blood tests mean for yourself and then try to educate your doctor about what is wrong with you, and perhaps ask to be prescribed some natural thyroid extract, which will supply a balanced amount of both T4 and T3.

If your doctor says your blood tests are fine, but you feel lousy, before you get totally depressed (a symptom of poor thyroid function) about how to sort out what is going on in your body, a great, "not too technical" explanation of thyroid testing and how it relates to thyroid function can be found at: www.ITookCharge.nz/ThyroidTesting

- The other route, which I would suggest is the only true route to wellness, is to follow the protocol I outline in Chapter 16 Your 'Rapid Reset' Plan

5.10
What Causes Thyroid Malfunction?

Before we can start to heal thyroid function, we have to understand the key factors that contribute to why thyroid malfunction is so common.

- **Distress:** the excess adrenaline and cortisol released when you are consistently stressed inhibit the balanced manufacture of all of your steroid hormones, including your thyroid hormones.

- **Nutrient deficiency:** adequate iodine, selenium and iron are the key nutrients required for thyroid function.

The thyroid has one of the highest concentrations of iodine in the body and is the most efficient organ in the body at scavenging iodine from your blood. Yet iodine deficiency is widespread throughout the world because many soils are inherently low in iodine and the widespread use of soluble fertilizers displaces iodine off the soil structure so that it becomes vulnerable to leaching out of the root zone. These two factors mean that most food contains low levels of iodine.

- **Toxicity:** the thyroid gland is one of the most susceptible organs in the body to toxicity from the food we eat, the air we breathe, the cosmetics and nail varnish we put on our skin and nails, and the hundreds of chemicals that are present in our everyday environment. Iodine is also one of the chemical family called the halides, which includes fluorine, chlorine and bromine. These other halides are widespread in the modern world, and compete with iodine for a place on your receptors, so their presence can lead to a functional deficiency of iodine.

- **Estrogen dominance:** this can come from being overweight since fat cells are very efficient producers of estrogen, but can come from natural sources in food as well. However, the widespread occurrence of xenoestrogens (literally, 'foreign estrogens', external compounds which have potent estrogenic effects) in our environment, food, and cosmetics are a common cause of estrogen dominance. Many synthetic chemicals that cause this estrogen response (such as PCBs (polychlorinated biphenyl), BPA (Bisphenol A), and phthalates) also act as thyroid disruptors (See Chapter 7 Why Your Sex Hormones Are Out Of Balance).

- **Thyroid disruptors:** like estrogen, thyroid disruptors can come from both natural and synthetic sources.

  Natural disrupters include a compound from the brassica family and isoflavones from soybeans. Synthetic sources include a wide range of chlorinated pesticides, and the BPA used to line food cans. The structure of BPA is almost identical to thyroid hormone – a key reason why BPA can trigger an autoimmune reaction.

- **Poor blood sugar regulation:** often from high levels of stress hormones, this causes weight gain and inflammation, which then places a strain on the thyroid.

- **Underlying infections:** such as bleeding gums or SIBO (See Chapter 9 Bugs Are Important).

- **Gluten intolerance:** your bowel lining opens in response to gluten, which will cause inflammation in your body (See Chapter 10 Bad Carbs Make You Fat and Sick).

- **Liver function:** The liver is responsible for producing the binding protein so that inactive T4 can be transported to the liver, where it is converted to active T3. Poor liver function can also contribute to the development of thyroid malfunction.

It is also important to realize that thyroid disorders seldom appear by themselves. There are nearly always other hormonal issues and imbalances like adrenal fatigue, estrogen dominance, and an excess of insulin.

CHAPTER 6

Thyroid – The Canary in Your Coalmine

*"Certain toxins are taken up via the thyroid iodide
pump and concentrated"*

Joseph E. Pizzorno ND

As I mentioned in the previous chapter, your thyroid gland contains a special 'pump' mechanism to scavenge iodine out of the blood supply. This makes your thyroid function particularly vulnerable to disruption by toxins from your food and your environment. At the same time, your thyroid is also exquisitely sensitive to a number of nutrient deficiencies and to disruption by your stress hormones.

Thus your thyroid function is probably the most vulnerable part of your body to disruption from all three legs of your stool of wellness – The Canary in Your Coalmine. Because of this, I will dig a little deeper than I have with the other 'Three Musketeers', into both the causes and remedies of thyroid dysfunction.

Various surveys from around the world suggest that the incidence of thyroid issues in women living in industrialized countries could be as high as 1 in 7 women but, more importantly, about half of those women have not had a diagnosis of thyroid problems.

It is also important to realize that thyroid disorders seldom appear by themselves. There are nearly always other hormonal issues and imbalances like adrenal fatigue, estrogen dominance, and excess of insulin.

My aim is to show you how to rebuild your thyroid function, not about how to prop it up, whether with a thyroid extract taken from the glands of animals or worse, a synthetic approximation of thyroid hormone, in the form of a drug that has some (but not all) of the functions of your own thyroid hormones.

We know that the body is constantly regenerating itself, replacing old cells with new in an ongoing cycle that lasts throughout your lives. NEW CELLS, DERIVED FROM HAMBURGERS, TV DINNERS, HIGH LEVELS OF WHITE FLOUR AND SUGAR, ENERGY DRINKS, COFFEE, ALCOHOL, MEAT GROWN WITH THE USE OF HORMONES, DRUGS, AND FRIES COOKED IN DAYS OLD VEGETABLE OIL, ARE LIKELY TO BE WORSE THAN THE OLD CELLS THEY REPLACE. These cells built from unhealthy building blocks can be the beginnings of deterioration towards degenerative diseases, such as diabetes, arthritis, heart disease, and cancer.

On the other hand, NEW CELLS CREATED FROM REAL FOODS that your grandmother would probably recognize, WILL BE HEALTHIER THAN THE CELLS GENERATED BY THE DIET DESCRIBED ABOVE. These are the cells needed to repair and rebuild healthy organs and tissues. There is a rapidly growing body of evidence supporting the beneficial effects of diets which emphasize the consumption of real foods on your overall health; for instance, the Ketogenic, Mediterranean and Paleo diets.

Like all the other hormone imbalances, repairing the thyroid requires working through a process, not taking a simple remedy. It's the same three basic steps:

- Detoxify the body.

- Detoxify the mind.

- Supply all the essential nutrients in natural form to provide the building blocks to build healthy cells. Your thyroid CAN NOT make your thyroid hormones without adequate iodine, selenium, and iron.

6.1
The Place and Role of Iodine

Iodine is accepted to be an essential mineral nutrient, and I just want you to focus on the word essential for a moment. An essential nutrient means - that your body has to have the nutrient to be healthy, so you MUST get it from your food or supplements, preferably on a daily basis. Otherwise, your body is deteriorating in some way.

A French chemist called Bernard Courtois discovered iodine in 1811 when he was working with seaweed ash. Since seaweed and sea sponge ash had commonly been used to treat goiter and lung disease for thousands of years, it was soon evident that it was the iodine in the sea organisms that was the active ingredient.

In the next few years, iodine was picked up by doctors for the treatment of many diseases. According to medical records in the early 1900s, iodine was considered almost a universal medicine and was used to treat conditions as diverse as:

- Goiter

- Atherosclerosis

- Uterine fibroids

- Mercury, lead, and arsenic poisoning

- Swollen glands

- Swollen prostate

- Scarlet fever

- Bronchitis and pneumonia

- Obesity/weight gain

- Depression
- Breast pain and fibrocystic breast disease
- Eczema and psoriasis
- Genito-urinary diseases, such as syphilis
- Malaria
- Ovarian cysts
- Rheumatism
- Gastralgia
- Tonsillitis
- Coughs

6.2
Current Status of Iodine

Researchers who have been studying the role of iodine in health in the past ten years or so estimate that somewhere between 95% and 98% of the US population is deficient in iodine. It's fair to say that this probably represents the situation in many other parts of the world as well, because many soils are inherently very low in iodine and this has been exacerbated by the widespread use of soluble fertilizers that do not contain trace elements. The high concentrations at which these soluble fertilizers are applied means that they displace iodine and other trace minerals from the soil structure, so the vegetables grown in such soils and the meat from the livestock that graze pasture grown on these soils, will also be low in iodine and other trace minerals.

6.3
Iodine's Decline

When patented antibiotics, such as penicillin, were developed after World War II, iodine came to be considered 'old-fashioned'. Gradually its traditional properties, other than its use as an antiseptic, came to be forgotten.

The disappearance of iodine from medical doctors' arsenals was hastened by the publication in 1948 of a paper by an eminent endocrinologist, who suggested that high levels of iodine could potentially be toxic, based on a rat study. More recently this so-called 'Wolff-Chaikoff Effect' has been shown to be, in the vast majority of people, a transient disruption of thyroid hormone production, in response to a large single dose, which is your body's way of avoiding a surge in thyroid hormone in response to the large dose.

Yet somehow the warning to avoid iodine supplementation became enshrined in medical practice. This may relate to the fact that a synthetic thyroid hormone came onto the market at around the same time. A combination of advertising to promote the new drug and to position iodine as being old- fashioned seems to have been very effective – to the point that synthetic thyroid hormones are now the most prescribed drugs in the USA.

In 2000 Dr Guy Abraham initiated a research project on iodine deficiency, including a comprehensive review of iodine research. This evolved over five years into what became known as The Iodine Project, which is re-looking at the science around the levels of iodine that your body requires. The key figures involved in this project have been Dr Abraham, Dr Jorge Flechas and Dr David Brownstein.

This trio, whom some call the Iodine Doctors, started to publish the results of their studies at medical conferences where they also talked about the often dramatic clinical results being achieved. These ideas were picked up by patient activists from these conferences and taken back to their groups and online forums. This rapidly turned into a patient-led movement where individuals, often scientists and doctors, dug deeper into the medical literature and experimented for themselves. This has led to a large number of people experiencing relief from a wide range of conditions, which had been having serious effects on their health and their lives.

This doctor and patient movement came together in 2007 in an Iodine Conference, where results and protocols were shared to maximize the healing benefits of iodine and minimize the potential detox symptoms that can sometimes be experienced when first using iodine.

The list of conditions which have been helped by the use of iodine from the participants in the Iodine Project is large and includes the previous list, plus a quite a few more. The take-home lesson from these findings is that ensuring you have an ongoing optimum iodine intake is important for your good health – it is an essential nutrient after all!

6.4

Why are you Likely to Need More Iodine?

So you say, "Well, I have my daily dose of iodized salt, I should be fine."

Sorry. The amount of iodine that you get from iodized salt doesn't even start to cover your body's needs for iodine. The notion that refined iodized salt is all you need is probably the most dangerous misconception about iodine.

The recommended daily intake (RDI) for iodine aims at preventing the development of goiter, so provides most of the requirement for your THYROID only, but the rest of your body needs iodine as well, particularly for your breast and brain health. So what we are looking for here is what is the optimum amount of iodine you need for wellness.

The RDI for iodine is currently 0.15 milligram, and if you're having the average intake of iodized salt, as it leaves the factory, you're probably consuming a little bit more than that. However the form of iodine in the iodized salt is very poorly absorbed and you're probably getting, at best, about three-quarters of the RDI into your tissues.

On top of this, from the time iodized salt leaves the factory until it gets onto the grocery store shelf, half of the original iodide content is lost by evaporation to the atmosphere. Once the salt is opened in your home the rate of evaporation increases, especially if you use it in cooking. After all that, only a proportion of the iodine in salt is absorbed into your tissues because of the high chlorine content of the salt.

The lack of iodine in our diet has also been exacerbated by the rise in the use of gourmet salts such as Celtic sea salt and Himalayan rock salt, which usually do not have any added iodine. Another exacerbating factor is that many people are using less salt, because their doctor mistakenly thinks a lower salt intake can lower their blood pressure – recent research has shown that this is not correct. The end result of these two factors is that estimates of the intake of iodized salt in western diets suggest that it halved between 1971 and 2000.

6.5
Bromine, Chlorine and Fluorine vs Iodine

Iodine, bromine, chlorine and fluorine are part of the chemical family called halides, and the most reactive members of the family dominate the receptors on your cells.

The chemical reactivity of the halide group goes like this:

Fluorine: the most chemically active member; widely used to (supposedly) protect your teeth (See Appendix B Take Care of Your Mouth), and it is also present in a substantial number of medical drugs.

Chlorine: the 2nd most chemically active member; widely used as a water disinfectant, so you inhale it pretty much every time you have a shower, or swim in a treated pool, or drink water from a tap. Chlorine is also widely used in making plastics, dyes, paper products, insecticides and in many industrial chemicals.

Bromine: the 3rd most chemically active member; widely used as a fire retardant chemical, and in many other industrial chemicals and, in some countries (i.e. USA), it is still widely used as a bread dough conditioner.

Iodine: the least chemically active, but the only one of this family that is an essential nutrient which your body MUST have to function correctly.

Because iodine is the least chemically reactive of the group, to force the potentially toxic fluorine, chlorine, and bromine from your cell receptors, the levels of iodine in your body have to be quite high. Thus chlorine, bromine and fluorine are iodine antagonists - substances that majorly interfere with or inhibit iodine's role in your body.

Calculation of the RDI doesn't seem to have allowed for the fact that since the 1970's the intake of iodine has halved, while the levels of fluorine, chlorine and bromine in our food and the environment have all increased substantially.

6.5.1
Bromine, Bread, and Iodine

There is a lot of evidence that suggests that a major contributor to the widespread symptoms of iodine deficiency in the population is a phenomenon known as bromine dominance. This can develop when bromine is acquired from your living environment, prescription drugs or dietary exposure, and causes bromine levels in the body to raise high enough to inhibit iodine metabolism.

The drop in urinary iodine levels in the population started when iodine was removed from use in bread and baked goods around 1970.

In the 1960s, the average slice of bread contained 0.15 milligrams of iodine in the form of potassium IODATE as a dough conditioner. Thus, every slice of bread used to contain around the RDI of iodine. So since most people would probably consume several slices of bread each day, the average intake of iodine was probably closer to one milligram.

There are a number of theories as to why potassium iodate was removed as a dough conditioner, but whatever the reason; unfortunately, the baking industry started using the much cheaper potassium BROMATE as the dough conditioner of choice, and so replacing iodine in the diet with a major iodine antagonist. Bad move for your health!

More recently, potassium bromate was deemed possibly carcinogenic to humans by the International Agency for Research on Cancer and has been banned from use in food products in New Zealand, Europe, Canada, and China, but it IS STILL USED in the USA (labeled as enriched flour) and some other countries. Fortunately in New Zealand, following the banning of potassium bromate in 1996, vitamin C has become the most common dough conditioner. A good move for your health!

6.5.2
Bromine in Your Environment

Currently the worst exposure to bromine comes from brominated fire retardant chemicals called BFR's. They can be found in rugs, cars, mattresses, upholstery, electronics, children's pajamas, draperies, and many other items including children's' toys. Bromide dust leaks from these items, is inhaled and gets into your bloodstream.

Bromide is also found in pesticides (methyl bromide), brominated vegetable oil (often added to citrus-flavored drinks like Mountain Dew), some asthma inhalers and prescription drugs, hot tub cleansers, plastic products, some personal care products, including permanent wave and hair dyes and some fabric dyes.

Exposure to bromine has been linked to skin disorders, mental conditions, low-frequency hearing loss and kidney cancer.

6.6
Chlorine

The second most reactive halide chlorine, is widely used to disinfect most urban water supplies. It is the active ingredient in most bleach because it is such a powerful oxidant that it kills organic molecules. This means that every time you drink, shower or swim in chlorine-treated water your body will be absorbing chlorine through your skin or gut. The best way to minimize this exposure is to install a good quality 'whole of house' water filter and, if possible, swim in the sea, clean rivers or ozonated swimming pools.

Another widespread source of chlorine is from the molecule perchlorate which is commonly used as a powerful oxidizer in rocket fuel, fireworks and matches, and as a contaminant in some fertilizers. While you might think that you are not likely to be exposed to much from these sources, the molecule is quite persistent, so it is a common contaminant of water, so can even be found in vegetables irrigated with contaminated water.

Perchlorate is so good at competing with iodine within your thyroid that for a short time it was used to treat hyperthyroid, although this was quickly discontinued when it was found that it also caused serious anemia. A 2006 study found that even very low levels of perchlorate exposure caused decreased thyroid function in women.

Chlorine is also widely used in many industrial processes to make plastics, dyes, paper products, insecticides and many other pesticides.

6.7
Fluorine

As the chemically most reactive member of the halide family, low levels of fluorine can have a significant impact on thyroid function. Regarding acute toxicity, fluoride is actually more toxic than lead and only slightly less toxic than arsenic.

Fluoride can enter the body from fluoridated water supplies; fluoride in toothpaste and fluoride is an ingredient in about 100 popular drugs.

Early symptoms of fluoride poisoning include stomach pain, nausea, vomiting and headaches. The dose required to produce these symptoms is estimated to be only 0.1 - 0.3 mg of fluoride per Kg of body weight. Thus a child weighing 10 kg (22 pounds) can suffer symptoms of acute toxicity by swallowing just 1 – 3 g of the toothpastes marketed specifically to children – that's about half a teaspoon. Because the symptoms outlined above may mimic other common childhood ailments, it's likely that many cases of fluoride poisoning go undiagnosed.

Although the USA Centers for Disease Control suggest water fluoridation is one of the 10 top public health achievements of the 20th century, it is worth noting that 97% of the Western European population drinks non-fluoridated water. The tooth decay rates in Europe have declined precipitously over the last 50 years, just as they have done in the USA.

Regarding acute toxicity, fluoride is actually more toxic than lead and only slightly less toxic than arsenic.

6.8
How Much Iodine do you Need?

As discussed earlier, the recommended daily allowance (RDI) for iodine is currently 0.15 milligram, which only aims to prevent goiter developing, but makes no allowance for the rest of your bodily needs for iodine, particularly for your breast and brain health.

The average Japanese on a traditional diet which is high in sea vegetables is getting somewhere around 10-12 milligrams per day. That's nearly a hundred times more than the RDI. Yet a study of the health of the population in seven different countries, published in 1989, showed that at that point the longevity and health of the Japanese population was the best in the world.

If you suggest to your doctor that you want to increase your iodine intake to a level similar to the traditional Japanese intake, they are very likely to say "Oh, that much is dangerous," or "the Japanese have a very different metabolism from Caucasians." However, when Japanese move to a Caucasian country and eat a typical Caucasian diet low in iodine they develop all the same diseases that are rampant in Caucasian society.

Because of the issues outlined in section 6.3 Iodine's Decline, the safety of consuming high levels of iodine is undoubtedly controversial and, according to the National Institutes of Health in the USA, the tolerable upper limit for iodine intake is 1.1 mg per day. However iodine is routinely used at quite high levels to disinfect water, particularly by the military, and by people traveling in areas where water treatment is unreliable. Thus the US military commissioned a study to clarify the safety of iodine at higher doses.

The authors concluded, "A review of the human trials on the safety of iodine ingestion indicates that neither the maximum recommended dietary dose (2 mg/day) nor the maximum recommended duration of use (3 weeks) has a firm basis". Backer and Hollowell 2000

They went on to say that there appears to be marked individual sensitivity but no clear safe threshold dose. Other studies highlight the importance of having an adequate intake of selenium if you are supplementing with iodine as this will minimize any potential for toxicity.

6.8.1
The Iodine Project

The Iodine Project has been looking at what the actual requirements are for iodine for about ten years, and they have done some human studies with a wide range of patients from North America.

Participants in the studies were given 40-60 milligrams of iodine per day and the iodine levels excreted in their urine monitored.

The studies consistently found that the participants needed to have that level of iodine intake for somewhere between four to six weeks before they got to the level where they start to excrete significant amounts of iodine in their urine. In other words, it takes four to six weeks before they have sufficient iodine in their bodies, since once a person has adequate iodine stores they excrete any they don't need in their urine.

The other interesting thing is that about two-thirds of the people in these trials KNEW when they arrived at the point of iodine excretion, because their brain fog disappeared and they felt well.

So most people need a very large amount of iodine to load their body to the point where they're saturated with it.

Some people suggest that when you start supplementing with iodine, that you take relatively high doses of iodine in the early stages to help detoxify your body, because you need high concentrations of iodine to displace the chemically more reactive bromine, chlorine, and fluorine from within your cells. Such an approach can potentially lead to unpleasant detox symptoms, so I favor a more gentle approach unless you are under the care of a very iodine knowledgeable practitioner who can help you manage any symptoms that arise.

Once you have reached saturation, the recommended daily intake that The Iodine Project is suggesting is in the range between 12.5 – 45.00 milligrams per day.

In fact, that is what the RDI before 1950 used to be.

"about two-thirds of the people in these trials knew when they arrived at the point of iodine excretion because their brain fog disappeared and they felt well."

6.8.2
Iodine and Breast Health

The amount of iodine required for your breast, brain and whole body health is many many times more than that needed for thyroid health – so it's not entirely surprising that the levels of breast health issues are also extremely high in women, and that breast cancer is the most common cancer for women. Research suggests that only about 5 -10% of the risk of developing breast cancer comes from your genes. The other 90 - 95% of the risk factors are all lifestyle, so are directly under your control, if you so choose.

Breast cancer develops slowly and benign breast disease is a high risk factor for cancer. Yet benign breast disease, where the breasts feel tender or swollen can be described by some doctors as normal, although how a condition with disease as its last name can be described as normal, I find hard to understand; common okay, but absolutely not normal. It is well known that breast cancers have typically been growing for seven or more years before being detected, but the myth of cancer striking instead of developing still persists.

Research at the Mayo Clinic found that one-third of the women diagnosed with benign breast disease progressed to invasive breast cancer within five years. Dr Jorge Flechas has reported that benign breast disease noted at autopsy has increased from 23 per cent in 1928 to 89 per cent in 1973.

We know that iodine deficiency is strongly linked to benign breast disease and breast cancer, and more women get thyroid cancer than men do, and the situation is getting worse. The risk of breast cancer had risen from 1 in 20 women in 1970, to 1 in 8 by 2006 and it remains at that level today. The incidence of thyroid cancer has risen 182% since 1975.

While the exact role of iodine in breast health is not yet fully understood, some of the things we do know include:

- When a woman with benign breast disease supplements with iodine, the breasts usually soften and return to normal.

- When dietary iodine was blocked in rats, they developed breast swelling, nodules, and benign breast disease.

- Rats given cancer-causing chemicals (DMBA) would not develop breast tumors if they were iodine sufficient.

- Iodine desensitizes estrogen receptors in the breast, making your breasts less vulnerable to estrogen dominance.

- When scientists gave iodine to a group of breast cancer patients, it caused cancer cell death, slowed cancer cell division, reduced the size and number of tumor-promoting blood vessels, and reduced estrogen production from the ovaries.

In the online forums there are many testimonies of women who have used high doses of iodine and have had a significant impact on their benign breast disease and even breast cancer.

For those who are curious to learn more about iodine than I can cover in this brief review, there are now a number of comprehensive books on the subject including "Iodine: Why you need it, Why you can't live without it" by Dr Brownstein, or "The Iodine Crisis: What You Don't Know About Iodine Can Wreck Your Life" by Lynne Farrow.

> *"Research suggests that some breast cancers may be an iodine deficiency disease"*
> *Lynne Farrow*

There are clickable links to several more detailed resources at www.ITookCharge.nz/Iodine Resources.

The links include access to a comprehensive database of research on iodine, breast cancer options, including the therapeutic use of iodine.

There are also links to several iodine forums. The accuracy of some of the posts leaves a lot to be desired in these online forums, but some are well moderated and, in my opinion, more accurate.

Working with what the 'Iodine Movement' calls an Iodine Literate Practitioner is obviously the most desirable course of action, however finding one of these in your area can be a challenge.

Sending an email to ffp_lab@yahoo.com, which is a lab which specializes in iodine testing, and asking for a referral to an Iodine Literate Practitioner.

6.9
The Role of Selenium

Selenium is not only essential for thyroid health; it's essential for a healthy immune system. It improves fertility, helps to fight viral infections, and reduces the risk of heart disease, cancer and arthritis.

Selenium is a part of the enzyme that converts inactive T4 into the active T3 form of thyroid hormone. While the majority of this conversion occurs in the liver and kidneys and cells in your body, some conversion happens in the thyroid.

Selenium has been shown to be helpful in treating autoimmune disease and inflammatory states, so having adequate selenium is important for people with autoimmune thyroid issues, such as Graves' disease and Hashimoto's thyroiditis.

The link between selenium and a healthy immune system is so strong that the recently published Selenium World Atlas (2002) used the incidence of HIV-1 (AIDS) in Africa as a surrogate measure of soil selenium levels because of a lack of data on actual soil levels. In the United States, a relationship between soil selenium and incidence of HIV-1 has also been demonstrated.

I started my family on a selenium supplement over 40 years ago, after I discovered that all the local vets were taking a Selenium supplement, because of the effects of low selenium they saw in all the livestock.

6.9.1
How Much Selenium?

Because most of the parent rock in New Zealand is inherently low in selenium, most soils are selenium deficient. Most livestock in NZ are routinely supplemented with selenium.

The decision to supplement with selenium or not depends on where you are in the world and your local soil selenium levels. Like most trace elements, selenium is required in a fairly narrow range for optimum health, and too much selenium has been shown to cause health problems where soil selenium levels are too high.

In New Zealand selenium is deficient on most soils (apart from around Mt Taranaki and parts of Northland). When the importance of selenium in human health was discovered in the early 1970s, scientists started monitoring the levels of blood selenium in people arriving in New Zealand from the United Kingdom. They found that within a month of arriving peoples' blood selenium levels had declined to one-tenth of their initial levels, which had been at the world norm. Recent research at Otago University has suggested that humans in NZ should be supplementing with at least 90 µg Se per day.

The incidence of selenium deficiency is on the rise because of the widespread use of simple soluble fertilizers in conventional agriculture. These displace trace elements like selenium from the soil matrix. The choice to eat organic foods can potentially reduce this problem because organic production avoids soluble fertilizers.

6.10
The Role of Iron

Having adequate iron levels in your body is also key to normal thyroid function. Like selenium, iron can affect several parts of the thyroid system, including the conversion of inactive T4 to active T3.

In fact, there is considerable overlap between the symptoms of low thyroid and low iron – weakness, palpitations, brain fog, fatigue, and low libido.

Too much iron, however, can cause overload problems, particularly in your liver.

It is best to get iron from food sources such as leafy greens, sea vegetables and grass-fed meats, since many women find that iron supplements can exacerbate constipation issues which are really bad for your detox systems.

6.11
What to Do First

I encourage you to try the nutritional and lifestyle suggestions outlined in Chapter 16 Your 'Rapid Reset' Plan, as a first step to correcting thyroid issues. I have seen people respond to this within days.

When I talked to a woman friend about thyroid issues she said:" I've been on synthetic thyroid hormone for years, and it seems to be working fine for me, so what's the problem?" If you are in this situation, I strongly recommend you go back and read the section on Iodine and Breast Health and have a rethink about how fine you really are.

6.12
Hormone Supplementation

The next step if you need more help, or need help faster, is to go to your health provider to get a prescription for a thyroid hormone supplement.

My first choice:

1. Start with natural desiccated thyroid

In many ways nature is very conservative, so once it finds an approach that proves successful it tends to be encoded into the DNA of every other successful species. As a result, the thyroid hormones produced by other mammals are identical to our own.

The original thyroid supplement was made from sheep thyroid but, since the early 1900s, desiccated thyroid from pigs has been widely available.

Some of the brand names available include:

Armour Thyroid, Nature-throid, and Westhroid, or you can get it made up to prescription by a compounding pharmacist.

The beauty of desiccated thyroid is that it contains both the inactive T4 and active T3 in the ratio that your body needs them, and also contains T2, T1 and other thyroid proteins about which little is known – but which are probably important to normal thyroid metabolism.

If your health provider is open to it (many may not be), I recommend that you start with the smallest dose because your body is probably not used to having freely available active T3, so anything but the smallest dose may put you at risk of developing hyperthyroid symptoms.

2. Synthetic T4 - Levothyroxine Sodium

While many sources claim that this is chemically identical to thyroxin (T4), this is not so, on two counts:

- The basic molecule is only the L-isomer of thyroxin and does not contain any of the D-isomer. While the chemical formula is the same for the two isomers, the molecular structure is different, so they perform differently in your body. A really good analogy for this is that your hands are isomers of each other – same basic structure, but they are mirror images of each other, so not identical.

- The basic molecule has been modified to turn it into a sodium salt, which means it has a sodium atom attached at one end of its chain. Your cell receptors work on shape; so the addition of the sodium atom means the shape is different, so its impact on your cells will be slightly different.

The key problem with using inactive T4 is that if there is any malfunction in your body's ability to transform it into the active T3, then it will not fully alleviate your symptoms. Many people who have been put on the synthetic, inactive T4 have not experienced full relief from their symptoms.

If this doesn't give you the response you are looking for, and you still can't convince your health provider to put you on natural thyroid extract, then the next best option is a combination of T4 and active T3.

3. A combination of T4 and T3.

You do need to be very cautious about taking T3, as it is very much more active than T4. How much you need of the active T3 is very dependent on how well your body is currently converting inactive T4 to active T3. This means that there is a relatively high risk of developing hyperthyroid symptoms, which can be quite scary and potentially nasty.

CHAPTER 7

Why Your Sex Hormones Are Out Of Balance

"Hormonal problems are the top reason I find for accelerated aging,"
Sara Gottfried, MD

You have three key sex hormones which basically drive all your reproductive functions and hence your libido.

The estrogens are the main feminizing hormones that drive the changes in your body as you reach puberty, and which drive your monthly hormonal cycle to prepare your uterus to receive an egg, and to prepare an egg ready for release. This monthly cycle for women is superimposed on the daily cycle of all the other hormones that are at play in both male and female bodies, and it is this monthly cycle that makes women particularly vulnerable to hormonal upsets.

The other feminine hormone is progesterone, which is the natural complement to estrogen and is mainly responsible for maintaining the pregnancy if fertilization happens. You also produce testosterone, in much smaller amounts than the other two, but it has an important role to play in your emotional well-being and your libido.

It is the balance of these three hormones that control your mental and emotional well-being and how well you are. As we saw with your stress and thyroid hormones, modern living is very good at messing up this delicate balance, and while there are a large number of potential causes for your sex hormones becoming out of balance, the most common ones are as follows:

7.1
Estrogen Dominance

Estrogen Dominance was first described by Dr John Lee in the early 1990s and is when the estrogen signaling at the cellular level is out of balance with the amount of progesterone your body is making. This can occur as a result of exposure to xenoestrogens, hormone replacement therapy, pre- and post-menopause, birth control pills, or a hysterectomy.

It is not uncommon for women in their twenties and thirties to have cycles where no egg is released, caused by hormonal imbalances, which can exacerbate PMT symptoms as no progesterone gets produced by the ovaries.

7.2
High Stress

If your life has lots of stress, either eustress or distress, then your body's demand for the stress hormone cortisol, results in cholesterol being preferentially used to make cortisol, rather than it being used to make progesterone, estrogens, or testosterone, which are the hormones that help to drive your libido. The main impact of stress tends to be a reduction in progesterone – the happy hormone for women.

In times of prolonged stress from famine, this has the desirable effect of preventing pregnancy when a woman does not have the food resources to carry a successful pregnancy, but this is no longer relevant to most women in the developed world.

7.3
Living in a Masculine World

In this modern world many women find themselves having to, or choosing to, work in roles in the workforce where you are exposed to a lot of masculine energy or competing with men. Since we all become like those we spend a lot of time with, when you work a lot with men, effectively you have to spend a large chunk of your day working in your masculine energy, being assertive and decisive and unfeminine. This has been shown to both drop your estrogen levels and raise your testosterone levels, which makes you behave more like a man.

This is fine, as long as when you get home you don't continue the whole evening feeling like you are still in a masculine environment while you go about organizing the family meal and getting them ready for the next day. At some stage you need to consciously come back into your feminine energy to raise your estrogen levels and drop your testosterone levels, which will attract the masculine energy from the man in your life, like the opposite poles of a magnet. See Chapter 14 - Take Charge of your Sexiness.

7.4
Your Estrogens

Estrogens are the main feminizing hormones in your body and, before menopause, your ovaries produce the majority of your estrogens, but your adrenal glands produce small amounts.

Fat cells are also little estrogen factories. They can contribute a significant amount of estrogen if you have lots of them, so particularly after menopause, your fat cells are likely to become your major source of estrogen.

Estrogen is not actually a single hormone. There are three different estrogens which are made in different parts of the body and have somewhat different activity.

They are:

Estradiol: During your reproductive years 10 - 20% of the estrogen made in your ovaries is estradiol. This is the estrogen responsible for developing secondary sex characteristics. It affects bone growth to give you the characteristic broader hips, and fat deposition as part of breast development, and around your butt to give you your feminine shape.

It is also the estrogen that prepares the lining of the uterus, triggers the release of the egg, and has some role in maintaining your pregnancy.

Estrone: Roughly 10% of the estrogen made in your body is estrone, but it is the major estrogen formed by fat tissue which means it can end up being the major estrogen produced after menopause. Estrone is more active in the body than oestradiol, and it may act as a reservoir that your body can use to convert to oestradiol as needed.

Estriol: Represents about 70 - 80% of the estrogen made in your body, primarily in the liver, and it is produced in significant amounts by the placenta during pregnancy to help maintain the pregnancy.

The amount of estriol produced by your body doesn't drop much after menopause, which is important because estriol is the most effective estrogen for maintaining vaginal and cervical health, and it also has some protective effect against breast cancer.

7.4.1
Estrogens in Action

When you hit puberty, estradiol is the main hormone that initiates all   the feminizing effects on your body: the development of your uterus, your breasts, your hips, your butt, and all your secondary sex characteristics which contribute to your feminine shape which is so attractive to men.

Estradiol is also the estrogen that initiates the first half of the menstrual cycle, the growth of the egg and building the cells of the uterine lining ready to receive a fertilized egg. Once the egg has shed the level of estrogen drops away, and the amount of progesterone increases dramatically in a beautiful crossover.

If conception does occur then the placenta starts to produce estriol to help maintain the pregnancy.

7.4.2
How do I get Estrogen Dominance?

For an estrogen molecule to do its job at a cellular level it needs to bind onto an estrogen receptor, which is 'kinda like' a key fitting into a lock. The parts of a woman's body that are most sensitive to estrogen are the ovaries, the breasts and the bowel (in guys it's the prostate, the breasts and the bowel). These parts of your body are very sensitive to estrogen because they have high levels of estrogen receptors.

Unfortunately, your estrogen receptors have an Achilles heel in that they are particularly vulnerable to being stimulated by a range of other chemicals from outside the body. These chemicals are called estrogen mimics and they are widespread in our food and our environment.

They can be grouped into three categories:

Phytoestrogens: compounds found in plants which have weak estrogenic effects in your body. These are widespread in nature, but are found in the highest concentrations in flax seed, red clover, or soya beans, so these are the sources most often used to promote health.

Synthetic estrogens: your natural estrogen molecules cannot be patented, so the pharmaceutical companies create slight alterations to the natural estrogen molecules so that they can be patented, manufactured, and used in birth control pills and HRT (hormone replacement therapy) at high prices.

Xenoestrogens: are a huge class of estrogen-like synthetic chemicals that also have the ability to lock into an estrogen receptor on the cell, and trick the cells of your body into responding as they do to estrogen. These chemicals are one of the key drivers of estrogen dominance. These estrogen mimics are particularly important because they can be dramatically more potent than the natural estrogen produced by our bodies.

If your estrogen receptors are getting stimulated by estrogen mimics this can throw your estrogen/progesterone balance out of whack, creating a state of Estrogen Dominance. This will mean that, to some extent, the crossover between estrogen and progesterone, which should happen at ovulation, doesn't happen, leaving you vulnerable to a range of, generally unpleasant, side-effects.

For instance, the brain is very sensitive to estrogen. It is estrogen that helps regulate the production of your feel-good chemicals, oxytocin, serotonin, and dopamine. Estrogen dominance also stimulates your body to retain copper, and copper and zinc antagonize each other so, if you are high in estrogen, the levels of zinc getting into your brain are reduced which can lead to serious mood swings, stress reactions and even depression (PMS anyone?).

The scale of the problem?

Your own estrogens do vary a little in potency, but let's assume for a moment that the estrogens you produce give a signal strength of 1 when they bind to a receptor.

By comparison:

Phyto-estrogens: send a very weak signal to your cells. When you take them at low levels, they can block more potent estrogens from binding onto your estrogen receptors and so, at the right daily intake, they can act to lower your total estrogen loading and reduce estrogen dominance. However, if you eat them at high levels, e.g. you eat a lot of soy products, they will still add to your total estrogen loading and contribute to estrogen dominance.

Synthetic estrogens: are not able to be metabolized and excreted easily by your body and so hang around for a lot longer and thus end up having substantially more potent effects on your body than your own estrogens.

Xenoestrogens: when these bind to an estrogen receptor they have the ability to send a signal strength of somewhere between 10 and 1,000 times that of natural estrogen. Thus, they are hugely powerful in their impact on your body and we all need to consciously reduce our exposure to them. These are the ones that significantly contribute to the development of the estrogen driven cancers such as breast, ovarian, uterine and bowel cancers.

7.4.3
The Xenoestrogen Problem

The problem is that these powerful estrogen mimics work at extremely low levels.

In most chemistry it is the size of the dose that determines the effect on a system, but new research has shown that sometimes the smaller the dose of these xenoestrogens (sometimes called endocrine disrupters) the bigger the impact they have on our bodies. There is also a growing body of evidence which shows that the effects of such chemicals on the body are not just additive, but actually work synergistically, so that 2+2 can equal 7 or a much larger number.

One of the first pesticides to be recognized as a xenoestrogen was DDT.

This was developed and first used extensively as an insecticide during the Second World War, mainly being put in soldiers' clothing to keep the nits and lice off their bodies. Because DDT was such an effective insecticide and was very persistent in the environment, the use of DDT spread very quickly, and it became widely used in agriculture during the 1950s and 60s.

In 1962 Rachel Carson wrote a famous book called 'Silent Spring', and it was she who first really alerted the world to the huge damage that pesticides like DDT were having on wildlife populations and the natural environment, by direct toxicity to animals and birds.

Many people think that her book was the beginning of the environmental movement. It was certainly the beginning of the move to ban or limit the use of pesticides like DDT from our food production systems. The use of DDT was banned in the USA in 1972, but it wasn't until 1989 that DDT usage was banned in New Zealand. DDT is still in widespread use in Africa, Asia and South America, so that worldwide production of DDT hasn't actually declined since the 1950s.

A sequel to the DDT story came out in 1996 by Theo Colborn called "Our Stolen Future", which looked at what had happened in the 30-odd years since Rachel Carson's book. Colborn found that, yes, the levels of pesticides like DDT in the USA environment had been drastically reduced, but the wildlife populations were not recovering as expected. The book goes on to link the cause of this to the impact xenoestrogens like DDT were having on the fertility of the wildlife. The book also detailed the research being done on the impact of xenoestrogens and endocrine disrupters on the human population.

A further concern is that agricultural pesticides tend to be reasonably well regulated in Europe and North America, but they are seldom well regulated in other parts of the world which is where an increasingly large proportion of our food is coming from. Also, many of the hundreds of other chemicals used by industry are very poorly regulated worldwide, and mostly they are assumed to be safe unless proven otherwise. By the time we are made aware of health issues, their use is firmly entrenched in the industry and getting them banned can be a long slow process – see BPA below.

It wasn't until the 1990s that we really had the technology to measure xenoestrogens at the very low levels they are active, and so we went on to find that even in regions where DDT is banned, it is still abundant in the environment. DDT is now so widespread that it is present in the fat of humans and animals throughout the globe – from the top of the Himalayas to the bottom of the oceans, and from the Arctic to the South Pole. There is nobody in the world that does not have some DDT in his or her body.

There is another issue with the testing technology itself. If you exhibit some symptoms of a hormonal imbalance, your health practitioner is likely to test the levels of your three sex hormones and may well come back with the answer that "they all look fine, so that's not your issue". Because so many different chemicals exhibit an estrogen response in your body at very low levels, it simply is not possible to test for their presence and thus assess the effect they may be having on your health.

This is why your symptoms really matter, as they are the only real signposts you have to indicate whether you have Estrogen Dominance or not.

7.4.4
Common Xenoestrogens in our Environment

Insecticides such as DDT, dieldrin, and endosulfan are still in widespread use around the world and are contaminants in our food supply. Although DDT is banned in New Zealand agriculture Diazinon is still being used, so chemicals like these still act as a major source of xenoestrogens in our food supply.

Herbicides such as atrazine, which is one of the most widely used herbicides in the USA and many other countries, has been shown to contaminate groundwater in New Zealand and around the world.

BPA (Bisphenol A) is the plastic used to manufacture polycarbonate drinking containers, and the epoxy resins used as the lining in most food and beverage cans. It is one of the highest volume chemicals produced worldwide. Scientists have found that even picomolar concentrations of BPA (concentrations of less than one part per trillion) can disrupt a cell's normal functioning, so the use of BPA in food contact is starting to be banned around the world. Canada was the first country to ban it from being used for lining cans. In New Zealand the selling of food in cans lined with BPA is still allowed.

Unfortunately, very recent research reveals that a common BPA replacement, Bisphenol S (BPS), may be just as harmful, so not eating or drinking from cans may be the only safe option at this stage.

In the future PET (#1 plastic) and a plant-based oleoresin may turn out to be safer alternatives for can linings. In the short term, buying food and drinks in glass jars or shelf-stable pouches can be a great alternative to cans. Aseptic packaging, like Tetra Pak containers (which are lined with a safe plastic called polypropylene), are also a good way to avoid BPA or BPS.

BPA or BPS are also used as part of the coating of thermal paper used in EFTPOS or credit card printers, so avoid them if possible.

PVC plastics, which are used to make plastic wrap, are widely used in the packaging of fresh food. Many food packers use them to cover their food before sale, but even worse is when they are used to cover food when it is put in the microwave. The steam from the heating food condenses on the plastic wrap and leaches large amounts of xenoestrogens out of it, which then drops down into the food.

Many 'factory farm' raised animals like beef cattle and pigs are routinely fed chemicals such as DES or Zeranol, which are hormonal growth promoters and act as powerful xenoestrogens. These work to increase animal growth rates because one of the key effects of estrogen is to increase rates of cell division.

The chemicals used by the cosmetics industry are also not well tested for safety or stringently regulated, and there are some very nasty chemicals used in cosmetics, which have not been tested for their impact on human health. In fact, many of the ingredients used in personal care products such as cosmetics, sunscreens, shampoos, and fragrances have been shown to be estrogenic. Many people have the very incorrect perception that your skin is an effective barrier to chemicals.

Pretty much everything that is put on your skin goes into your body. The only variable is just how rapid the absorption rate is - if you wouldn't eat your cosmetics, why would you put them on your skin?

Yet surveys have shown that on a daily basis the average consumer (whoever that might be) uses personal care products that contain over one hundred different synthetic chemicals.

7.4.5
How to Avoid Xenoestrogens?

There are some steps you can take to reduce your exposure to xenoestrogens:

- Eating as much certified organic food as you can access or afford would be a great start.

- Eating animal products from free-range or grass-fed animals are less likely to have had exposure to hormones and antibiotics.

- Limiting the amount of food that you use from cans until safer can linings are in widespread use – which is starting to happen.

- Buy processed food that is packaged in glass, plastic pouches, or aseptic packaging (i.e. Tetra Pac).

- Put a plate over food you are microwaving, rather than using plastic wrap.

- Choose your cosmetics and personal care products with great care. Read the labels. There is a good chance that if you can't pronounce the names of the ingredients, then you shouldn't be buying it.

- Regularly use small amounts of phytoestrogens in your diet to help reduce your estrogen dominance from the exposure you can't avoid.

7.4.6
Phytoestrogens

Phytoestrogens can be a very powerful tool to modulate the estrogen signaling in your body to a healthy level. While the estrogenic effect from plants is weak, they are just as likely as the xenoestrogens to bind to receptors. Thus they can block more potent estrogens from binding to your estrogen receptors. This means they can be used to lower your total exposure to estrogenic effects at the cellular level.

However, it is important to remember that they are still estrogens, so if you take them in large quantities you can expect them to exacerbate symptoms of estrogen dominance. This is likely to be happening if you routinely consume significant amounts of soy-based foods (See below).

The three most widely used phytoestrogens that are used in low doses as therapeutic tools to block the inevitable exposure to xenoestrogens are:

Lignans

Many plants contain lignans in relatively small amounts but flax seeds are unusual in that they contain substantial levels of lignans. Like the isoflavones in soybeans, the lignans in flax seeds are not directly active in your body and, before they are active, need to be converted to human lignans by the beneficial bacteria normally present in your gut.

Lignans also act as powerful antioxidants so, on a per serve basis flax meal is right up there with such antioxidant-rich foods as blueberries and chocolate.

I used to assume that the beneficial bacteria in your gut would naturally reassert themselves, over time, to become dominant again after a course of antibiotic treatment. However, there have recently been two studies that have shown that in one case two months and, in another, four months after treatment with antibiotics, women's ability to make human lignans from flax lignans had not been restored. The message I take from these studies is that it will be important for your health to take probiotics once you have finished any course of antibiotics (See Chapter 8 Bugs Are Important).

My experience over the last 25 years of dealing with customers using flax meal is that around one tablespoon per day can give a useful reduction in estrogen dominance effects, but people vary considerably in the amount they need to consume to achieve any useful effect.

Coumestans

Coumestans usually refers to a combination of four different isoflavones found in red clover.

Red clover is a widely used pasture legume and contains the isoflavones at levels substantially greater than soya beans.

These are widely extracted to provide a dietary supplement that can be taken to reduce the symptoms of estrogen dominance, especially around menopause. Most of these provide 40 mg per dose in a pill form, which are well tolerated by most women, but it can be a bit hard to fine-tune your personal dose when taking a pill.

Isoflavones

Isoflavones are compounds found in many plants, most of which act as phytestrogens. Foods that contain high amounts of isoflavones include soya beans, peanuts, chickpeas, alfalfa, fava beans, and kudzu. Some isoflavones are termed antioxidants because of their ability to inhibit the oxidation of other molecules and thus prevent the production of free radicals that can lead to chain reactions that may damage cells.

The isoflavones in soya beans need to be converted to human isoflavones by the beneficial bacteria in your gut before they are active.

A word of caution on Soy Products

They are found in high concentrations in soya beans so drinking two glasses of soymilk per day can be sufficient to alter the timing of your menstrual cycle. It has been estimated that children raised exclusively on soymilk formula are being given the estrogenic equivalent of five birth control pills every day.

The soya industry claims that mature soya beans have been eaten for thousands of years as a mainstay of Asian diets, which is a key factor in why these Asian populations are healthier than modern Western civilizations.

However, the reality is way more complex than this. The soya plant has been widely used since ancient times as a green manure crop to enhance soil fertility as the soy plant is a legume that adds nitrogen to the soil system.

This meant that it was not planted principally as a food crop, although the immature green beans were harvested and eaten as edamame. The mature soya bean only came to be more widely used as food around 1000 years ago, when the Chinese developed the fermentation process to turn the mature dry bean into a paste, now best known as miso.

The other key issue, which is seldom talked about by mainstream media, is that soya beans contain a number of anti-nutritional factors which are at lower levels in the immature green beans but occur at high levels in the mature dry bean used to make most soy-based foods.

These include:

High levels of trypsin inhibitors - which block protein digestion and are not deactivated during ordinary cooking. Their presence in your food can produce serious gastric distress and reduced protein digestion and absorption by your body.

Hemagglutinin - which promotes clot formation causing blood cells to clump together.

High levels of phytates – which block the uptake from your digestive tract of the essential minerals: calcium, magnesium, copper, iron, and zinc. If you want a recipe for a woman's health disaster, regularly eating food with high levels of phytates is right up there. Phytates are present in all seeds to help protect against insect damage, however, soya beans have one of the highest levels known.

I have had customers with supposedly unresolvable anemia which has been completely resolved by stopping their regular use of soymilk.

Goitrogens - which depress thyroid function.

While the soya bean processors have done their best to reduce the impact of these powerful anti-nutrients, even the highly complicated industrial processing required to make soy protein isolate does not eliminate them.

The most effective way of reducing the levels of these anti-nutrients in soya beans is the traditional long-term fermentation and precipitation techniques used to make miso, tempeh, and traditionally made tofu. Even these techniques may not be sufficient to eliminate these anti-nutritional factors. Indeed, some nutritionists claim that the use of these fermented soy products in the traditional Asian diet is probably the reason why many Asians are quite small in stature. Given that many young Asians on a more European-type diet can grow to be very tall, this suggests that there could be more than a grain of truth in this claim.

If you decide that you want to use soy supplements as a source of phytoestrogens, then it is important to limit your intake of isoflavones to no more than 30 to 40 mg per day. If you want to eat soy-based foods, there is no easy way to find out the isoflavone content, as there is no requirement to include this information on a label and the growing region and processing method can have a major impact on how much is in your soy food.

Just be aware that a small amount of phytestrogen-rich food can be good for your health and a lot can have damaging effects on your health, so consume in moderation.

7.4.7

Synthetic Estrogens

Contraception

The development of the contraceptive pill was seen as a major advance because of its ease of use and the efficiency with which it prevents unwanted pregnancies. However, because contraceptive pills use synthetic versions of your estrogen and progesterone, they can cause infertility and problem periods after stopping them. They can also cause loss of vital nutrients like zinc and magnesium, and have side-effects such as increased blood pressure, migraines, weight gain and risk of blood clots.

It is quite usual that it takes at least a year, and possibly longer, for a woman's hormonal cycle to resume a stable normal rhythm after stopping birth control pills. This is because the synthetic estrogens and progestins used in birth control pills are oil soluble, and so are very difficult for your body to detoxify and eliminate.

Infertility treatment

Synthetic estrogens are given as part of treatment during an infertility program to stimulate ovulation in infertile women, (which is much more common in those who have previously used the contraceptive pill).

These can further exacerbate any deficiency of zinc and magnesium and potentially decrease fertility even further.

Menopause and Peri-Menopause

In more primitive societies, where women tend to be physically active and are often short of food, there is often not even a word to describe menopause. The end of your fertile years and the ending of your monthly periods is something that just happens naturally, as part of your transition to your 'crone' or your wisdom years.

Yet, in developed societies, the unpleasant symptoms of estrogen dominance are widespread leading up to and during menopause. While the production of estrogen does decline during pre- and post-menopause, the reality is that the levels of progesterone usually decline more contributing to symptoms of estrogen dominance.

The initial hormone treatment used around menopause was ERT (Estrogen Replacement Therapy) that started in the 1960s. The high levels of side-effects from the use of ERT, and the fact that within ten years multiple studies showed that ERT increased the rate of uterine cancer by a factor of 4 to 8, meant that the use of ERT was relatively short-lived.

Drug companies were quick to come out with a replacement: what is now called HRT (Hormone Replacement Therapy), where a synthetic estrogen is opposed by a synthetic progesterone, more correctly called a progestin (or sometimes a progestogen). This new form of therapy did reduce the risk of uterine cancer, but by early in the new millennium, several large-scale studies had demonstrated an increased risk of risk of deep vein thrombosis, stroke and breast cancer from the long-term use of HRT.

These findings led many physicians and women on HRT to abandon its use, but some doctors do still prescribe HRT for short-term use when menopausal symptoms are severe.

Measuring your hormone levels in saliva is a simple process and they are often tested before administering hormone replacement therapy. Unfortunately measuring the impact of your total xenoestrogen load is not technically possible, so you could well be prescribed with an estrogen-based hormone replacement therapy, which is just going to exacerbate the potential for estrogen dominance.

There are much safer and more effective alternatives. See Section 7.5.2.

7.4.8
Osteoporosis

Osteoporosis is a condition of excessive bone loss and decreased bone density so your bones get lighter, more porous and more easily fractured.

Firstly, there are a number of myths about osteoporosis that I need to correct so that you can understand how to prevent yourself from developing osteoporosis.

Myth 1: Calcium Deficiency

Most women with osteoporosis are getting adequate calcium in their diet, which is not difficult to do on even a relatively poor diet.

The issue is that calcium is being lost from the bone faster than the bone is gaining calcium due to an acid-forming diet, low in plant-based foods, which is a process largely independent of calcium intake.

Myth 2: Estrogen

Supplementing estrogen will not build new bone, it just slows down the loss of bone.

Like every other cell in your body, your bones are continually being renewed and replaced in an ongoing process. Within your bones, cells called osteoclasts reabsorb the bone structure, and then bone-producing cells called osteoblasts grow new bone.

The decline in estrogen levels that occurs with a hysterectomy, or leading up to and during menopause, stimulates the activity of the osteoclasts and so causes the loss of bone density that is the basis of osteoporosis. Supplementing estrogen will not build new bone, but can slow the loss of bone mass for a few years after menopause.

This increased osteoclast activity usually occurs for a period of 5 to 8 years around menopause. This is often a key reason why your doctor might recommend HRT around menopause, but this recommendation ignores the health risks associated with estrogen dominance, and the potential role of progesterone outlined below.

Myth 3: Menopause

Osteoporosis is not a disease of menopause.

Osteoporosis usually begins its insidious march long before your estrogen levels start to decline around menopause, usually between five and twenty years before menopause. As you will read in the next section, the decline in progesterone levels leading up to and during menopause is proportionately much greater than the decline in estrogen.

The great news is that new bone growth is stimulated by progesterone and testosterone because they stimulate the osteoblasts that you need to have working efficiently to regrow new bone cells and restore your bone strength.

So if you are starting to have a decline in bone density because of estrogen dominance, or lack of progesterone around menopause, then enhancing your progesterone levels using the techniques I recommend later, is likely to help your body to restore your bone strength.

7.5
Progesterone – Your Happy Hormone!

"If you only hate your husband two weeks out of four, then the chances are it's not your husband that is the problem" Anna Cabeca DO.

Progesterone is the other side of the sex hormone balance required for fertility and pregnancy, so is the natural complement to estrogen. There is some background production of progesterone by the adrenal glands, but the primary producer of the progesterone that regulates your menstrual cycle is your ovaries.

Progesterone starts to be produced in the ovaries just before ovulation, and the amount produced increases rapidly after ovulation to reach a peak around days 13 to 15 of your menstrual cycle. This happens because, once the egg gets shed from the little sac it develops in at ovulation, the sac changes into a little yellow body (corpus luteum), which becomes a powerful progesterone factory.

The name progesterone comes from pro- (supports) -gestation (pregnancy). If fertilization does not take place, your levels of progesterone then start to decline, to the point where menstruation occurs and the whole beautiful dance of the hormones, which is your monthly cycle, starts again. If, however, the egg is fertilized the placenta takes over from the corpus luteum as the progesterone factory that is designed to maintain the pregnancy and stop further egg production.

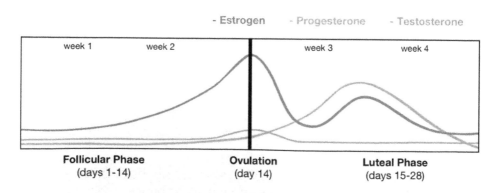

Figure 7.1 The monthly dance of your sex hormones

7.5.1
Your Feel-good Hormone

The high levels of progesterone you produce during pregnancy are the reason that many women find that being pregnant feels wonderful (in spite of some of the discomforts). Progesterone is your natural antidepressant which is calming, even sedating, and helps you feel content with the way you are.

Progesterone, testosterone and estrogen all contribute to you having a normal healthy libido, so that sex is something you look forward to with pleasure. Notice the little surge in testosterone around ovulation time which helps enhance your libido. Having these three hormones in the right balance is really important for your sexiness.

Progesterone is also important for healthy brain function. Your brain concentrates progesterone to levels twenty times higher than in your blood. Many emergency rooms recognize this and will routinely administer natural progesterone to any head injury cases that come in. If you're unfortunate enough to have someone close to you in this situation you may wish to ask if this has been done as it can make a major difference to how well the brain heals.

7.5.2
Progesterone Supplements

A way of synthesizing progesterone from plant extracts was developed in the 1940s. It is this progesterone, which is chemically and physiologically identical to the progesterone you produce in your body, which I shall refer to as 'natural progesterone'. Natural progesterone is NOT the same as the synthetic progestins used HRT or birth control pills.

There has been long-established clinical use of natural progesterone for the relief of estrogen dominance symptoms during menopause. The pioneer in this field was Dr Katharina Dalton in Great Britain in the 1950s, and this was followed up by the work of Dr Ray Peat in the 1970s. The most widely known author in this field is probably Dr John Lee who, in the 1990s proposed the term Estrogen Dominance as an explanation for the unpleasant symptoms that can arise when your hormones get out of balance, particularly around menstruation.

While there have been many significant studies published demonstrating the safety and efficacy of natural progesterone, there is not the depth of published research that is a feature of synthetic HRT (which start with natural progesterone's, which are then modified to form synthetic progestins). The major reason for this is that natural hormones cannot be patented, so there is no commercial advantage to be had from research in this field. However, the published studies on natural progesterone that have been done do not contain the bias often seen in the studies of synthetic HRT using progestins, which are financed by the drug companies.

The compelling nature of the evidence of the safety of natural progesterone for treating hot flashes, protection from heart disease, the reduction in risk for breast and ovarian cancer, and for the protection of endometrial tissue has led to a surge in the use of natural progesterone. There are now many practitioners familiar with the use of natural progesterone and who are available to tailor a progesterone supplementation regime to your specific needs. Everyone is different.

In many countries natural progesterone is available over-the-counter, however, in New Zealand, you require a doctor's prescription to be able to purchase it. Getting such a prescription can sometimes be an issue, as many doctors are not familiar with natural progesterone. I have prepared a paper outlining the published research demonstrating the safety and efficacy of natural progesterone aimed at informing doctors, so they may be more comfortable about prescribing progesterone. This eBook is freely available from my website: www.ITookCharge.nz/Progesterone

There are some nutrients, such as cholesterol, zinc, magnesium, Vitamins B6 and C, which are crucial to providing the environment needed to support your body to boost your own progesterone production. My recommendations in Chapter 16 Your 'Rapid Reset' Plan are designed to provide this support.

7.5.3
Fertility

During your normal cycle, if you are not overly stressed, you will produce around 20-25 mg of progesterone per day but during pregnancy your placenta produces up to 300-400 mg of progesterone per day, which means that supplementing with natural progesterone is extremely safe. The same cannot be said for the synthetic progestins which are widely used in birth control pills and conventional HRT. Both treatments come with very nasty side effects like increased risk of breast cancer, stroke, and deep vein thrombosis.

If you regularly have unpleasant symptoms of PMS before your period, there is a high probability that your body is not producing enough progesterone to balance your total estrogen loading and that you have some degree of estrogen dominance.

If you are also trying to have a baby and having difficulty maintaining your pregnancy, even to the extent of having a miscarriage, then it is likely that your estrogen dominance is to some extent counteracting the effect of the increased progesterone your body is producing. In this situation, knowledgeable practitioners will suggest supplementing your own production of progesterone with some extra natural progesterone to help you maintain the pregnancy.

7.5.4
Perimenopause

From about age 35 on, many women start to have menstrual cycles where you don't produce a ripe egg which, as you can imagine, starts to play havoc with your normal hormone patterns.

Progesterone levels drop, because there is no corpus luteum formed to produce the progesterone, and the levels of estrogen you produce can also fluctuate. If progesterone from your corpus luteum does not balance the estrogen you are producing, then the estrogen can continue to stimulate your uterine lining. This can contribute to increased endometrial thickness, lots of breast tenderness and heavy bleeding. You might not completely shed your uterine lining during one period, which would look like a very light period, followed by a very heavy period next month.

One of the other key indicators for low progesterone is a shortened menstrual cycle; so if your cycle is around 24 days or less you should probably look at getting your health practitioner to test your progesterone levels at day 21 of your cycle.

Low levels of progesterone may also lead to irritability, mood swings, loss of libido, or even migraines. Low levels of progesterone and/or estrogen dominance also tend to drive the formation of cysts around this time, such as breast or ovarian cysts and possibly PCOS (polycystic ovarian syndrome).

7.5.5
Sleep and Progesterone

One of the common effects of perimenopause is not sleeping well. Not enough sleep can severely disrupt your whole hormone system, as I mention in every chapter of the book. If you are not sleeping well because of decreased levels of progesterone in your system, for some women supplementing with natural progesterone works like a charm to give you a deep and restful sleep.

If the way your body is behaving suggests that you are low in progesterone or are estrogen dominant and you are not sleeping well, then you should probably do something about it without delay. A good sleep is so fundamental to your progress along the path to wellness, that I would recommend you seriously consider the option of supplementing with natural progesterone while you work on the other solutions later in the book.

It can be as simple as dabbing some progesterone cream or oil around your neck or face if you wake in the night. Just rub it in and for most women off to sleep you go!

7.5.6
Menopause and Progesterone

During menopause the amount of progesterone your body produces declines to less than 1% of the amount you produce while you are ovulating. The relative drop in progesterone production at menopause is more extreme than the decline in estrogen production, which also happens during menopause,

This is why paying attention to potential progesterone deficiency or estrogen dominance symptoms during menopause is one of the keys to sailing gracefully through a healthy normal menopause.

It is important to remember that menopause is not a disease that should be treated with a drug. It should be a natural progression of your body and being towards your 'crone' years when you have accumulated some of life's wisdom. That said, the widespread occurrence of unpleasant symptoms related to estrogen dominance around menstruation and menopause means that many women are desperate for a solution.

Implementing the recommendations I make in Chapter 16 Your 'Rapid Reset' Plan, can correct or minimize these symptoms over time. However, many women could need a solution right now to restore some balance to life. The short-term solution may be to work with an experienced practitioner to get additional natural progesterone into your hormonal system to balance out the excess estrogen. This strategy usually gives rapid relief from unpleasant symptoms.

It is important to remember that hormonal imbalances seldom occur in isolation so while it is fine to get symptomatic relief by using natural progesterone, to move forward towards real wellness requires implementing strategies to balance your diet and do a physical and mental detox, such as I outline in Chapter 16 Your 'Rapid Reset' Plan.

7.5.7
Stress and Progesterone

Progesterone is one of the precursor hormones produced from cholesterol. Not only are the other sex hormones, estrogen and testosterone produced from progesterone, but so is the stress hormone cortisol, so progesterone is an extremely important hormone to have in balance for your hormonal health.

Cortisol is essential (without any you will die within seven days) for your body to manage the stress response, inflammation, sugar balance, blood pressure and general survival. So if your body gets stressed it will use whatever progesterone it needs to convert into cortisol. Your body regards survival as being way more important than your reproduction or your happiness.

This mopping up of all your progesterone to make cortisol is a phenomenon sometimes called 'cortisol steal', and is a key reason why progesterone deficiency or estrogen dominance symptoms can be a key indicator of your body being chronically stressed.

There's another nasty little twist in the cortisol story. High levels of cortisol will block the progesterone receptors in your cell walls, so that what little progesterone you do make can't get into your cells. If you are really stressed just before your period, then lack of progesterone getting into your cells means your mood may get even worse; you may feel anxious and unable to calm down, and since progesterone acts as a diuretic you may also notice fluid retention and breast tenderness. So it is worth getting serious about doing something to reduce your stress levels.

7.5.8
Exercise and Progesterone

Studies have shown that women described as recreational athletes can have a high incidence (around 50%) of subtle disturbances to their menstrual cycle. In these studies, a recreational athlete is described as a woman who exercises for one to two hours, four times a week, so we are not talking about a whole lot of exercise here.

Such menstrual cycle disturbances can mimic the symptoms of low progesterone or cycles where no egg is shed. Even in quite young women this can cause unpleasant symptoms similar to those of perimenopause or PMS and can also cause thyroid issues.

One of the key effects of 'more than moderate exercise' is an increase in cortisol production, a key indicator of stress. This has been shown to be due to a chronic energy deficiency because of the exercise, which your limbic brain thinks is a famine and so it tells your body to pump out more cortisol, which steals from your production of progesterone, which then plays havoc with your menstrual cycle and your happiness.

The other effects of your body thinking there is a famine is that it tries to store fat whenever possible, which can make it really difficult to exercise off any excess weight you might be trying to lose.

I'm not trying to suggest that you shouldn't exercise, but that it's really important to exercise in such a way that you don't trigger this response in your body (See Chapter 13 Move Your Body).

7.5.9
Endometriosis and Progesterone

Endometriosis happens when some of the inner lining cells of the uterus migrate into places they don't belong, typically around the fallopian tubes, but they can implant anywhere around your pelvic cavity.

Unfortunately, these cells are still bathed in the same hormonal brew as when they were part of your uterus, so they still respond in the same way. They swell up with blood in response to the estrogen in the first part of your cycle and, then some seven to twelve days before menstruation, they start to bleed into the surrounding tissue which causes inflammation and pain, which can become excruciating during menstruation.

Endometriosis can be a symptom of estrogen dominance, and many women find that endometriosis can be resolved over time by the use of natural progesterone. Many health practitioners use synthetic progestins to try to achieve the same result, but these commonly come with potentially dangerous side-effects. If this section applies to you, I recommend you search out an experienced practitioner to help you work out a natural progesterone regime that works for you.

7.6
Testosterone

Testosterone is the key player in a group of masculinizing hormones called androgens. Most of the others have much weaker effects than testosterone so, for the sake of simplicity, I will refer to all the androgens as testosterone. You make some testosterone in your ovaries but mainly in your adrenal glands at roughly one-tenth of the levels produced by males. While having lots of testosterone is responsible for masculinizing effects, having it at optimum levels for women contributes to your libido, emotional wellbeing, assertiveness and your sense of belonging, so having enough testosterone is important for your health.

If your stress and cortisol levels are high, both your testosterone and progesterone levels will be low. Adding some strength training into your exercise regime can help boost your testosterone levels.

7.6.1
Testosterone and Libido

As you go into menopause, the levels of estrogen and progesterone produced from your ovaries decline drastically. However, because your adrenal glands produce most of your testosterone, your testosterone levels do not drop proportionally as much as your estrogen and progesterone levels. This is why after menopause you may start to lose some of your feminine hourglass shape and start to have a body shape more like a man's.

As you age, it is common for the levels of all the three sex hormones produced by your body to decline, usually because of a degree of adrenal exhaustion from ongoing stress. However, it can also happen earlier in life because of disruptions to your monthly hormonal cycle from stress and/ or estrogen dominance, which can really mess with the hormonal output from your ovaries.

Both these reasons for disrupted hormonal balance can contribute to loss of libido.

Is this necessary? Absolutely not!

We used to think that testosterone and estrogen were the key hormones for female libido, but we now know that progesterone also has an important role to play. Like pretty much everything else in your body, it's the overall balance that's important for you to retain your juiciness, playfulness, and sexiness.

While the drug industry is spending a lot of time trying to find a hormonal cure for loss of libido in women, they ignore the fact that the biggest sexual organ in a woman's body is in her head, and that your libido is primarily a function of your brain. There is a multitude of mental factors that can affect your libido; from the subtle effects of the 'tend and befriend' response to stress, to the relationship you have with your lover becoming a bit stale (See Chapter 17 Take Charge of your Sexiness).

7.6.2
Excess Testosterone

One of the nasty side effects of insulin resistance is that the high levels of insulin in your body can drive your ovaries to make excessive levels of testosterone. This is bad enough, but the high levels of insulin also cause the liver to make lower levels of the protein which binds sex hormones, so that you end up with a lot more free testosterone floating around your body wreaking havoc.

A very high proportion of women with excess testosterone end up with a condition known as PCOS, which is a leading cause of infertility in women. PCOS is where a series of eggs produced by your ovaries fail to develop normally and end up as small cysts on your ovaries. As you can imagine, this messes with your estrogen and progesterone balance and, also makes your body vulnerable to the effects of excess testosterone.

High levels of testosterone can lead to effects such as a long time between periods, acne, a deeper voice, increased pubic or facial hair, male pattern baldness, depression and anxiety, or weight gain.

Because of the strong association between high testosterone and insulin resistance, developing any symptoms of testosterone excess or PCOS should be seen as a powerful warning sign that diabetes and even dementia may be looming in your life.

The symptoms of PCOS are very variable but, as you might imagine from the insulin link, it's associated with being overweight and with you having a lot of difficulties losing weight. Having hair where it doesn't normally occur on the female body is another powerful indicator. Because of the wide range of symptoms, PCOS is quite seriously under-diagnosed, so that while PCOS probably affects nearly one in five women in the USA, many are completely unaware that they have it.

7.7
Menopause

I have already talked about the way that your levels of estrogen and progesterone drop substantially during menopause and also about the impact of stress on your monthly cycle, because stress also drops your levels of estrogen and progesterone. In practice, this means that menopause feels a bit like a programmed stress response where you have gone almost overnight from being able to handle stress, well - sort of, to not being able to handle stress at all well.

Maybe up till now you have been able to feel good and maintain the shape you want to be by reducing your calorie intake a bit and doing a bit more exercise. However, as you go into menopause, you suddenly find that the things have that have worked for you until now, DON'T ANYMORE, and you may well find that you start to gain some unwanted belly fat. So your natural response is to cut calories more and exercise some more, which doesn't work at all as it used to - it just makes it worse.

I go into a lot more detail about why this happens in the next chapter, but the practical implication of this for you is that instead of going for an intense workout at the gym you should now look at going for a gentle walk in nature – anywhere where you are exposed to green. The Japanese realized the healing power of walking in nature in the 1980s and coined the term Shinrin-yoku, which means literally 'bathing in the forest'. Such activity still burns calories but, far more importantly, it will reduce your levels of stress hormones and their impact on your belly fat. There are lots more techniques for reducing your stress hormones discussed in Chapter 14 Detoxing your Mind, like soaking in a spa or having a massage.

CHAPTER 8

The Hormonal Reasons Why Diets Don't Work

"Eating for vibrant health often has the stunning side-effect of dramatic weight loss"
Tana Amen BSN, RN

Let's face it, weight loss is a big deal for many people, in fact so much of a big deal that the weight loss market in the USA is estimated to be around $60 billion each year. Unfortunately, that means many in the industry don't have a lot of scruples about what is really going on in your body, they are more interested in what sells. My aim in this chapter is to help you understand your body's workings so that you are better able to work with it to achieve your size goals.

The number one reason people give as to why they want to lose weight is to feel healthier. The old idea of how to lose weight and become healthy was that it was the result of lots of hard work and deprivation. That way is no fun at all, and many studies show it doesn't work. The new revolution is that being healthy, lean and loving your life is the by-product of being at peace and in sync with the world around you and eating the right food.

I will try to help you to understand that the solution to achieving your ideal size is actually to become healthy first. Once you choose to take care of your body and move toward wellness, the fat will naturally fall off.

If you are carrying more fat than you would like and have FLC syndrome and go to your doctor, their likely response is to put you on the scales, measure your height and say "your BMI is ... so you are overweight". They will then tell you - "you need to eat less and exercise more". This is doctor speak for "stop eating like a pig and get off your lazy butt and move".

There are two major problems with this approach. Firstly, nobody consciously chooses to be overweight, so such advice is very judgmental and makes you feel even worse about yourself than before (if possible).

Secondly, the traditional 'eat less and exercise more' approach to creating a calorie deficit and therefore losing fat, rarely works. Many studies have shown that well over 98% of those who take this approach to weight loss are unable to continue the diet long-term and, at least two-thirds of those end up weighing more long-term than when they started the 'diet'.

8.1
So what is really happening here?

Eat less; lose fat – sounds simple doesn't it? Well, it sort of is simple, because you only need a certain number of calories to get through your busy day so anything above that number makes you gain fat. As long as your gut is healthy, this works most of the time. The problem is that the reverse effect of eating fewer calories than you need almost never works to make you lose fat in the long term.

What is actually happening is that your lifestyle and some poor food choices are driving a hormonal cascade that makes you crave comfort foods, full of refined carbohydrates, sugar and bad fats (Big Food uses this effect all the time). At the same time, you will have really low energy and the idea of going out and exercising feels impossible.

Your brain only comprises 2% of your body weight, yet because it is so active it consumes around 20% of the energy your body produces. So if you go on a calorie restricted diet, then your brain will not be performing optimally, which makes it hard for you to function well and make good food choices.

This triple whammy makes it highly unlikely that you will be able to white-knuckle it through a sustained fat loss program that does not include making radically better food choices for the long haul.

The reality is that, yes, you are making some bad food choices unconsciously from lack of knowledge, but it is the resulting changes in your hormones and biochemistry that are driving your behavior, not your lack of willpower.

However, lack of willpower is what your doctor and most of our society (if they are really honest) tend to think is behind your fat gain. This outdated thinking is driven by the false idea that all sources of calories are created equal. We now know that your food provides powerful information that drives your hormonal cascade and switches your genes on and off very quickly.

In this chapter, I aim to empower you with the knowledge you need to get your hormones back in balance, so they're working for you, not against you – to allow you to take charge of your belly fat!

As I have said before, your limbic system is all about survival, so it really doesn't want you to waste any food in case it gets scarce anytime soon (not likely). As a result, your body's default setting is to store as much energy as possible in your fat cells, mostly around your belly, just in case! Four key hormonal systems are doing their level best to make this happen:

8.2
Cortisol

Your body's cortisol response to you going on a diet is a key reason why, if you want to lose fat, the conventional diet of eating less and exercising more simply doesn't work. Sure, you initially lose some water and body weight and fat, but the intense exercise and food deprivation actually raises your cortisol levels. This is really bad news, as the stress hormones cortisol and adrenaline work together in four different ways to help you gain weight.

The first key impact of cortisol is that it has a very strong tendency to cause you to store fat on your belly and around your organs (belly fat is sometimes called your visceral fat or your muffin top). What you see on the outside of your belly is a powerful indicator of the amount of fat stored inside your belly, around your organs, particularly your liver. Belly fat is the fat that is really dangerous for your health and which commonly makes up about 20% of your total body fat.

Raised cortisol levels results in your rate of fat loss slowing dramatically, because the elevated cortisol level is telling your body to slow down your metabolism and to store fat, so you will survive the 'famine' that it believes is happening because of your lower food intake.

The other unpleasant side effect of excessive exercise and raised cortisol levels is that this combination is quite powerfully aging, which nobody wants.

The inevitable result is that you get disheartened and, with your new low metabolic rate caused by the dieting, it's highly likely that you will rapidly regain all the fat you lost and maybe even more. Many published research studies demonstrate how frequently this pattern happens.

For many women this seesaw of dieting and fat gain starts to feel like losing a battle with your body to keep it the way you would like it to be. This can be an immense source of mental stress for women and, of course, adds another layer of stress hormones which can easily end up with you having feelings of hopelessness and "why should I bother?"

The second nasty effect of elevated stress hormones is that one of the first impacts of adrenaline on your system is to minimize the blood flow to your gut, as digesting food is not a priority when your life might be in danger. This has a direct impact on your gut's ability to properly digest foods and manage the balance of bacteria, which hurts your digestion and poor digestion makes you feel more stressed – another vicious cycle. Stress also has a direct impact on your gut microbiome by changing the balance more towards the types of bacteria which help you gain weight more easily – welcome to more belly fat (See Chapter 9 Bugs Are Important)!

The third nasty effect of having long-term stress and elevated cortisol is that you develop a strong tendency to develop pleasure seeking or compulsive behaviors. This can take the form of eating lots of high-energy junk foods, compulsive exercise, or the use of alcohol or other drugs.

While these behaviors have been shown to blunt the feelings of stress and make you feel better in the short term, the fat gain that goes with such behaviors actually makes you feel more stressed. Hence it is very easy to get into a vicious cycle, making it very difficult to lose fat.

The final nasty little twist your body has in store for you, and why diets seldom work, is that, of course, in this modern world, there is no famine! But the high levels of cortisol in your blood that your 'diet' creates will mean that, when abundant food is in front of you in the form of a chocolate bar or bag of crisps, the limbic system in your brain is screaming at you "I see food – eat it now", because your limbic system is all about survival. Especially at the end of a bad day it becomes really, really, really hard not to scoff the lot, despite your best intentions. This can then add another layer of mental stress as you tell yourself "I have no willpower, I am so hopeless".

The reality is that there are simple and effective techniques to destress the body and detox the mind. Applying these simple techniques is infinitely preferable to giving up and letting the fat pile on, and your health deteriorate.

8.3
Thyroid

Your thyroid is also conspiring against you in your mission to take charge of your belly fat. When you restrict your food intake and go on a diet you also get poor conversion of the inactive thyroid hormone T4 to the more active T3, which slows your metabolic rate.

Your body again assumes that you must be in the middle of a war or a famine so it must slow down your metabolic rate to conserve those precious fat stores – exactly what you didn't want to happen.

8.4
Estrogen

Because your fat cells are very efficient producers of estrogen, there is a very close connection between the estrogen signaling in your body and your total body fat levels.

You can very easily become caught in a cycle where increased body fat raises estrogen levels, and estrogen works with cortisol to help accumulate belly fat.

8.5
Your Energy Balance Hormones

There is also a part of your limbic system which controls the intricate hormonal balance required to maintain the energy balance in your body.

This group of hormones includes the following:

8.5.1
Leptin

Leptin was only discovered 1994 and, for a brief time, it was thought that this was the magic ingredient in fat control and that all you would need to do to lose fat would be to add a bit more leptin into your system. There are very rare cases where the inability to make enough leptin is the reason for fat gain, but for most people, it is, unfortunately, not that simple.

Leptin is less well known than insulin, but they kind of work in concert. Leptin is a complex protein made mainly in your white fat cells, so the amount of leptin you make is normally directly proportional to the total amount of fat in your body.

Your white fat comes in two types:

• The highly undesirable 'belly fat' that you store around your belly and internal organs

• The relatively neutral 'bum fat' that you store under the skin, particularly around your butt and thighs.

Your white fat used to be thought of as something you could happily liposuction out of the body, but we now know that these fat cells are one of the most important hormone factories in the body (and liposuction is purely cosmetic and does nothing to improve the metabolic markers that signal the status of your health anyway).

Leptin's key role is to maintain your energy balance by controlling your metabolic rate, fat storage, and eating behavior. This means that to 'take charge of your belly fat', it's really important to understand how to keep your leptin levels in the ideal range.

However, leptin is much more than just about fat control. The latest science is showing that leptin connects your gut, brain and your individual cells' requirements for energy at any moment into a highly complex system. Moreover, having optimum leptin levels in your brain has now been shown to be critical to your ability to think, remember things, and to protect your brain from the effects of aging.

Leptin is the hormone that allows your fat stores to communicate to your limbic system on how much total energy you have stored away and, thus, what your metabolic rate should be. As your limbic system is totally about survival, if your leptin levels indicate that your fat stores are about right

Are you leptin resistant?

I can imagine you saying, as I did when I first discovered this information, "Oh my God, am I leptin resistant".

The biggest clue to this is to look in the mirror and ask yourself, "am I carrying more fat that I would like?" If the honest answer to this question is "Yes", then you probably have some degree of leptin resistance.

If you have an unusually large appetite, crave carbohydrates before you go to bed, have high reverse T3 in your blood (See Chapter 5 Your Energy Hormone - Thyroid) or higher cortisol levels later in the day, then these are also powerful indicators that you have leptin resistance.

then your limbic system will instruct your thyroid to keep your metabolic rate up, and your body hums along nicely.

Maintaining your energy balance is one of the most complex systems in your body, and it is fundamental to your survival. If your metabolic rate is too high, you burn through all your fat stores and may in fact run out of energy and die (this is what your limbic system thinks anyway). Conversely, if your leptin signal doesn't reach your brain, your brain interprets this as a famine and will instruct the rest of your body to do whatever it can to lay down more fat stores.

When your body is working properly your fat cells start to produce more leptin as you eat, and when your leptin levels reach a certain point, that tells your brain that your tummy is getting full, so it sends the signal to stop you overeating. This means that you will stay in energy balance, burn energy at a normal rate, maintain a stable weight and feel great.

If, however, you were to go into a famine (not likely with the supermarket just down the road) or go on a diet to try to start burning fat, then your leptin levels will fall rapidly and your limbic system will instruct the thyroid to slow down your metabolic rate. Even worse, leptin will increase the production of a hormone called Ghrelin which increases your appetite to send you looking for more food NOW.

So it's not your lack of willpower that sends you sneaking to the fridge in the middle of the night - it's likely to be some combination of this very powerful trio - Leptin, Ghrelin and Cortisol.

Ongoing overeating causes excessively high levels of leptin in your blood, which you would think would tell your brain to keep your metabolic rate up and to stop eating. Unfortunately, overeating carbs also causes you to produce more insulin, which tells your liver to produce high levels of triglycerides (a large fat molecule your liver makes with any excess energy), which is designed for later storage in fat cells. However, triglycerides have a nasty habit of clinging to the leptin receptors in your brain, which then blocks the leptin you are producing from telling your brain that you should stop eating.

So even though the amount of leptin your body is producing is directly related to the size of your fat tissue, these blocked leptin receptors create what we now call 'leptin resistance', preventing the message to stop eating getting through to your brain.

Leptin resistance is a major cause of excessive belly fat. This is because the signal not getting through to your limbic system translates into you having to eat excessively large amounts of food before enough leptin gets into your brain cells to tell you that you are not starving, that you should stop eating now, and that your brain should keep your metabolic rate high.

As a result, overeating has strong potential to turn into a vicious cycle in that overeating promotes leptin resistance, which turns into a very powerful compulsion to overeat because your brain is not receiving the signal that you have eaten enough.

A big contributor to leptin resistance is fructose. Fructose is the molecule that has the really sweet taste we love so much and is found at high levels in HCFS (high fructose corn syrup), sugar, and fruit juices like apple and orange. Because fructose can only be digested in the liver, any excess fructose you eat is going to be made directly into triglycerides which will contribute to your potential to develop leptin resistance.

As you have seen above, this can turn into a compulsion to overeat. Minimizing your intake of all soda drinks and fruit juice is crucial to getting your leptin levels under control so that you can maintain a healthy weight (See Chapter 10 - Bad Carbs Make You Fat and Sick).

Leptin resistance nearly always precedes insulin resistance, so it really is the beginning of the cascade of ill health towards high blood pressure, heart disease, diabetes, cancer and dementia known as metabolic syndrome or Diabesity (See Section 8.9)

Leptin's discovery is still so new that it's still not fully understood, but its relationship with the limbic system means it not only regulates thyroid function, it also directly affects the function of your stress and sex hormones and insulin. Getting your leptin levels right can have a major impact on your health.

I believe it's useful to think of leptin as your body's team coach. Leptin's job is to make sure the whole team is working together to keep your body humming. Leptin doesn't take orders from anyone but does take feedback from all your body systems. This then gets synchronized into beautiful action which is the daily dance of the hormones in your body.

8.5.2
Leptin and Sleep

An important example of this synchronization is what happens when you sleep. Besides your leptin levels increasing as you eat, your leptin levels also follow a diurnal rhythm, which sees your leptin levels peaking during the evening as it prepares your body for you to go to sleep to allow for night-time repair, which it does by controlling your pattern of hormone release during the night.

Leptin co-ordinates the release of your sleep hormone (melatonin), the repair and rejuvenation hormone (human growth hormone), your thyroid hormones and your sex hormones. It's also part of leptin's job to give your body the wake-up call that comes in the form of a surge of cortisol to get you bouncing out of bed and into your day.

If, on the other hand, you're not getting to bed early enough then your leptin levels plummet, which seriously disrupts your body's repair processes during the night. It also tells your brain you're hungry and that you need to raid the fridge, and to take steps to store anything you eat as fat.

Even worse, being overtired dulls the part of your brain responsible for decision-making and impulse control, which makes it difficult to make good decisions (a little bit like being drunk). Also, being overtired makes you look for something to help you feel good, like high-carb snacks. There is good evidence to show that an overtired brain tends to crave junk food, but an overtired brain also lacks the impulse control to say no.

All of which translates into a very strong tendency to gain fat if you are not getting enough sleep. So important is getting enough sleep, that in one study the participants lost almost three times as much fat when they slept 7.5 hours per night, compared to when they slept just 5.5 hours per night.

Getting at least seven to nine hours sleep is absolutely fundamental to you waking up feeling like bouncing out of bed, ready for your wonderful day.

I will be talking much more about how to achieve this (See Chapter 14 - Detoxing your Mind).

8.5.3
Leptin and Light

If you have leptin resistance, then one of the factors that help to reset both leptin, dopamine and also give yourself a normal early-morning cortisol level is that you really need to be exposed to natural daylight for around 15 to 60 minutes in the early morning, depending on your sensitivity to light.

Exposure behind glass doesn't count because the glass causes a big reduction in light intensity. Typical levels of light indoors usually range from 200-500 lux, whereas research suggests that most people will need more than 10,000 lux to mimic the daylight response. Within an hour of sunrise, daylight will be around this level, and will typically rise to at least 70-80,000 lux around midday.

Any exposure to the natural light first thing in the morning is better than nothing, but to fully normalize your hormones it's ideal to combine light therapy with getting your body moving. Try a brisk walk, a more gentle walking meditation, or doing a Tai Chi routine out on the grass in bare feet (to also ground you).

If this is simply not feasible for you, then you may want to consider buying a light-box that is capable of putting out more than 10,000 lux, which is a lot of light. The spectrum of light doesn't seem to matter very much; it's all about the intensity. You could potentially sit in front of this while you eat your breakfast - it's quite important not to be staring directly at the light.

People who are affected by low mood in midwinter and low-light conditions usually find that they achieve the best relief of their symptoms by the use of their light-box quite early in the morning.

8.5.4
Ghrelin

Ghrelin works very closely with leptin so is almost its alter ego and is often called 'the hunger hormone'. Ghrelin is produced mainly by the stomach and small intestine, and it is the rise in Ghrelin levels that tells your brain when you need to eat, when your body should stop burning calories and when it should store energy as fat. Ghrelin also stimulates your HGH (human growth hormone) production which helps with the build-up of muscle.

The key role of Ghrelin is to control when you eat so, if you have any routine around eating, then Ghrelin levels will increase at your normal eating times to give you hunger pangs so that you are ready for your meals.

Unfortunately, there are a few other things that can impact on your Ghrelin release patterns.

If you are achieving healthy levels of sleep, then your level of Ghrelin will decrease naturally at night because sleeping requires less energy than being awake. If, on the other hand, you are not achieving your required 7 to 9 hours sleep, you end up with too much Ghrelin in your system so your limbic system thinks you're hungry. This means you have a strong tendency to store anything you do eat as fat because your brain thinks that there is a shortage of food.

What you do for breakfast is key to managing your Ghrelin levels for the rest of the day. If you skip breakfast you have a very strong tendency to crave sweet, fatty foods for the rest of the day.

Having a relatively high protein breakfast helps to set you up for the rest of your day because Ghrelin levels stay low for longer after a high-protein breakfast. The complex carbs found in whole grains and pulses have a somewhat similar effect to protein in helping to keep Ghrelin levels down for longer after breakfast. On the other hand, a breakfast high in refined carbohydrates, like sugar, has the initial effect of lowering Ghrelin levels but after a couple of hours they rebound to even higher levels. Having a high- fat breakfast doesn't have much impact on your Ghrelin levels after the meal, but it does have other important effects (See Chapter 11 Good Oils Make You Slim and Healthy).

If you want to control your cravings for sweet fatty foods throughout the day, it's a really good idea to have a high-protein breakfast, combined with plenty of good fats and maybe a limited amount of complex carbohydrates.

As in many areas, the Omega-3 fats have a different impact from other fats, so having your daily dose of flax seed oil or fish oil can help moderate your Ghrelin levels and your appetite.

8.5.5
Insulin

Your pancreas produces insulin in response to stimulation by the limbic system, which happens when the levels of glucose in your blood rise after a meal, because your liver has more than it can cope with.

It is the job of insulin to allow the glucose produced from the digestion of your food to be transported into your cells to either be burnt as energy or, if you have a surplus, to store it. Where? - In fat cells around your belly, so it can be accessed readily in case of an emergency.

While most people associate insulin mainly with diabetes, in fact insulin is way more than this, and one of its key jobs is to be your fat storage hormone. This means that managing your insulin levels is vitally important for controlling your good health and belly size.

The insulin receptors on all your cell walls are a bit like locks that insulin opens to then let glucose into your cells.

Insulin resistance can develop over time when you consume a diet rich in refined carbs (like white bread, bagels, white rice or pasta), sugar (in all forms) and potatoes. These types of 'foods' are pretty much just pure energy, and they are digested and absorbed into the bloodstream very quickly which creates blood sugar spikes. This results in your pancreas having to produce spikes of insulin to clear the excess glucose from your bloodstream and store it in your fat cells

The Myth of Bad Fat

I know that the health star system now being brought into New Zealand and Australia says that saturated fat is bad for you. Unfortunately, such systems are not perfect because they are heavily influenced by the food industry and politics. The reality is that government agencies and government committees are extremely vulnerable to lobbying by industry groups. For example, the recommendation to eat more polyunsaturated vegetable oils and more grain-based foods have been an absolute goldmine to the huge soya bean, corn, vegetable oil, and wheat industries, both in the United States and around the world. So in spite of large amounts of research showing that these original Dietary Goals were based on bad science, there is still a huge amount of money being spent by such industries to promote these Dietary Goals.

After these Dietary Goals were published, the majority of people were heavily conditioned by aggressive promotion from the food industry to see fat as the root of all evil. At the same time, the food manufacturers flooded the market with all kinds of low-fat foods and promoted them as 'low-fat health foods'.

The major unforeseen consequence of the low fat craze, is that because it is fat that makes food taste good and feel good in your mouth, the simplest way of making low-fat food appealing is to use lots of sugar and refined flours. Thus low-fat foods are almost all loaded with refined carbs, sugar and High Fructose Corn Syrup (HCFS), which are all strongly associated with diabesity and heart disease.

In recent years there have been numerous excellent books written detailing the latest research which shows that a high carb diet is actively bad for your health, especially refined carbs and sugar, but the power of Big Food to influence Big Media means that such research gets very little mainstream media attention.

– mostly as the dangerous belly fat - where it is readily accessible to provide fast energy for fuel in the future.

These spikes in insulin levels can cause the insulin receptors on the cell walls to get desensitized, so then they don't 'open up' to allow glucose into the cells. The pancreas responds to the resulting high blood sugar levels by pumping out more insulin. Perhaps calling 'insulin resistance' by the name 'carb intolerance' might help you to understand how this works.

Eating lots of refined carbs and sugars which spike your insulin levels can create two vicious cycles in your body.

The first cycle happens when high blood sugar levels induce high insulin levels in the blood but, because of insulin resistance, this isn't effective at actually reducing the blood sugar levels. This means the pancreas has to pump out more insulin to get the surplus energy or glucose out of your blood and into your fat cells. This cycle can result in a rapid rise in insulin resistance, and is usually the beginning of the metabolic syndrome or diabesity cascade that can eventually result in type II diabetes or dementia, as the pancreas gets worn out and is unable to produce enough insulin.

The second related vicious cycle is that a blood sugar spike induces an insulin spike to reduce the dangerous levels of blood sugar as quickly as possible, by pumping it into your belly fat cells. This usually means that the blood sugar spike is followed not long after by a blood sugar crash, which of course makes your brain start screaming "I'm starving - feed me now". It's really difficult to resist such a powerful biochemical urge, so you usually binge on some more carbs or coffee to get rid of the food cravings and the unpleasant symptoms of a blood sugar crash. Welcome to even more fat storage!

Lack of sleep can contribute to insulin resistance. Only four days of insufficient sleep is enough to decrease your insulin sensitivity by over 30%, so your body has trouble processing glucose from your bloodstream and ends up storing it as fat.

Getting glucose into your cells is only one of insulin's jobs. It also stimulates growth, promotes fat cell formation (cells which then want to be filled) and encourages inflammation. If insulin levels are high long-term because of insulin resistance, this disrupts all your other hormonal systems which can magnify the nasty side effects that can go with diabetes.

As you learnt in the previous chapter, one of the sex hormones most affected is testosterone, because high levels of insulin long-term and/or insulin resistance can cause your ovaries to make more testosterone. This can lead to acne, greasy skin and polycystic ovarian syndrome (PCOS).

8.6
The Diabesity Epidemic

The whole phenomena of leptin and insulin resistance, obesity, diabetes, heart disease and dementia is all part of a continuum which many people are starting to call metabolic syndrome or diabesity. There is a common thread between all these conditions that are strongly related to the now disproved idea, that a high carb intake is the basis of a healthy lifestyle.

Now I can hear a fair proportion of you saying "I've never heard of a high carb diet being good for you", which is probably true, yet the common food pyramid has carbohydrates as the biggest proportion of your recommended daily intake.

What you will have heard lots of is that a low-fat diet is good for you, which only happened after the US Congressional Committee chaired by Senator George McGovern published "Dietary Goals for the United States" in 1977. This report recommended that people eat a low-fat diet and particularly avoid saturated fat, as this was thought to be a significant cause of heart disease.

As you can imagine, with this being official US Government Policy, there was substantial funding to research these ideas. Fortunately, subsequent studies have failed to show any link between saturated fat intake and heart disease or any other degenerative disease.

What is worse, is that a very recent analysis of all the research available AT THAT TIME, to guide this Congressional Committee to make these recommendations, showed that even in the 1970s there was zero evidence that increased saturated fat intake was linked to increased risk of heart disease. So saturated fat has never been, and never will be, actively bad for your health. It's generally not particularly good for you either; it's more of a neutral fat that you shouldn't eat too

Identifying the correct fat to be concerned about

While being obese does increase the risk of developing diabetes, heart disease, some cancers and dementia, most people fail to differentiate between the different types of fat and treat all fat on your body as bad.

However, as I have already pointed out, it's all about where the fat is situated – in other words, how much belly fat you have.

I am not trying to suggest that the widespread occurrence of being overweight is not a problem. The reality is that nearly 10% of the US population has diabetes, nearly 30% of the population has pre-diabetes, and nearly 2% of the US population has dementia, with nearly two-thirds of those being women.

much of because it's a very concentrated form of energy.

It's very sad, but hardly surprising given the above situation, that the latest data from the WHO shows that globally the incidence of obesity has more than doubled since 1980, just after the McGovern report was released. The sad fact is that nearly 30% of the world's population is now classified as being overweight or obese and this trend has now got to the point where being overweight is credited with causing more deaths worldwide than being underweight.

In the US, one-third of the adult population is now classified as obese, and another one-third are classified as being overweight. Unfortunately, the data for New Zealand is very similar. However, I have some major issues with the classifications used, as I explain below.

Having just given you a bit of an overview of the politics behind what is being called the 'obesity epidemic', which is affecting a very high proportion of people around the world (The power of the 'Big Three' in action); I now want to bring it back to the personal level.

8.10
Your BMI Lie

I have heard many women refer to a desire to have "a flat sexy belly", as though the only belly that's sexy is a flat one. On the other hand, I think I can safely say that most men feel that a woman has to have a few curves to be really sexy. Beauty really is "in the eye of the beholder", not in what your ego is telling you when you look in the mirror. So how do you determine if you really should do something about your fat for your health's sake?

The most common indicator used by professionals to measure obesity is your BMI (Body Mass Index - which is a person's weight in kilograms divided by the square of their height in meters). This index was developed by a mathematician to give some indication of public health trends on a population basis. There is no physiological reason behind the choice of the numbers in the formula, but on a population basis it picks up trends in fat levels reasonably accurately.

Using your BMI to indicate your fat level was never the intention of the guy who developed it because, at a personal level, it is a long way from being the perfect indicator. Because muscle, bone and body fluid all weigh more than fat, a relatively high BMI can be either the result of a high level of body fat or a high lean body mass with lots of muscle and bone, so not all weight is created equal.

To put this in perspective, the BMI of the film stars Tom Cruise and Alexander Skarsgard are right on the margin between 'normal' and 'overweight' – do they look overweight to you? Even sillier is that the BMI for the former All Black Captain, Richie McCaw is 30 and film star Dwayne Johnson (The Rock) comes in at 31 so they are both technically obese according to the BMI index. Get the picture?

It gets even more complicated because not all fat is created equal, so that the fat around your butt and thighs (sometimes called your subcutaneous fat) doesn't seem to be bad for your health. Many people have a BMI of over 25, which is theoretically overweight. However, several studies have shown that it is the people with a BMI of 25 – 30 who actually have the longest lifespan.

So you definitely need some fat to be healthy, as long as it's in the right places. Even 20% of the technically obese adults (BMI> 30) have a completely normal metabolic status, with no evidence of disease, and can live a normal lifespan.

The other default measurement commonly used by doctors, and people in their own home, is to jump on a pair of scales. Because body fluid levels normally change dramatically during a woman's monthly hormonal cycle, any changes measured could be just a loss of body fluid. Even more depressing, any sudden weight gain is almost certainly just some fluid retention, but such gains can really do a number on your head and your self-esteem and bump up your stress levels.

Probably the best, easily measurable indicator of your current state of wellness is your waist size, or your waist to hip ratio, because these measurements are directly measuring your belly fat.

These measures are very seldom taken by professionals, partly because it's quite an intimate measurement to take because it's not that easy to standardize where to measure, without intimate contact. Also, most doctors probably don't know what useful comment they can make, other than "eat less and exercise more" which, as you now know, very seldom helps at all.

American studies have suggested that a waist size of greater than around 90cm (measured over your belly button) for women and/or a waist to hip (measured over your hip bones) ratio of greater than around 0.85 are both correlated with an increased risk of insulin resistance and metabolic disease. Your metabolism is likely to be pretty healthy if your waist to hip ratio is around 0.8 or less.

The great thing about these particular measurements is that they are measurements that you can take relatively easily in the privacy of your own home. This also means that you are much more likely to be able to honestly and openly take on board any negative message this measurement might give you, rather than going into denial or shame. The first thing you have to do before you can make any change in your life, is to accept that you need to change or want to change.

For your health's sake, if your ego is busy telling you that you're overweight, then I urge you to get a tape measure to check out whether you have the dangerous belly fat or not. Please understand that your belly fat can originate either from a very stressful lifestyle, including your egos input (the cortisol path) or from poor food choices (the insulin path) or both. This chapter has aimed to give you some clues about how to start the process towards taking charge of your belly fat.

If changing your overall body composition to less fat and more muscle becomes one of your key goals, then it is really important for your progress towards this goal to have a 'before' photo and note down your measurements. Use a tape measure to measure your waist, your hips, and it's also a great idea to measure your upper arms (mid-bicep) and both legs (mid-thigh). You can then easily calculate and track your waist to hip ratio and your total centimeters. A handy little device called an 'Orbitape' can help you simplify and standardize taking these measurements because it has a built-in tension system, which will give you a very repeatable measure, so you can more easily chart your progress.

"Probably the best, easily measurable indicator of your current state of wellness is your waist size or your waist to hip ratio because these measurements are directly measuring your belly fat."

8.8
Exercise

There is no doubt that getting some exercise is probably the single best thing you can do for your wellness, because exercise works at so many levels. The one thing it won't do, by itself, is cause you to lose weight. There is not a single study that shows that exercise alone causes significant weight loss.

Part of the reason for this is that you actually have to do a lot of really hard work to burn a significant number of calories. For example, if you do an hour of strenuous running or tennis or pushing weights in the gym, you maybe burn 600 – 700 calories, which is roughly equivalent to one cup of sugar (or roughly 2 liters of soda).

To lose 0.45 kg (1 pound) of fat, you need to burn 3500 calories more than you take in as food. So if you cut 500 calories from your diet every day, you will lose your 0.45 kg (1 pound) in a week. To achieve the equivalent result with just exercise is a whole hour of hard sweat nearly every single day. Personally, I think looking at the way you eat is a much better option.

The other reason that exercise doesn't help you lose weight is that it causes you to build muscle instead of fat, which is really great for your health but doesn't change your weight a lot. True, the proportion of fat in your body declines, but that's mainly because you have built up the amount of muscle in your body so that you may have lost some centimeters but not some weight – measure, don't weigh.

When you exercise, one of the first things to happen is that you burn off your stores of liver fat giving you an immediate improvement in your insulin sensitivity, which has several positive flow-on effects on your metabolic hormone balance – great? Unfortunately, the other effect of exercise on your metabolic hormones it is not so helpful. Your limbic system wants to keep your fat cells full in case of famine, so in response to a decline in leptin production, because you have burned some fat, your body reduces your metabolic rate. So, again, your hormones are working against you if your goal is to reduce fat by eating less and exercising more.

If, in spite of all of you have read so far, you are still continuing to try to reduce fat by eating less and exercising more; then there is one completely counterintuitive tweak that you need to incorporate into your program, which is actually quite fun because it involves a 'cheat' day.

It works like this. If you restrict your food intake, it takes several days for your overall leptin levels to decline to the point that it starts to affect your metabolic rate and reduce your rate of fat loss. On the other hand, if you overeat, your leptin levels rebound again in the space of a few hours. This lag in your leptin levels dropping is why it's important that if you must go on a 'diet', you should have a cheat day once a week when you can eat absolutely everything that you love.

This has the effect of resetting your leptin levels, but probably just as importantly, it helps to reset your mind, as if you know that your binge day is only a couple of days away you are much more likely to be able to resist those urges to eat when you shouldn't. Your cheat day is best done by having your normal high fat, moderate protein breakfast, but from then on there are no rules for the rest of the day – eat whatever you like. It's probably a good idea to do this on a Saturday as it's highly likely that you will not feel that great the next day after such a binge.

In Chapter 16 Your 'Rapid Reset' Plan, I talk about my recommendations for a complete program that will get your hormones back into balance so that you are working with your body towards wellness rather than working against it.

"When you exercise, one of the first things to happen is that you burn off your stores of liver fat which gives you an immediate improvement in your insulin sensitivity, which has several positive flow-on effects on your metabolic hormone balance."

8.9
"It's my Glands"

I'm sure you've heard people say "it's my glands; I eat nothing, and yet I gain weight. Whatever I eat goes straight onto my waist (or thighs)". You're probably like I used to be, and think "what a load of rubbish they're just kidding themselves".

However, it's not uncommon for this to be true, with what appears to be similar people eating the same diet, but one person gains weight relentlessly while the other does not. This can be very hard to live with, if nothing you do seems to shift the belly fat.

In this Chapter I have explored how the hormones produced by your 'glands' contribute to the problem. If these explanations don't fit the way your body is – don't panic yet, there are still other potential reasons why this can happen:

One potential answer to this puzzle is not in your glands, but it's in your gut (See Chapter 9 Bugs Are Important).

A second reason could be that, because your liver is the primary starting point for fat burning, if your liver is overloaded by trying to detox your body from chemicals in your food and environment, then it will not have spare capacity to burn fat (See Chapter 12 Detoxing Your Body).

A third reason could be from hidden stress, created by your ego from happenings from your past that you have not yet come to terms with. You may think you are dealing with your current stress levels, so that your weight issues have nothing to do with stress, but your past can still come back to haunt you. For instance, a not uncommon side effect of sexual abuse is unexplained weight gain and difficulty losing weight much later in life.

A fourth reason could be because your sex hormones progesterone, estrogen and testosterone all help to counteract the fat storage effects of cortisol. When your levels of these hormones decline during menopause, you become a lot less able to handle stress, so don't go for a run, go for a massage (See Chapter 14 Detoxing Your Mind).

CHAPTER 9

Bugs Are Important

"All disease begins in the gut" – Hippocrates

which means that,

"All healing begins in the gut" - Me

9.1
An Introduction to Your Microbiome

We are currently in the middle of a quiet revolution in the way science, and some innovative medical practitioners, view how our body works, how disease states develop, and how to heal the body. This includes healing from what were previously thought to be untreatable conditions, such as diabetes, autoimmune disorders, superbug infections dementia and Alzheimer's

I know that sounds a pretty extraordinary statement, but much of it comes from our very new understanding of what is called our 'microbiome': the vast number of bugs that live on our skin, in our gut and mouth, and actually inside our organs, such as our brain, our blood vessels and our tissues. We are in fact, very far from the sterile organisms we thought we were until very recently.

Your body's bug population consists of about 100 trillion cells, made up of a wide array of species of bacteria, archaea, fungi (mycobiome), protozoa, bacteriophages, viruses (virome) and even parasites. All up, they weigh about 1-3 kg, and they're not just hanging out randomly. They are effectively a living 'organ' or ecosystem, which is communicating actively both within the organ and directly with the cells of your body.

To give a perspective on your bug population, it is estimated that about 90% of the cells (by number) in and on your body belong to your bugs and not directly to you. Similarly, over 99% of the genetic material – the DNA in and on your body – actually belongs to your bugs. So only 1% of the genes in and on your body are those you inherited from your parents!

What's more, it's becoming increasingly obvious as the research progresses, that interactions between your body's cells and your bug's cells are happening all the time and have major consequences for how you feel and how your body behaves. They do, to a fair extent, run the show.

Some people believe, that because our own DNA has changed hardly at all since we were hunter-gatherers, that to be healthy we need to eat only the foods that were available at that time (e.g. the Paleo or Primal Diets). On the other hand, we now know that bugs are highly promiscuous in swapping their DNA, so they are changing and evolving all the time - very rapidly. So while your own DNA has changed very little in the last 10,000 years, the DNA of your bugs has changed a lot, which means that if you have a healthy bug population, you are always evolving and adapting to your modern environment, which can have a huge influence on your health.

Yes, you need to pay attention to what your ancestral diet was, especially when you are trying to heal your body and get it back in balance. However, once you have achieved balance, you need to be acutely conscious of what your body is telling you about how you are treating it, to help you find a regime that suits your personal state of evolution, or stool of wellness.

As an example of this, it seems that most Japanese people have certain strains of gut bacteria that have picked up the genes for seaweed digestion, from bacteria that normally live on seaweed. These seaweed bacteria didn't actually colonize the gut, but their genetic material transferred to the rest of their bugs. It turns out that if you don't have the right genes within your bug population, you can have trouble digesting some of the potentially beneficial compounds found in seaweed.

If you are healthy, then your relationship with your bugs is a mutually beneficial relationship. You provide the food and a nice, cosy environment for your bugs and, in return, your bugs protect you against bugs that could potentially produce disease. Your bugs can also produce really important goodies that help keep your body healthy, such as Vitamin C, the B Vitamins – particularly B1, B2, B5, B7, B9, and B12 – and Vitamin K2. They also ferment soluble dietary fiber into short chain fatty acids, such as butyrate, which is a very healthy fuel for the cells of your gut lining, which can have a major impact on reducing inflammation around your gut and throughout your body.

If you are healthy, then your relationship with your bugs is a mutually beneficial relationship.

However, if your gut bug population gets out of balance (often called gut dysbiosis), then you are set for conditions as nasty and diverse as weight gain, diabetes, heart disease, autoimmune conditions, depression, brain fog, and cancer. These little critters can also become a bit demanding, and it seems that they are often responsible for driving food cravings. So if you try to cut sugar out of your diet, they can tell your body "hey, you can't cut off our sugar supply, we need sugar NOW", which can make it very hard to get yourself onto a more healthy diet. Fortunately, when your bugs are in balance, they will lead you to crave healthy foods, feel hungry and full at the right times, and speed up your metabolism to help you burn fat instead of storing it.

We are now starting to understand that your bug population is so influential on your health that it is like an extra organ. It's the unseen force that regulates how you process food, your immune system (80% of your immune system is in your gut), the production of your brain hormones, and generally keeps you working like a healthy, well-oiled machine.

To get your head around this requires a complete reversal of how we have been trained to view bugs (or germs or micro-organisms). For most of us, the idea until now has been that most bugs are bad for us. At best there are some neutral ones, but most of them need to be avoided at all costs, or zapped with sanitizers or antibiotics as frequently as possible. So, you do things such as encourage your children not to play in the dirt (which is something they instinctively want to do) and to wash their hands with antiseptic soap before they eat.

The new understanding completely disrupts this reality, and we now know that the number of beneficial organisms in our bug population greatly exceeds the number of neutral or harmful organisms and that the bug population of a healthy body has somewhere in the vicinity of 85 - 90% beneficial organisms. It also turns out that many bugs, which can cause disease states when their numbers get excessive, can also be important contributors to your wellness when your bug population is balanced. This concept even applies to viruses, some of which attack potentially damaging bacteria, so using vaccines to get your immune system to attack viruses like measles or HPV can potentially damage your body's ability to fight serious bacterial infections.

So, which are the bad bugs? There may not be any; your microbiome may just be out of balance! I'm sure you have all heard of the bacteria, E.coli, which has been used for years as an indicator of fecal contamination, which is bad, right?

Well, no actually, only some strains of them. We now know that there's a whole range of E. coli strains, and now that we can readily measure their genetic expression, we find that some of them can be very toxic and dangerous, but some of them are quite beneficial. Some of them can even be involved in the detoxification of toxins in your gut, rather than your liver having to do it all for you.

We now know that up to half of the detoxification of drugs and environmental toxins actually takes place in your gut and is done by your bugs, rather than by your liver, which can greatly reduce the load on your liver. Also, some problem plant compounds like oxalates (high in such foods as spinach, beet greens and almonds) cannot be broken down by your body, but requires the presence of specific bacteria in your gut bug population to detoxify them.

This new understanding requires a complete about-face in the way we think about bugs, and also requires some important changes in the way we live our lives. For instance, the science is now showing that it's really important for your children to play in the dirt; it's a really key part of them developing a healthy immune system. We also understand that the overuse of sanitizing products in the home is contributing to antibiotic resistance and an imbalance in your bug population, which contributes to serious health issues.

"This new understanding requires a complete about-face in the way we think about bugs, and also requires some important changes in the way we live our lives."

I am not suggesting that personal hygiene is not important for your health, but it is important not to get extreme about it. It's really important that you get regular exposure to the bugs in your environment from stroking your dog, working in your garden (preferably without gloves), or rolling around on the grass with your children (as long as it hasn't been sprayed with pesticides). In other words, exposure to dirt is good.

For example, in the USA, the Amish and Hutterite dairy farming communities share a very similar diet, genetics and lifestyle, with no pets or television. However, a recent study showed that the Amish children have extremely low rates of asthma, whereas the Hutterite children have similar rates of asthma to the general population.

It seems the key lifestyle difference is that the Amish homes are situated very close to their farm animals, and the woman and children frequently go between house and barn, inadvertently tracking dust rich in bugs from the barn into the home. In contrast, the Hutterite families live some distance from their animal barns, and the woman and children seldom visit. The researcher's theory is, that the early exposure to a diverse bug population that comes from living in close contact with farm animals, conditions the immune system not to develop allergies such as asthma.

9.2
Where Did the 'All Bugs are Bad' Idea Come From?

From the time of Hippocrates until the end of the 19th century, the 'humoral theory' was the central theory of Western medicine, based on the idea that the human body contained a mix of four humors. Each person had a particular balance of humors, and it was the development of an imbalance that caused disease. A part of this theory was the idea that the bugs that caused a wound to go septic, or bread to go moldy, were spontaneously generated from whatever they were growing on.

It wasn't until the 1870s when Pasteur proved that bugs caused decomposition, that science started developing the tools to start to understand the role of bugs in causing disease. The germ theory, which is the way we have been trained to think since then states, 'specific microscopic organisms are the cause of specific diseases'. This theory was developed between about 1870 and 1920 and encouraged the idea that diseases are just a simple interaction between the bugs and the host.

This theory essentially did away with the need for attention to environmental influences such as diet, climate, and lifestyle, which were part of our earlier understandings of health and disease. It also fitted perfectly with the evolving thinking of the time, which was increasingly around the values of mass production, mass consumption, standardization, and efficiency.

Central figures in the development of the germ theory were scientists such as Lister, who promoted the concept of antiseptic surgery, and Koch, who showed that specific bugs caused diseases, such as anthrax, cholera, and tuberculosis. Pasteur also developed the first laboratory vaccines for cholera, anthrax, and rabies.

The germ theory required a new public awareness around how bugs were transmitted between people, with a new emphasis on the importance of hygiene and sanitation. This paved the way for the development of antibiotics in the 1940s, which meant that the diseases caused by bugs could now be cured. This was also the beginning of the pharmaceutical industry and the concept that there was a quick fix antibiotic or chemical drug for every condition – a pill for every ill.

For most people this was seen as a godsend in their increasingly busy lives, as they could eat what they liked (increasingly this was packaged, convenience food), and give responsibility for their health to their doctor, who could prescribe a pill for anything, and that was the end of that. Or it was, until people developed a side effect from the first pill, which necessitated a second pill to fix that, and so on.

We did not understand until very recently how all these antibiotics and widely prescribed drugs, such as statins (to control cholesterol) and PPI's (proton pump inhibitors to control acid reflux) were damaging our bug population. This means that such drugs are contributing in some way to the development of chronic conditions such as heart disease, cancer, diabetes, dementia, depression, and an increasingly wide range of autoimmune conditions. Recent studies have shown that use of PPI's increase the risk of stroke, heart disease and death and a 44% increase in the risk of Alzheimer's.

Unfortunately, the current practice of 20th-century medicine, which evolved around the germ theory, is very badly equipped to deal with such chronic conditions, although it does a brilliant job of dealing with acute conditions such as a mangled hand, a breech birth, or a lung infection.

We are now starting to see situations where the over-prescription of broad-spectrum antibiotics in the recent past is increasingly leading to the development of infections that no longer respond to antibiotics. To give you some idea of the scale of this problem, in the United States around 80% of all antibiotic use is on factory farms, to promote faster animal growth rates, rather than being used for curing infections in humans. A recent USA study, looking at over-prescription of antibiotics, also found that at least 30% of human prescriptions for antibiotics were for viral conditions, which do not respond to antibiotics at all.

The transfer of antibiotic resistance from the bugs from factory farms, and from people given antibiotics inappropriately, has led to a situation in the USA where at least 2 million people per year become infected with bacteria that are resistant to all antibiotics, and at least 23,000 people die each year as a direct result of these infections.

An example of this is the development of infectious diarrhea in hospitalized patients, caused by the organism Clostridium difficile. In the USA this is now the leading cause of hospital-acquired infections, affecting over 500,000 people annually, with a death rate of up to 4%. Because of the appearance of resistant strains, the most effective antibiotics available now have a reinfection rate of 20-25% in treated patients, even up to 50% in some situations.

However, because of the new understanding of how the bug population works, which is part of 21st-century medicine, the use of a fecal transplant; to restore diversity to the bug population is rapidly becoming the accepted treatment. One large study reported cure rates of 98%, which is unheard of for other medical treatments.

Fortunately, in the 21st century, we are starting to see a rapid rise in the number of Functional Medicine and other Integrative Medical Practitioners, who look at the 'WHY' and take a more holistic view in trying to treat the causes of ill health, rather than just treating the symptoms. Many of them incorporate our new understanding of the microbiome into the way they treat their patients.

9.3
Where Does Your Microbiome Come From?

Before birth babies are probably mainly sterile in the womb, although we are not sure about this as your bug population is being discovered in more and more organs in your body all the time. Certainly, as soon as a baby is born, they become colonized by bugs. Babies born via a normal vaginal birth become covered in a film of bugs from your birth canal.

The vaginal bug population has recently been shown to change markedly in preparation for the birth, to make sure the baby gets all the bugs it needs. Of course one of the first things they do is put their hand in their mouth or on to your nipple. This is the beginning of their gut being colonized by bugs, which includes the bacteria they need to digest their first meal fully.

Babies born by C-section (caesarean birth) are a completely different story, and their lack of exposure to their mother's vaginal bug population can have profound effects on their health for the rest of their life. The WHO (World Health Organization) estimates that the rate of C-sections required to achieve optimum overall mother and baby health is somewhere between 5 and 10%. Similarly, they estimate that rates of greater than 15% do not improve overall mother and baby health, and may result in more harm than good.

A survey done by the WHO in 2009 showed that Brazil, China, Turkey, and Mexico all had C-section rates more than 40%, the USA 32%, the OECD average was 26%, and the New Zealand rate was 24%. The average ANNUAL growth rate of this number was 3.2% over the whole of the OECD.

This recent rise in the use of C-section to deliver the baby is of major concern, because this means that the baby's body is colonized first by the skin bugs of those handling them and other bugs present in the hospital environment. This is a very different set of species from those present in their mother's vagina. The problem is exacerbated further by the fact that the mothers are routinely treated with antibiotics as part of the procedure, which further reduces the chances of a C-section baby developing a normal, healthy bug population and immune system.

Some well-informed doctors are using procedures such as incubating gauze in the mother's vagina for an hour, before wiping it on the baby's mouth, face, and body after the C-section. This has been shown to double the diversity of the baby's bug population, but vaginal delivery contributes to a six-fold increase in biodiversity compared to C-section.

Breastfeeding also helps to develop an optimum bug population, as the babies are exposed to a wider diversity of bugs from the mother's milk, and breast, so breastfed babies have been shown to have a more diverse bug population than formula-fed babies.

"This doubled the diversity of the baby's bug population, but vaginal delivery contributed to a six-fold increase in biodiversity."

Contact with their family continues to be an important source of a baby's bug population, as illustrated by a fascinating study from Sweden. It turns out that picking up your child's pacifier and sucking it clean, rather than rinsing it under the tap or boiling it, has a measurable effect on the child's oral bug population. While the idea of sucking clean a pacifier that has been on the floor may gross you out, doing this was associated with a one-third lower risk of the child developing eczema (which is a good indicator for developing other allergies). It seems the effect is additive, since normally delivered babies whose parents sucked their pacifiers had only a 20% incidence of eczema, compared to C-section delivered babies whose parents didn't lick their pacifiers, who had the highest rate of eczema at 54%.

The other major source of your bug population comes from the 'dirt' in your local environment, home and the soil. However, importantly, it also comes from your exposure to nature, so every time you go for a walk in the woods and smell the beautiful smells, you are in fact inhaling virus particles and bacterial and fungal spores.

Similarly, the ocean contains about 10 million viruses in every drop of seawater, so every time you breathe in the spray from the waves or get a little bit in your mouth when a wave dumps you, you are enriching your bug population. There is increasing awareness that the state of your outer ecology – your home, your garden, and the farms or factories where your food comes from – all have a major impact on your inner ecology or microbiome.

Your exposure to nature is so important to your health, that if you are like most people and spend very limited time in natural surroundings each day, you might want to consider budgeting some time in your day or week to make this happen. Maybe you could go outside and sit on the grass to eat your lunch or go for a walk outside rather than going to the gym. Alternatively, make an effort to spend a chunk of time in nature on one of your days off.

9.4
Biodiversity and Your Microbiome

Because this is such new field of research and the science is rapidly evolving, there is not a lot of hard data to go on. Various estimates suggest that we in urban communities have lost some 60 - 80% of the biodiversity present in the bug population of surviving hunter-gatherer populations around the world. The key reason why this has happened is that the diet of these populations is very diverse, with them often eating around 100 – 120 different plant species each year. Spend a minute or two to recall how your diet compares to that?

It would be helpful to start thinking of the bug population on and in your body as your personal organic garden. It is part of an interconnected ecosystem, which is in a continuous state of flux as it responds to various inputs from your body, from your environment, and from your food. We know that in complex ecosystems such as this, a relatively small change can end up having a profound effect on the whole system. (I'm sure you've heard of the story of a butterfly flapping its wings on one side of the world initiating a cyclone on the other side).

We also understand that the more diverse an ecosystem is, the more stable it tends to be, so having as much microbial diversity as possible in your bug population is going to be good for your health in the long term. Estimates suggest that for a reasonably healthy person some 10 - 15% of your microbiome consists of bugs that could potentially be damaging. The other 85 - 90% are either neutral or actively contributing to your state of wellness, and very importantly, keeping the potentially bad bugs in balance. Thus, the more diverse your bug population is, the less likely you are to succumb to an infection, and the better your state of wellness will be.

We are also starting to understand that it's all about the ecosystem balance, so that bacteria that could potentially cause a disease state in your body can also have a beneficial role to play. For example, most of the family of Corynebacterium are considered benign, but one species has been shown to be able to produce vitamin C in your body yet its presence has also been linked to urogenital infections. So one theory is, that this species grows into 'infectious' proportions that could contribute to urogenital infections when the body is starved of vitamin C. At other times it is just part of the normally balanced bug population doing its job.

Food produced by industrial agriculture has devastated the diversity of the soil bug population by the use of chemical fertilizers, fungicides, herbicides, and pesticides, with intense tillage systems and little or no return of organic matter to the soil. If most of your food comes from such sources you are likely to have a low level of diversity in your personal bug population. The produce from such farming systems is usually then washed in chlorinated water to render it as sterile as possible, enabling it to sit for days on the supermarket shelf and in your fridge. Or 'Big Food' heavily processes it into shelf-stable 'food' products, which renders it sterile. Such 'food' will contribute to a very low level of biodiversity in your internal bug population.

All plants are covered with a film of bugs which has come from the air around them and from the soil they are growing in. Just ponder, if you will, the difference between the bugs on a lettuce grown with the use of hydroponics – its roots bathed in a sterile solution of nutrients and its leaves probably bathed in filtered air – and a lettuce grown organically in a soil that has been fed with compost and is teeming with bugs. So, which lettuce do you think will contribute more to the diversity of your bug population? How your food is grown, and the diversity of your diet, can have a profound effect on your state of wellness.

A lack of diversity in gut microbial populations from these factors and such factors as C-section births, formula feeding, and multiple exposures to antibiotics has been shown to be linked to infants and children becoming more prone to conditions such as autism, inflammatory bowel disease, asthma, obesity and diabetes.

9.5
Leaky Gut

The lining of your gut, which controls what moves from your gut into your body, is only one cell thick but has roughly the area of a tennis court. The gap between each cell is normally a 'tight junction' which does not allow undigested food particles into your bloodstream. Chronic irritation from stress, processed foods, alcohol, antibiotics and other medications and bacterial imbalances can allow these tight junctions to open up to leak undigested food particles, bacteria, and toxins into your bloodstream –

hence the term 'leaky gut'.

Even a small leak will set up an immune response that is likely to lead to chronic inflammation and, if the damage is bad enough, it can wreak havoc on your health. The list of conditions associated with leaky gut includes acne, allergies, arthritis, and autism, and many, many more. In fact, the latest research is showing that leaky gut is involved in the development of over thirty types of autoimmune conditions.

Symptoms of a leaky gut vary from more minor gut issues, such as bloating, gas, cramps or diarrhea. If the leakiness is more pronounced, then you are likely to have body-wide symptoms including fatigue, joint pain, asthma, all sorts of mental health issues, and even autoimmune conditions.

"If you use a full therapeutic dose of NSAIDs (painkillers) for two weeks, there is a 75% chance you will develop a leaky gut, that doesn't go away when you stop taking the drug," Leo Galland MD.

The good news is that the cells lining your gut wall turn over pretty quickly, being completely replaced about every three weeks. One of the key objectives of the program I have designed for you in Chapter 16 Your 'Rapid Reset' Plan, is to heal any leakiness in your gut wall and dampen down the inflammatory fire in your belly. Keeping a balance between the good bugs and the bad bugs in your gut has been shown to have a profound influence on the silent inflammation in your gut.

9.6
Your Skin Microbiome

You may be surprised to learn that you have a wide range of bacteria and other organisms living on your skin, that they are usually different species from those in your gut, and that the balance of your skin bug population has a lot to do with your skin health.

Even more surprisingly, we now know that some of these bugs actually live quite deep in your skin. These bacteria have a crucial role in re-colonizing cuts and other wounds which helps to make for rapid healing – and you thought it was important to keep a wound completely sterile!

A study done in Sweden several years ago compared the healing of wounds from minor surgery when preventative antibiotics were routinely used, or not used. The rate of infections and other complications was substantially lower when antibiotics were NOT given routinely, and this latest research finally explains why - using antibiotics killed off the good bugs in your skin as well.

A few years ago I started to get uncomfortable with the lack of non-toxic deodorants and the fact that in my early 60s my skin was starting to show my age. I reasoned that water is a very powerful solvent for everything but oils, and that my regular use of soap was probably leaching the natural oils from my skin. I started showering without the use of soap and saw an immediate improvement in my skin condition. Great.

I happened to be making goats' milk cheese at the time, so I had access to lots of whey. I also decided to try applying that to my body after my shower to see if that would rebalance my skin bacteria and if that would help alleviate the resulting body odor problem. This approach worked a treat, so for the last ten years or so, with great success, I have not used soap for anything but greasy, dirty hands, nor any deodorant.

More importantly, I started to smell of me, which my partner thought was wonderful, so she quickly followed suit in dropping the soap and I now think her natural smell is wonderfully erotic.

A couple of years later I was visiting Istanbul with my son and we decided to try out a Turkish bath as a way to spend our last evening together.

As part of the process I was very thoroughly lathered with soapsuds all over, which felt great at the time. However, the next morning, I got straight onto several long-distance flights, which meant I was 22 hours from hotel to hotel, and by the time I got to Bangkok I stunk – even to me.

A good shower fixed the immediate problem but, of course, I didn't have any deodorant with me or access to whey, so I went looking for some natural yoghurt and slathered that all over myself for 10 min, before I washed it off, just to see what that would do. That worked very effectively to restore some healthy skin bugs, and in spite of the heat in Thailand and a very busy schedule over the next few days, I had no further issues with my smell.

That is the only time I have had to repopulate my skin bugs in the last ten years.

It's now becoming clear that what we have done to our gut with the overuse of antibiotics, sanitizers and antiseptic cleaning products, and showering and swimming in chlorinated water, we have also done to our skin. At the same time, we have also drastically reduced our exposure to the outside air, reduced swimming in rivers and the sea, and reduced our contact with soil which, in the past, have been the source of our diverse skin bug population. At this stage there is little research to tell us what effects skin products such as lotions, cosmetics, cleansers, and deodorants have on the health of our skin bugs and epidermal barrier, but the chances are it's not good.

We're now starting to understand that healing your skin can be an inside-out process, and there is now compelling evidence that taking probiotics internally is a promising treatment for the skin conditions, acne and rosacea. While the research on applying probiotics directly to the skin is in its infancy, there are already studies showing beneficial effects from topical application of probiotics to the skin in situations as diverse as wound healing, acne, dermatitis, and even in psoriasis.

"for the last ten years or so I have not used soap for anything but greasy, dirty hands, nor any deodorant..."

9.7
Your Mouth Microbiome

We also now understand that a very important part of maintaining your oral health is looking after the bug population in your mouth. While it is obviously connected to your gut bugs, your oral bug population is actually a unique ecosystem in its own right. It is an essential component of the salivary immune system, which is the first line of defense protecting us from potentially deadly viruses and bacteria entering via our food or through the mouth and nose.

Because the mouth is the main place where air and food from the outside environment enter the body, your mouth is a constant battleground where external viruses and bacteria can most readily get a foothold. They are more easily able to do so when you have a distorted oral bug population or oral dysbiosis, which is often caused by oral care products. Most of these products were developed while we had the understanding that all bugs are bad and that your mouth should be as sterile as possible, but this is changing.

Plaque is actually a deposit produced by a distorted bug population, which builds up around the gum line and between your teeth. A healthy oral bug population is just a very thin biofilm that acts as a protective layer for your teeth and actively remineralizes your teeth from nutrients in your saliva. We now know that maintaining a healthy bug balance is the secret to having a healthy mouth, free of gum disease, plaque, and tooth decay.

For instance, there are species of bacteria in your mouth that are responsible for tooth decay and plaque development, if oral care products distort your bugs. Yet, the same species of bacteria have also been shown to have an important role to play in maintaining a healthy, balanced bug population in your mouth.

Gum disease is caused by a build-up of plaque and tartar on your teeth, which irritates your gums, causing chronic inflammation and bleeding when you brush your teeth. Factors which increase the risk of you developing gum disease include oral care products that distort the oral bug population, but obviously includes lack of care around brushing and cleaning between your teeth, smoking, stress, and poor diet, which can all contribute to a challenged immune system, potentially leading to gum disease. The most common source of low-grade chronic inflammation in your body is from your mouth, and such inflammation puts a major strain on your immune system. Estimates of the incidence of gum disease and gum bleeding in the adult population put the incidence at around 70 - 90%.

As an indication of how important this can be for your overall health, advanced gum disease can raise your risk of a fatal heart attack by tenfold, and if you have a heart attack related to your gum disease, nine times out of ten, it will be fatal. One study showed that just by brushing your teeth twice a day reduces your risk of a fatal heart attack by 40% - who needs statins anyway? Advanced gum disease also raises your risk of developing any cancer by 24% and doubles your risk of developing lung or colorectal cancer.

The most common advice given by a dentist if you have gum disease is to send you to a session with a dental hygienist, who will use ultrasound and physical scraping to remove the plaque and tartar that has built up on your teeth – great. However, this will usually be accompanied by advice to routinely use antimicrobial mouthwashes or toothpaste, or both, to reduce the bacteria associated with gum disease. Such advice is from the old 'all bugs are bad' paradigm.

Given the high incidence of gum disease in the adult population, it's probably not that surprising to find that most oral care products kill some of the bacteria in your mouth, and so distort your mouth bug population.

As an example of the old way of thinking, I was recently at my (supposedly) holistic dentist for a check-up, and I objected to the pink, chlorhexidine mouthwash he wanted me to use as a rinse.

He said "there are no good bugs in your mouth. It's really important that you keep your mouth as sterile as possible".

So I pointed out some of the information above, including that a group at Otago University have isolated Streptococcus strains which are very effective at treating gum disease and sore throats, and if used as a preventative can also reduce the incidence of lung infections.

Not surprisingly, he was rather taken aback at this new idea, which was completely contrary to his training in dental school, but he was very happy when presented with some of the research.

These products include:

Detergents – such as sodium lauryl sulfate, and similar soap-like products in toothpaste, many of these are derived from coconut oil, which sound all natural and good for your teeth but actually contribute to oral dysbiosis.

Antibacterial agents - Synthetic types, such as triclosan (an endocrine disruptor) and chlorhexidine (which damages the DNA in your mouth) damage your bugs, but so too do the antimicrobial essential oils such as Peppermint, Tea Tree, Holy Basil and Oregano.

Mouthwashes – These contain a wide range of ingredients, but most of them contain alcohol, which dehydrates the bacteria, thus damaging your bug population. They often also contain the active antibacterial agents outlined above.

It turns out that the best things you can do for your overall health also support your oral health, so what you eat and, perhaps rather surprisingly, how you exercise, are both important for your oral bugs.

Since your oral bugs would benefit from you avoiding nearly all toothpaste, there are three strategies you can adopt that have been shown to support your oral health.

1. Coconut oil 'pulling'. This is an ancient Ayurvedic practice, which science has confirmed works to improve your oral health when done occasionally. It involves rinsing your mouth with a small amount of coconut oil (or sesame oil), much as you would with mouthwash.

Work the oil around your mouth and between your teeth for at least five, but desirably up to 20 minutes. Once the oil turns thin and becomes milky white it's time to spit it out and rinse your mouth. Do not swallow it.

2. Use a prebiotic (supports the growth of

your bugs) nutritional toothpaste designed to support a balanced oral bug population, e.g. Revitin products. If you have patches of gum that bleed rub some on the gum after you have finished brushing – it is actually desirable to absorb the nutrients direct or swallow it.

3. Use a probiotic (supplies you with beneficial bugs) formula specifically designed for the mouth.

Most probiotic formulas are ineffective at changing the mouth bug population. However, work at Otago University has shown that specific strains of the bacteria, Streptococcus salivarius, are effective against tooth decay, gum disease, sore throats, and upper respiratory tract infections, - e.g. the Blis M18 or K12 products.

9.8
The Gut-Brain Connection

In recent years, over 25 diseases or syndromes have been linked to gut dysbiosis or an altered gut bug population.

Not surprisingly, many of these relate to the gut directly such as IBS (Irritable Bowel Syndrome), colon cancer, and Crohn's disease. Perhaps more surprisingly, many of these relate directly to the brain so that conditions as diverse as Alzheimer's, autistic spectrum disorders, anxiety-depressive disorders, chronic fatigue syndrome, dementia and Parkinson's disease have also been linked to gut dysbiosis.

We now realize that there is continuous two-way communication along the vagus nerve, which runs between your brain in your head and what is increasingly being called the gut-brain. This is the enteric nervous system which contains extensive neural circuits that are capable of acting independently of your head brain (Yes, those gut instincts are real).

Your bugs are a very active participant in this crosstalk. It turns out that your bugs are responsible for the production of the majority of your brain hormones. Yes, you did read that right – there are more 'brain' hormones produced by the bugs in your gut than by the whole of the rest of your nervous system. For example, your gut produces about 90% of the serotonin and dopamine produced in your body. Note that both of these are happy hormones, so looking after your gut is vital for your sense of happiness.

New research shows that your bug population not only plays an important role in brain development, but it also has a major impact on brain function and fundamental behavioral patterns, including social interaction and stress management. So, conditions such as autism, anxiety, depression, and

OCD (Obsessive-Compulsive Disorder) have been shown to respond very positively to treatments that aim to rebalance the bugs. As I told someone recently diagnosed with Alzheimer's, "if you have a constipated gut (which she did) you will have a constipated brain."

All this now makes total sense with the very recent discovery of a bug population in your brain; the composition of which is quite closely related to your gut bugs. I'm sure your initial response to this was a sense of disbelief "surely the blood-brain barrier means your brain is sterile". Well, that is the case for most animals, but a brain bug population has been found in all the primates, and we now know that the bugs present in your brain enhance the ability of your brain cells to make new connections, or learn, which is a finding with some pretty profound implications.

So how do the bugs get into your brain? There is a part of your white blood cell immune system called macrophages (big cells) whose usual job is to engulf infectious bugs and digest them to neutralize them. It now seems that they also engulf SELECTED bugs picked up from your gut, and then escort them around your body and through the blood-brain barrier and into your brain - Wow!

Exposure to stress has also been shown to be a major predictor of inflammatory bowel disease. One of the first impacts of elevated stress hormones is to minimize the blood flow to your gut, as digesting food is not a priority when your life might be in danger. This restricted blood flow has a direct impact on your gut's ability to manage the balance of your bug population and properly digest foods.

The direct impact of stress is by changing the balance of your gut bugs towards the types of bacteria that help you gain belly fat more easily – the Firmicutes (See below.). The restricted blood flow also disrupts your digestion, and poor digestion makes you feel more stressed – another vicious cycle.

Research so far has shown the bacterial families, *Bifidobacterium* (*B. longum, B. breve, and B. infantis*) and *Lactobacillus* (*L. helveticus, L. rhamnosus, L. plantarum, and L. casei*) are associated with improved brain function, but there are potentially thousands of bacterial species involved so, at this stage of our knowledge this list should not be seen as a definitive guide.

Does this mean that taking antibiotics will negatively impact on your brain health and mental state? Almost certainly. So, if you're feeling a bit low after dealing with an infection that necessitated you taking a course of antibiotics – did you follow up with a course of probiotics? You should.

9.9
Obesity and Your Microbiome

Two of the major families of micro-organisms in the gut are the Bacteroidetes and Firmicutes. It turns out that overweight people are much more likely to have higher levels of Firmicutes compared to Bacteroidetes.

In animal studies it's been shown that you can transform skinny animals into fat animals just by transferring some of the gut bacteria from fat animals. It has also been shown that there is a bacterial toxin that induces obesity in animals by promoting inflammation.

One of the bacteria that produces this toxin was found at very high levels in the gut of a morbidly obese, Chinese man, making up 35% of his bug population. When he was put on a diet of whole grains, traditional Chinese medicinal food, and prebiotics, he lost 51.4 kilograms over six months (nearly 1/3 of his body weight), and the toxin-producing bacteria were no longer detectable in his gut. Furthermore, when the offending bacteria was isolated and used as a fecal transplant into animals they became obese, confirming the link between the bacteria and the obesity.

There was also a very small study done in China with children who have a 'genetic' disorder that causes them to be compulsive eaters. (If you have one of these children in your family then you may need to have a padlock on your fridge and pantry doors, otherwise, they are likely to become morbidly obese). The microbial ecologist in charge of the project gave Chinese herbs that swung the balance in favor of Bacteroidetes which, for most of them, resulted in massive weight loss. This was in children who supposedly had a 'genetic' disorder, not a 'microbiome' disorder. I'm sure we're going to find some very interesting developments in this field over the next few years.

All very fascinating, but how can I use this knowledge to influence my belly fat?

At this stage of our knowledge, it doesn't seem as if it is going to be as easy as taking a probiotic with lots of Bacteroidetes in it. Oh, that the human body was so simple.

However, it turns out that there are several things that you can do to promote a more healthy balance towards more Bacteroidetes in your bug population.

- Bacteroidetes love the family of antioxidants called polyphenols that you will find at high levels in spices, fruits, vegetables, seeds, and nuts. The highest content of polyphenols on a per serving basis come from the dark colored fruits, such as blackcurrants, blueberries, cherries,

I'm sure you've all heard that you should have a probiotic supplement after a course of antibiotics to restore your bugs. I used to assume that "surely your bug population would restore itself over time", so I never got around to taking the probiotics. I was also aware that for the lignans in flax seed to be active in your body as phytooestrogens, they need to be converted by the beneficial bacteria in your gut into human lignans However, during my research for this book, I discovered two studies that showed that even three or four months after a course of antibiotics, no human lignans were being produced after eating flax seed. In other words, the bug population had not been restored to effective balance even after a long period. In fact, we now know that with every course of antibiotics, you take your bug population gets less and less diverse – really bad news.

strawberries, blackberries, plums, raspberries, and apples. Coffee, black and green teas and cider vinegar also have quite high contents of polyphenols, as do artichoke hearts, spinach, and red onions. Some of the surprises high on this list include flax seed flour, dark chocolate, chestnuts, hazelnuts, and black olives. So it's a great idea to eat a wide range of these colorful foods to help diversify and shift your bug population in the right direction.

- Avoid all forms of sugar and processed carbs, which spike your blood sugar.

- Firmicutes are so well suited to grow on sugar that they are a major problem in factories that process sugarcane into sugar.

- Increase your intake of beans and lentils as Bacteroidetes also love these. If you can't digest beans very well, this is a strong sign that your bug population is low in Bacteroidetes. Rather than avoid them completely, I suggest you add a few beans, that you have soaked for two days before cooking, into your diet slowly, maybe a tablespoon a day with your evening meal, and try and stick with it. For most people, the bean- induced gas and bloating problem will go away after a couple of weeks.

- Eat a high fiber diet, rich in good carbs, which means, eat lots more 'above ground' vegetables.

- Eat and sleep in a regular pattern, as we now know that even your bug population has a daily rhythm. If your lifestyle includes shift work, jet lag, or erratic mealtimes on a regular basis, this can significantly disrupt your bugs' balance, enough to cause glucose intolerance and a shift towards obesity.

Eating and living in the ways suggested by the list above will help to tip your bug population towards Bacteroidetes dominance, and help you to get your body into a state that will help you to take charge of your belly fat.

Such foods are also very rich in antioxidants that have other multiple benefits on your health, particularly heart health and the rate you age, so eat lots of them.

9.10
The IBS – SIBO Link

We now understand that IBS (Irritable Bowel Syndrome) is very strongly related to a condition now called SIBO (Small Intestinal Bacterial Overgrowth), which is a chronic overgrowth of the small intestine by bacteria that normally reside in your colon or large intestine.

The most common symptoms of SIBO and IBS are very similar: gas and bloating shortly after eating, diarrhea, constipation, leaky gut, poor fructose digestion, and excessive fermentation of a class of carbs called FODMAPs (Fermentable Oligosaccharides, Disaccharides, Monosaccharides, and Polyols).

FODMAPs are complex sugars that are very poorly digested by some people but don't cause any issues for others because they can happily digest them and they help feed the bugs in their colon.

The grains that are high in gluten: wheat, barley, rye, and oats, are also high in FODMAPs, so it can be difficult to separate out FODMAP intolerance from gluten intolerance. Amaranth is the only other grain high in FODMAPs, and this is gluten-free. Other 'gluten-free' grains, such as rice and corn which contain gluten-like storage proteins that can affect some people with gluten intolerance, do not contain FODMAPs, so there is no crossover between them.

There is, however, a wide range of other foods which are also high in FODMAPs. The list includes vegetables such as onions and cauliflower; fruits such as apples and peaches; protein foods such as beans and cashew nuts; dairy products such as milk and kefir; sweeteners such as HFCS and honey; and juices from apples and tropical fruits. Because such a wide range of foods can cause problems for people intolerant of FODMAPs, it's pretty hard to keep track of them all but, fortunately, there are some apps available for smartphones that can be used to keep track of what you can eat.

It's important to realize that if you have FODMAP intolerance, this is a very powerful signal that you almost certainly have SIBO, which will be contributing to chronic inflammation and will be damaging your health. There are many, very healthy foods that you should be consuming as part of a healthy diet and to feed your bugs, but which happen to be high in FODMAPs.

In practice, this means that if you have had a lot of gas or bloating shortly after eating, so you try a low FODMAP diet, which drastically reduces your symptoms. Great, but then you need to take active steps to correct your SIBO as soon as possible. You will need to work directly with a practitioner knowledgeable in this area to get the best results. There is good research comparing targeted antibiotics and herbs, and both approaches have similar effectiveness, so the choice of whom you go to for help is up to you.

Being on a restricted diet is a recipe for making life very difficult, and greatly enhances the risk of you developing allergies to foods you are frequently eating, which is absolutely not what you want to happen. For instance, you may have a minor allergic reaction to some foods that you are not aware of, but this minor reaction starts to train your immune system to mount a full response to these foods, so it can become a new food you are allergic to. You may find my recommendations in Chapter 16 Your 'Rapid Reset' Plan are sufficient to correct the problem of food allergies, but you may also need to find a Functional Medicine practitioner or herbalist to give you a hand.

"It's important to realize that if you have FODMAP intolerance, this is a powerful signal that you almost certainly have SIBO."

Some of the likely reasons for you developing SIBO are:

1. Not chewing your food sufficiently which means your stomach is trying to deal with food particles larger than its capacity to break them down. When they move through into your small intestine undigested, they become the perfect food for the bugs in your small intestine to grow on and ferment into gas. Remember - there are no teeth in your stomach.

2. Damage to the muscular activity of the wall of your small intestine by toxins from a food poisoning episode. This can be a tricky one to assess, as you may not easily recall having such an episode in your past, but the effects can be very long lasting.

3. Another likely reason is lack of digestive 'fire', which means that either your stomach is not producing enough acid, or your pancreas is not producing enough digestive enzymes – both will result in poor digestion. This can allow undigested carbs, proteins, and fats to pass into your small and large intestine where they will get fermented by your bugs, usually resulting in lots of gas (because that's what fermentation produces).

Lack of digestive 'fire' is also likely to mean that you will be suffering from acid reflux and thus you potentially take some medications to help with that. The widespread use of PPIs or antacids to alleviate the symptoms of acid reflux is closely linked with dysbiosis conditions, such as SIBO, and the potentially fatal C. difficile diarrhea. PPI's were never intended to be taken long term because they are also linked with poor nutrient absorption, heart and kidney problems and osteoporosis. Knowing this, you may choose to work with your medical practitioner to get off such medications, which may be an important step towards wellness for you (See Chapter 16 Your 'Rapid Reset' Plan).

9.11
How to Balance Your Microbiome

I hope this brief review of a huge and rapidly changing subject has given you a sense of the need to look after your bugs, both in and on your body.

So which comes first - get healthy so your bug population improves, or improve your bug population so you will become healthy? Your bug population and gut health are so fundamental to your health that being able to achieve wellness without actively supporting your bugs seems highly unlikely.

It turns out that one of the key effects of eating healthy carbs and good fats (as described in Chapters 10 and 11) is the effect they have on your gut health, via your bug population. So, eating plenty of a diverse range of above ground vegetables and other rich sources of dietary fiber, like mushrooms, supplies the prebiotics necessary to support the growth of a wide range of the good bugs in your gut.

The other important thing for you to do is to get plenty of probiotic foods into your diet on a regular basis, particularly home produced or locally produced fermented vegetables, yoghurt or kefir. Recent research has highlighted the effectiveness of using such food sources, rather than just relying on a probiotic supplement. However, using a probiotic supplement can be beneficial in some circumstances.

When it comes to restoring your bug population, there is no such thing as one size fits all. Probiotic supplements that work for most people, don't work for some, so at this stage of our understanding, a fair amount of trial and error needs to be involved. Having said that, probiotic supplements based on soil micro-organisms are usually well tolerated, as are those that contain *Bifidobacterium* (often found in yoghurt).

The trial and error process can take the form of trying out a new fermented vegetable brew or a new probiotic supplement and monitoring the amount of gas and/or bloating you experience over the next few days. A day or two of such symptoms is not uncommon as your bug population adjusts to the new guys on the block but, if your symptoms persist for longer than this, then you probably need to switch to another source of probiotics.

It turns out that your inner ecology is organized in a way that parallels your outer ecology. Your bugs are loosely organized in groups of different species that work together, but the behavior of the group is usually dominated by one or two species. One of the most common dominants in your gut are the species which live on plants, as the bacteria which live on plants are extremely hardy, so they more actively colonize your gut and have a multitude of beneficial effects which are hard to get in any other way.

This makes fermented vegetables one of the most important sources of healthy probiotics, as the fermentation process encourages the build-up of large numbers of the beneficial bugs. In the ideal world you would make these yourself from organically raised vegetables from your garden (which is pretty easy to do). Otherwise, you should try to source organic vegetables grown as locally as possible so that they contain strains that are more likely to be compatible with your local ecology, or purchase locally produced fermented vegetables.

Other fermented foods such as miso and tempeh, and fermented dairy products such as yoghurt and kefir can also be very important sources of very beneficial bacteria. Variety is the spice of life for your bugs, so the more fermented foods you can incorporate into your diet the better your health will become. Kombucha may be an exception to this, as the main fuel for the ferment is sugar. The resultant brew can contain significant amounts sugar, alcohol and caffeine so, unless you make it yourself, it's probably best avoided in the early stages of your 'Rapid Reset'.

CHAPTER 10

Bad Carbs Make You Fat and Sick

"My definition of 'Hangry' is a sugar burner (glucose-adapted) who has skipped two meals in a row"
Mark Sisson

It's unfortunate that most people still work on the theory that a calorie is a calorie, no matter what food the calorie comes from. When I am calculating the Energy Value to put on a food label, I am required to calculate that each gram of fiber contributes 8 kJ of energy, each gram of carbohydrate and protein contributes 17 kJ, and each gram of fat contributes 37 kJ of energy. These values are technically correct, in that if you burn each of these in a little furnace, that's how much energy would be released.

However, your body is not a simple furnace. You are an incredibly complex, living organism, which has to digest your food to convert it into potential energy. How and what your body does with this energy is driven by two things:

Firstly, the state of your stress hormones. If you are stressed, then your digestive system is largely shut down, which disrupts your whole gut microbiome.

Secondly, the state of your metabolic hormones, as is illustrated by the differing insulin responses below.

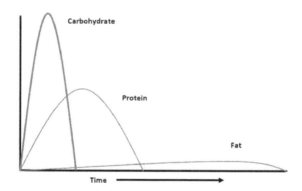

Figure 10.1 Blood sugar and insulin response over time to different foods

Carbs, as a group, are primarily quickly broken down into glucose creating a blood sugar spike, which provokes an insulin spike, released to get the excess glucose out of your bloodstream and into your cells.

Proteins do contain the same amount of potential energy as carbs, but they are initially broken down into amino acids which your body uses as the building blocks for new proteins as you require them. Only when there is a surplus of amino acids do they get converted into glucose, which then provokes a small insulin response. Because proteins take a lot longer to digest they help you to feel full for longer, and any insulin response takes a lot longer to develop.

Fats contain over twice as much energy per gram as carbs and proteins but they are digested into individual fatty acids, which are used, either as building blocks for cellular membranes or burnt to provide energy. They do not usually get converted into glucose so only provoke a small insulin response and, like proteins, they are also very slowly digested compared to carbs, helping you to feel full for longer.

10.1
What are Carbs?

Carbs, as a group, are the most abundant organic compounds on earth and are made up of carbon, oxygen, and hydrogen atoms (hence, carb-O-hydr-ates). They come in a huge range of structures. Simple sugars such as glucose and fructose are simple chains of just six carbon atoms and are used by both plants and animals as a means of storing energy. There are more complex 'sugars' that also function as energy storage, such as starch and glycogen, which are still digestible by your body. At the other extreme there are highly complex, three-dimensional structures, which form structural carbs such as cellulose in plants, and chitin that forms the exoskeleton of shellfish, insects, and some fungi. These are not digestible by humans.

Of the three macro-nutrient groups (fats, proteins, and carbs) only the fat and protein groups contain nutrients that cannot be made by the human body. So, you require them in your diet to be healthy, thus they are called essential nutrients. Your body, on the other hand, can make all the carbs you need from either fats or proteins, so there ARE NO ESSENTIAL CARBOHYDRATES.

This is not meant to suggest that you should not eat carbs, because many of the complex carbs can have a beneficial effect on your body and health. How many carbs you need depends very much on your personal body type and what you are currently trying to achieve in relation to your wellness but, for normal day-to-day living, most people probably do well on somewhere around 30% of complex carbs, mainly from vegetables.

However, (contrary to the belief of most children) you will not die if you don't get any sugar, and sugar is definitely one of those carbs that you should be actively avoiding for your health's sake.

So let's drill down into this a little further - are all carbs created equal?

10.2
The Bad Carbs – Avoid These

10.2.1
Glucose/Starch

Starch is a carb comprising a long chain of glucose molecules. It is produced by most plants as an energy store and is the most common carb in modern human diets. It is found in large amounts in foods such as potatoes, wheat, corn, rice, and cassava.

Glucose is one of the primary molecules your body burns as fuel in your mitochondria. Mitochondria are the little powerhouses in each of your cells, which convert the energy from food into a form of energy that your cells can use directly to power the multitude of activities going on.

Dietary glucose only exists alone in nature (without fructose) when it is in the form of starch, which is made of very long chains of glucose all linked together. One of the enzymes in your saliva starts the breakdown process, but because starch contains so many complex bonds it digests relatively slowly, which can help stabilize your blood sugar because it doesn't spike your blood sugar quite as badly as a simple sugar like glucose (which you digest very rapidly).

Once the glucose enters your bloodstream it triggers an insulin release that drives the glucose into your cells, to either be burned as energy or stored as fat - see Figure 10.1. About 20 per cent of it goes directly to your liver where most of it is stored as glycogen, but some may be converted into fats called triglycerides and get carried by your bloodstream to be stored in your fat cells.

This is why sugar and starch are the primary cause of high triglyceride levels in your blood tests. The amount of fat you eat has only a minor impact on your triglyceride levels.

In general, eating moderate amounts of starch/glucose in the form of pasta, white bread, white rice, or potatoes doesn't have any direct negative impact on your health. However, because it triggers an insulin response, sending glucose for storage in your fat cells, usually as belly fat, if you eat too much starch, long term it will take its toll on your health because it enhances inflammation. This can take the form of diabetes, dementia, and related conditions.

There's one little caveat to this starch story. Recent research is suggesting that if you combine carbs (even if they are relatively healthy carbs) cooked with fats, your body's 'I'm full' response doesn't work as well. Even worse, before very long you are likely to have a strong tendency to crave the fatty, starchy foods combination again.

Everyone is likely to react to this fat/starch combination in slightly different ways. So you should be aware that if you have a tendency to overeat on French fries and then crave some potato crisps later in the evening, then this food combination is probably not great for you with your current hormonal balance. Even once you make progress on your road to wellness, this particular combination may continue to be a problem for you.

10.2.2
Sugars

What we commonly call sugar is technically sucrose, which is a very different beast to starch, as it combines a glucose molecule with a fructose (sometimes called fruit sugar) molecule. Glucose and fructose have the same chemical composition ($C_6H_{12}O_6$) but have very different physical structures, so they are absolutely NOT the same in the way your body handles them.

Because the sweet taste of sugar stimulates the pleasure centers in your brain to some extent, you are wired to crave some sweetness in your foods. This is to help drive you to seek more quick energy in the form of naturally sweet plant foods, particularly in autumn and early winter

What many people don't realize is that the insulin spike/liver stress that comes from drinking fruit juice is actually no better for your health than the effect of drinking sugar-sweetened fizzy drinks.

and during childhood. However, we are not wired to handle the current prevalence of sugar in so many of our foods which can often translate into unhealthy food cravings and even addiction – sugar is eight times more addictive than morphine. The normal sugar craving in children should wane during adolescence. However, it can be converted into a sweet addiction, potentially giving them ongoing problems with belly fat control.

Recent studies have demonstrated that the dopamine response in your brain to the sweet taste and your dopamine response to a blood sugar spike are actually independent. Because of your instinctive response to the pleasure hit from the dopamine, there is potential for you to become independently addicted to both the sweet taste and the blood sugar spike.

The blood sugar spike comes because a simple sugar molecule is very quickly broken down in your body to release both glucose and fructose into your bloodstream.

The resulting glucose spike in your blood triggers your pancreas to release insulin to drive the glucose into your cells, where, if you don't need it for immediate energy, gets stored as glycogen for medium-term use or as fat for long-term use. This is a similar story to starch, except that it happens a lot faster, so the resulting insulin spike is much larger.

Because of its different chemical structure, fructose cannot be used directly in your cells in the same way that glucose is. The fructose portion of the sugar has to be processed by the liver before it can be utilized by your cells for energy. Your liver turns the fructose into fat precursors, some of which can then be used by your mitochondria for energy, but some likely go straight to storage as belly fat.

The production of fat precursors in the liver also makes your liver vulnerable to fatty liver disease, which now affects about 20 – 30% of the population in developed countries. Fructose is actually a lot like alcohol regarding the stress it puts on your liver. Apart from the name, fatty liver disease is identical to alcoholic liver disease.

Fruit juices, such as apple, orange, and grape juice mostly contain about the same amount of total sugar as Coke and other sodas.

Also, like regular sugar, orange juice, grape juice, and pineapple juice all contain about equal amounts of fructose and glucose, while apple juice contains about 75% fructose.

All forms of plant sugar, including the sugars in fruit, contain this dangerous duo of glucose and fructose, but the proportions do vary. Cane sugar contains roughly equal amounts of glucose and fructose, as do ALL the alternative sugar sources such as beet sugar, coconut sugar, palm sugar, brown rice and maple syrups. They ALL do nasty things to your metabolic hormones!

HFCS (High fructose corn syrup) usually contains about 60% of fructose. Because it is the fructose that contributes most to the intense sweetness your taste buds crave, so the sugary drink manufacturers can cut their costs by using a little bit less HFCS than if they were using regular sugar. However, the fructose and glucose are already separate molecules in the syrup so your body doesn't need to digest them to separate them, thus your blood sugar spike from HFCS happens even faster than with sugar.

Both glucose and fructose, when they reach high levels in your bloodstream can also cause the formation of damaged (or glycated) proteins or fats (most commonly seen as the browning reaction when you cook food). Glycated proteins are new molecules that can cause a lot of oxidative damage in your cells by turning on inflammation and forming free radicals. Your brain is particularly vulnerable to these.

On the other hand, eating whole fruit is a much better thing to do because the natural fiber content in the fruit slows down the release of sugar into your bloodstream, and adds a good dose of healthy fiber and antioxidants to your diet.

"fructose is the most likely carbohydrate to turn into belly fat and an important 'liver loader'."

10.2.3
Fructose – the Real Bad Guy

You may have come across literature from the sugar and corn syrup refining industries suggesting that because fructose doesn't affect your insulin levels, it is actually better for you than glucose. This ignores the fact that, as far as your liver is concerned, processing fructose puts a similar strain on your liver as does processing alcohol.

Fructose is the real bad guy, because it is metabolized almost exclusively by your liver and cannot be broken down directly into glucose or stored as glycogen. Instead, most of it gets turned into fat precursors in your liver, then goes to your cells, some to be burned directly by their mitochondria, but if supply exceeds immediate demand, the excess gets transformed directly into new fat. This makes fructose the most likely carb to turn into belly fat and an important 'liver loader'.

An unpleasant side effect of overloading your mitochondria with something like fructose is that they can start to shut down and you start to feel tired. If you're feeling ongoing fatigue in some shape or form, then your mitochondria are not functioning properly and could do with some nurturing.

Fructose also triggers an inflammatory reaction in your liver which can lead to liver insulin resistance. Liver insulin resistance means that your pancreas has to release more insulin to clear your liver of glucose, which will then force extra energy into fat cells, particularly around your belly.

Moreover, since fructose does not stimulate an insulin response and helps to generate liver insulin resistance, both of which interfere with your normal Leptin response, you tend to keep eating. Furthermore, fructose consumption doesn't decrease your Ghrelin levels so your tummy doesn't get the "I'm full" message. Together, these mean that the normal processes that limit your food consumption don't regulate your consumption of fructose. Not good.

Fructose also speeds up the inflammation and free radical formation from glycated proteins, making it happen seven times faster than glucose, which seems to contribute to the development of a leaky gut. This is where the single cell layer lining your gut becomes permeable, allowing potentially inflammatory molecules into your body. This probably happens partly because of the increased formation of glycated proteins which can easily damage this fragile layer.

Leaky gut syndrome can also be exacerbated by uric acid, which is a waste product generated when your mitochondria are turning fructose into energy. You might recognize uric acid as the bad guy that can accumulate in your joints and in your soft tissues as needle-sharp crystals, which cause the inflammation, swelling, and excruciating pain known as gout. Uric acid can also contribute to increased blood pressure.

Because uric acid is also a breakdown product of purine compounds in protein, it's been wrongly assumed for the last 130 years that meat was the primary culprit. It turns out that, just like having a low cholesterol diet has negligible effects on your blood cholesterol levels, having a low purine (meat) diet has minimal effects on your uric acid levels.

Only now that we better understand the metabolism of fructose is it emerging that fructose is the most likely culprit, which is probably why gout, high blood pressure, and diabetes are commonly associated conditions.

10.2.4
Alcohol

A bit of the alcohol you drink goes straight to your brain – whee! However, about 80% of it ends up in your liver where, like fructose, it cannot be broken down into glucose or glycogen. Instead, your liver turns it into fat precursors and, if supply exceeds demand, the excess gets transformed directly into new fat. Welcome to the beginnings of alcoholic liver disease.

Alcohol, like fructose, also triggers an inflammatory reaction in your liver which can lead to liver insulin resistance. As previously discussed, liver insulin resistance means that cells fail to respond adequately to circulating insulin so that blood glucose levels rise and your pancreas has to release more insulin to try to clear your liver of glucose. Persistent high levels of sugar and insulin in the bloodstream eventually leads to type 2 diabetes. Since insulin is the primary hormonal signal for energy storage into fat cells, it stimulates the formation of new fatty tissue and accelerates belly fat gain.

The final similarity between alcohol and fructose is that they both work on the reward pathway in your brain to make you crave more of them. So, the very popular alco-pops or pre-mixed spirits, which combine alcohol and lots of fructose, provides a double whammy to your liver and your brain which is why many teenagers tend to consume them in large quantities and end up very much the worse for wear. This trend has seen a rapid rise in admissions to hospital for alcoholic liver disease in the under-30s which, in the UK, has increased by over 100% in the last ten years.

10.2.5
How Much Sugar is Too Much for You?

Like most things, how MUCH sugar you have is really important.

The triple whammy of fructose not triggering an insulin response, interfering with Leptin response and not decreasing Ghrelin levels, makes it very hard not to keep eating when you have a high sugar meal or drink of soda. On top of this, a glucose spike in your blood directly triggers the release of your brain hormone dopamine – one of your pleasure hormones. This is also the hormone responsible for addictive behavior so, if you have any addictive tendencies, you can easily find yourself becoming addicted to sugar or the sweet taste.

If you struggle with sugar cravings or your belly fat and find it really hard to stop after just a couple of chocolates, then the amount of sugar you are eating now is definitely too much for you.

The good news is that your blood sugar is under your direct control because it is totally governed by what you eat. If you currently struggle with your belly fat and with sugar, and your blood test numbers are getting a bit high, you can relax, as in Chapter 16 Your 'Rapid Reset' Plan, I'm going to show you how you can get back 'In Charge' by losing your reliance on fueling your body with carbs.

10.2.6
Sugar Substitutes

The recently developed sugar substitute Truvia, is an extract of only one of the active ingredients in Stevia, combined with erythritol, so it may cause gut upset or diarrhea in some people. At this early stage there is no evidence to make a realistic assessment of its safety.

The natural response to realizing that the amount of sugar you are eating is impacting on your health and belly fat is to seek to replace sugar with low- calorie sweeteners so you can still feed that sweet addiction you might have unwittingly developed. Surely drinking a 'Diet Coke' is going to help with any belly fat or health issues?

Unfortunately, that's not what the science is telling us.

Artificial Sweeteners

Several studies around the world have shown that switching to foods containing artificial sweeteners dramatically increases the risk for both obesity and diabetes, even if you are eating more healthy foods.

A very recent Canadian study followed nearly 1500 adults for an average of 10 years and tracked their consumption of the artificial sweeteners aspartame (Equal, NutraSweet), saccharin (SugarTwin, Sweet'N Low), acesulfame K(Sunnett, Sweet One), and sucralose (Splenda). The results were quite shocking in that those consuming the artificial sweeteners had over 50% higher incidence of excess belly fat and, on average, a nearly 3 cm larger waist circumference.

Such counterintuitive results beg the question of 'why this should be happening'?

Some results suggest that low-calorie sweeteners confuse the brain because they do not produce satiety (feeling of having had enough food) so people using low-calorie sweeteners compensate by overeating.

Another likely explanation is that artificial sweeteners contribute to belly fat gain and decreased insulin sensitivity by changing your microbiome towards species associated with obesity, which reduces your body's ability to break down glucose. It's probably a bit of both!

Sugar Alcohols

There is a whole family of sugar alcohols (their names all end in 'ol') such as xylitol, sorbitol, and maltitol. These are not as sweet as sugar, and they do contain fewer calories, but they're not completely absorbed by your body so can often cause gas or even diarrhea if you use more than a little.

Xylitol is probably the best of these, in that its effect on your blood sugar is the smallest, so using some of these in moderation can help you wean off your sweet addiction but, for most people, this doesn't work.

The safest sugar alternatives are the plant extracts of Stevia, and Luo Han Guo (monk fruit).

Natural Sweeteners

If you are hooked on the need for your sweet taste, doing the 'Rapid Reset' Plan will likely change that as your taste buds do adapt reasonably quickly to you reducing your 'sweetness' intake by becoming more sensitive. The safest sugar alternatives are the plant extracts of Stevia, a South American herb, and Luo Han Guo (monk fruit), the fruit from a Chinese vine. These both have long histories of traditional use in their countries of origin, are hundreds of times sweeter than sugar, and are probably safe to use.

Honey contains roughly 50% fructose, depending on which flowers the bees have been working, so using a little bit of raw, creamed or crystallized honey might be justified because studies have shown limited health benefits, presumably because of the useful levels of antioxidants, enzymes and bugs present in raw honey. Generally speaking the darker, more flavorsome honey like Manuka and thyme tend to have the highest levels of goodies.

ALL the liquid honey in your store has been heat-treated to keep them liquid which destroys many of the healthy properties of the honey. Unfortunately, they are also often adulterated with either sugar or HFCS. They then become little more than pricey sugar syrup.

Agave nectar is often touted as a healthy alternative to sugar because it does not cause such a dramatic blood insulin spike, but this only happens because it contains about 75 - 90% fructose which makes it really hard on your liver. Agave nectar is basically HFCS on steroids; so don't get sucked in by the advertising.

The bottom line is that you can try to use sugar substitutes to help wean your body off sweet addiction, but given the highly addictive effect of the components of sugar on your brain hormones you may want to consider going 'cold turkey' for a while. Research has shown this is the only reliable way to tame your addictions and help get your belly fat and health under control (See Chapter 16 Your 'Rapid Reset' Plan).

10.2.7
Gluten

Is the whole gluten-free thing just a fad or is it something you should pay attention to?

Most people, including many doctors, assume that the only adverse reaction to gluten that is real is the autoimmune condition called coeliac disease where your gut lining is severely damaged by gluten. This disease can be so bad that you have major difficulty in absorbing nutrients into your body and have major gut issues such as bloating, gas, diarrhea, or acid reflux.

Unfortunately, most people fail to realize the difference between coeliac disease and gluten sensitivity. This can mean that even if you tested negative for coeliac disease, it doesn't mean you have no negative reactions to gluten.

"recent research from Harvard University is now suggesting that gluten stimulates your body to produce a protein called zonulin, which opens up the tight junctions in the gut lining and the blood-brain barrier of ABSOLUTELY EVERYBODY."

The science is getting more and more compelling that gluten is probably something you really want to avoid. Less than 1% of the population have been diagnosed with coeliac disease, but the latest research is suggesting that at least 30% of Caucasians have a moderate degree of gluten sensitivity and so would be healthier if they avoided gluten completely. In fact, recent research from Harvard University has now shown that gluten stimulates your body to produce a protein called zonulin, which opens up the tight junctions in the gut lining and the blood-brain barrier of ABSOLUTELY EVERYBODY.

If you are not aware of any reaction to gluten, these junctions will only be staying open for a relatively short time; however, if you are highly sensitive to zonulin, as coeliacs are, these tight junctions will stay open for an extended time causing massive inflammation.

Whenever this happens, even if it's only for a very short time, gluten will be allowing gut contents into your bloodstream causing an allergic reaction and an inflammatory response. Given that the gut lining has the same surface area as a tennis court; it doesn't take much leakage to cause a problem. While the science on this is changing very rapidly, the picture that is emerging is that there is a wide spectrum of sensitivity from transient and minor gut lining inflammation to full-blown autoimmune coeliac disease. However, estimates suggest that for at least a third of the population, their inflammatory response to gluten is having a negative impact on their health.

This explains why more than fifty-five diseases have been linked to eating gluten. However, the worrying statistic is that estimates suggest that 99% of people who have either coeliac disease or gluten sensitivity are never diagnosed as such.

This means that the vast majority of people have some adverse reaction to gluten, yet have no idea that their bodies are reacting negatively to gluten and creating inflammation.

10.2.8
How Does Gluten do This to Us?

We used to think that all our cells were tightly glued together. We now know that there is normally a small space or junction between cells. This becomes critical in places like the gut lining and the blood-brain barrier, which are only one cell thick. In response to your eating gluten, your body produces a messenger protein called zonulin, and it turns out that this is the messenger protein that controls how tight the junctions between your cells are.

If you are very sensitive to gluten, so much zonulin is released that it causes the tight junctions in your gut to open up, allowing food particles, toxins and potential pathogens through into your blood. This can create massive inflammation in your gut (a condition known as 'leaky gut'), throughout your body, and particularly your brain, and this can cause the autoimmune response of coeliac disease. If you are much less sensitive to gluten, the tight junctions will only open very briefly in response to eating gluten, so there is little or no leakage into your blood, and your immune system can deal with the problem WITHOUT YOU BEING AWARE that anything has happened.

I know a bread maker whose daughter developed a troubling gluten intolerance. In looking for solutions to help her, he wondered if the change in processing methods was part of the problem. He started making a 24-hour fermented white bread, which she (and nearly everyone else in our small town that had gluten intolerance) was able to tolerate without any noticeable gut disturbance.

If you think a leaky gut sounds bad, you really don't want to develop a 'leaky brain'. Few people recognize that zonulin will also open up the blood-brain barrier so you can get an inflamed brain as a result of eating gluten, which is not a good situation as this can potentially translate into a range of mental conditions including depression, dementia or Alzheimer's.

10.2.9
Gluten Intolerance Symptoms?

The symptoms are many and diverse which is why people often fail to get diagnosed with gluten sensitivity, particularly as health practitioners are often unaware of the extent of the problem and the diversity of the symptoms. People's reaction to gluten can range from headaches (often migraines), congestion, skin, and bowel issues, to quite severe mental reactions and muscle tics.

The understanding that gluten intolerance may not manifest as some sort of gut disturbance is a relatively new one. Some doctors noted that neurological disorders often accompany coeliac disease, but attributed this to poor absorption of essential nutrients. However, your brain is particularly sensitive to any form of inflammation so, if gluten sets off an inflammatory response in your body, this is likely to manifest as a silent attack on your brain. The latest thinking is that gluten intolerance always affects your brain in some way.

The inflammatory molecules that a reaction to gluten sets off have been found to be elevated in conditions such as Alzheimer's, Parkinson's, multiple sclerosis, ADHD, and autism. Some research is suggesting that gluten sensitivity is common in patients with neurological conditions that have no apparent cause, ranging from headaches to multiple sclerosis. Some Functional Medicine practitioners are putting such patients onto a gluten-free diet with amazing results – in some cases even reversing dementia and multiple sclerosis.

It's important to remember that nobody else in the world has your unique combination of the three legs of wellness, so while my body might respond to ongoing low-level inflammation with a heart attack, yours may respond with some form of autoimmune condition or dementia.

How this allergic reaction manifests in your body is totally dependent on your diet and lifestyle, how well you are and, to some limited extent, on your genetics. Your reaction to the unchecked inflammation that can go with gluten sensitivity may be the deterioration of your bowel, otherwise known as the autoimmune condition - coeliac disease. In your partner, this may result in obesity and heart disease, while in your children it may manifest as ADHD, depression, or learning difficulties because they have an inflamed brain.

Your brain does not cope with inflammation at all well and considering its very rapid metabolic rate, it doesn't have great systems to protect against brain inflammation. (Your brain burns a staggering 25% of the energy in your body although it's only about 2.5% of your weight). So it's hardly surprising that your body's inflammatory response to gluten can have such a dramatic effect on your brain.

We used to think the mental deterioration that so commonly goes with coeliac disease later in life was due to poor absorption of nutrients because of the bowel damage. A recent study showed that this was definitely not the case. They highlighted changes in brain structure, evident in brain scans, which looked very similar to multiple sclerosis or small strokes, yet they showed that this was due to gluten sensitivity. What is even more telling, is that several of the people in the study showed significant improvement in their brain function when they went on a gluten-free diet.

What is so exciting about these findings is that there is a rapidly growing body of evidence showing that a whole range of mental conditions ranging from headaches, brain fog, and depression, to Alzheimer's, schizophrenia, autism, ADHD, multiple sclerosis, epilepsy and bipolar disorder that are, in many cases, responding to people going on a gluten-free diet and changing the types of fat they eat and also increasing the amount of fat they eat, such as I recommend in Chapter 16 Your 'Rapid Reset' Plan

10.2.10
But We Have Eaten Bread Forever?

You may well ask why gluten is becoming such an issue now when grains started becoming an increasing proportion of our diet about 10,000 years ago, as we transitioned from being hunter-gatherers to being farmers.

There are four potential reasons for this:

Plant breeding

Changes in plant breeding techniques have allowed us to increase the amount of gluten in wheat up to fortyfold in the space of a few decades. This has been driven by the consumer demand for ever lighter, fluffy bread, bagels, and doughnuts.

Bread making techniques

Bread used to be made by a long, slow process that involved mixing and kneading the dough and then putting it aside, usually by the fire overnight, for the yeast to ferment and introduce carbon dioxide to make it light and fluffy. This long fermentation also released enzymes that broke down some of the anti-nutritional factors from the wheat grain.

Most modern bread processing involves a process called MDD (mechanical dough development) that beats the dough to introduce air to make it light and fluffy. This process makes bread very quickly and cheaply, but it allows no time at all for the enzymatic breakdown that used to happen in the traditional bread making process.

Exorphins

Gluten breaks down in the stomach to form chemicals that cross the blood-brain barrier and attach to your brain's opiate receptors – similar to the effect of your own endorphins (hence the term exorphins - from outside the body). These induce a mild euphoria, which can be quite addictive, so when a drug blocks this effect or people go on a gluten-free diet, some people can experience distinctly unpleasant withdrawal symptoms.

Of course, Big Food are very aware of this addictive effect of gluten so they try to pack as much gluten into their products as they can to encourage you to buy again. The use of gluten has become so widespread that it is hidden in literally all sorts of products ranging from seasonings, condiments, and ice cream, to soy sauce and soups. It's even being used in hand creams, cosmetics, and nutritional supplements. You need to be acutely aware of this contamination if you are trying to avoid gluten.

Low Stomach Acid

People who take PPI's to lower their stomach acid production are much more likely to develop coeliac disease or gluten intolerance. You need high stomach acid to digest protein completely, so it makes total sense that you have more problems with gluten if you have low stomach acid. About 80% of acid reflux is caused by low stomach acid, and acid reflux is widespread in this modern world. This is a complex subject, so I have written an eBook called 'Acid Reflux 101. How to Test For and Treat the Cause'. If you need this, you can order from www.ITookCharge/AcidReflux.

10.2.11
Surely Whole Grains are Good for You?

Our bodies evolved on a diet of wild game, seasonal plants and vegetables, and very occasional sweet treats such as berries and honey. The advocates of the Paleo, GAPS, or SCD diets, which all do wonders for some people's health, suggest that this means we shouldn't eat grains at all.

Some recent science does tend to support this view for some people, in that it's been discovered that there is a whole range of storage proteins called prolamines (about 35 different ones). These are structurally very similar to the gluten present in wheat, barley, and rye. Prolamines are also found in many other grains and seeds.

This means that if your body does not heal when you switch to a gluten-free diet, consuming rice, corn, quinoa, amaranth, or other high carb foods from the gluten-free aisles, then you could be actually reacting badly to these more exotic members of the gluten family and you will need to eliminate them from your diet until you heal.

There is no doubt that most people consume far too many refined carbs, which consist of little else but starch, which breaks down quickly to give a surge of blood sugar after you eat them. If a food has a high carb level, you will get a dramatic surge in blood sugar – even if it's 'Gluten-free' or 'Paleo' – See Figure 10.1.

The magnitude of the surge in blood sugar can be expressed as what's called GI (Glycemic Index), which measures the amount of, and timing of, the blood sugar released from a measured amount of carbs. This is expressed on a scale of 0 to 100, where pure glucose is 100.

While there are some fairly predictable high glycemic foods like a white baguette at 95, cornflakes at 93, and white rice at 89, factors like fat and fiber content, particle size, and how things are cooked have a big impact. So a boiled white potato comes in at 82, whereas French fries have a GI of only 64 because the fat content slows the rate of digestion.

Similarly, brown rice comes in with a GI of 50 – a lot less than white rice at 89 because of the fiber content. Rice flour has a higher GI than white rice because of the finer particle size, and a traditional bread made with stone-ground flour can have a GI as low as 35, whereas white bread is over 70. Popcorn can vary between 55 and 85, depending on how it's prepared. The average muesli is around 66, and All Bran is 55.

Raw carrots have a GI of only 20. However, boiled carrots have a GI of 50 because of a change in starch structure. The extruding of wheat pasta to make spaghetti lowers the GI to around 40 because of the formation of some resistant starch, whereas ravioli and fresh pasta can be as high as 70. Cooking pasta al dente helps to keep the GI lower compared to cooking it to mush.

Because of the fructose content, white sugar only has a GI of 68, yet as you have read above, sugar can do nasty things to your body. So GI is just an indicator of your blood sugar spike from any given food, and as indicated, the way you prepare food can have a big impact on the GI and the impact on your blood sugar and your health.

The bottom line is being aware of how the carbs you are consuming is affecting your hormonal balance and your wellness, but the probability is that the refined carbs and gluten you are eating are having a significant impact.

10.2.12
Other Troublemakers in Grains

All grains naturally contain chemicals that are designed to help protect the seeds from being eaten by predators, including us. These chemicals can include phytates, which block the absorption of important nutrients such as calcium, magnesium, zinc, and iron. Another important group are ATI's (amylase trypsin inhibitors) that can reduce the production of digestive enzymes from your pancreas. ATI's can lead to poor digestion of your food leading to fermentation in your gut and more inflammation.

Does this mean you should never eat any grains again?

I don't believe the real science supports this, particularly because everyone is different. As I have demonstrated above, many factors contribute to how your body reacts to any given food source; including what you eat with it and how it is prepared.

There is a world of difference between bread baked with very fine white flour at high temperatures, and Essene-style bread made from whole grains that have been sprouted for several days. The sprouting process minimizes the anti-nutritional factors such as phytates, which block you from absorbing minerals, and also starts to break down the gluten proteins into amino acids. It also tastes sweet and nutty and, to me, very delicious, but it's absolutely not light and fluffy.

I suggest one of the key reasons that some people get a dramatic response to the Paleo diet (which eliminates all grains) is because of the hormonal reset that happens when you eliminate sugar from your diet. When you look at all the successful diet regimes from around the world that create health – and there are many of them, such as the Atkins diet, the Paleo diet, the traditional Japanese and Mediterranean diets – the one factor they have in common is the very low levels of sugar consumed.

Does this mean you should never eat sugar or bagels again? Again, I don't believe the real science supports this because everyone is different. Once you have done the 'Rapid Reset' to balance your hormones, have become fat- adapted and are on the route to wellness, then you will likely be able to tolerate some sugar and white flour again. This is because you are in the wonderful state of being metabolically flexible, so your body switches effortlessly between burning fat or sugar.

How much can you tolerate? That depends on how steady the legs are on your stool of wellness.

10.3
The Good Carbs - Eat More of These

10.3.1
Fiber

The coarse structural fibers that occur in the stems of plants like flax, hemp and corn, or in cotton bolls are completely indigestible to humans. The dietary fiber that we used to consume in large amounts are the much finer structural components of vegetables, fruits and seeds, which all have major beneficial effects on your health.

Sadly, the amount of fiber that most people consume is only a fraction of the amount we used to eat in earlier times – probably not much more than a tenth of the amount. Studies have shown that modern hunter-gatherers probably eat around 120 to 150 g of fiber a day, whereas the US Institute of Medicine recommends eating 25 to 40 g per day. However, someone living in urbanized society and eating a relatively healthy diet is likely to be getting just 20 to 30g per day, and the average consumption is only 16 g per day.

There is a very popular misconception that the key role of dietary fiber is to keep your bowels regular and prevent constipation. While that is very important to help your body from becoming toxic, how much fiber you consume has other major implications for your wellness.

The big difference from other carbs is that fiber is not digested in your stomach and then absorbed by your body to burn as fuel. Fiber is the fuel for your bugs, so eating dietary fiber has a major impact on the health of your gut microbiome and your insulin response, which together probably have a bigger overall impact on your health.

So it's important that you increase your intake of fiber, from vegetables in particular.

There are actually two different types of dietary fiber that have quite different functions. Having a combination of both types of fiber in your food will have a major impact on the way you feel and your wellness.

Soluble fiber

Soluble fiber will absorb large amounts of water to create a gelatinous mass, which greatly slows down the rate of digestion and absorption of nutrients from your stomach and small intestine. This particularly affects carbs, so that it dampens down your insulin response. It also binds up many of the waste products produced in your liver which have been excreted in your bile and into your small intestine. Once soluble fiber reaches your colon, much of it is fermented by the microbiome in your gut as their food so it acts as a very important prebiotic.

Good sources of soluble fiber include oats, flax seeds, all the pulses, apples, berry fruit, carrots, oats, and psyllium.

Insoluble fiber

Insoluble fiber is not digestible, even by your microbiome, and does not absorb water, but it's very important role is that, like soluble fiber, it also binds up waste products from your liver so that they can be eliminated from your body. It also has a laxative effect because it speeds up the passage of waste and food through your colon.

Good sources of insoluble fiber include wheat, flax seed, barley, brown rice, most fruit and vegetables, especially root vegetable skins – don't peel your potatoes.

Many of us consume a significant amount of fruit juice, probably based on the assumption that this is much healthier for us than drinking soda drinks. However, fruit juice does not contain any fiber, so it merely adds to your sugar load and does little to contribute to your health. On the other hand, whole fruit inherently contains plenty of fiber, and usually loads of antioxidants, so fruit in moderation can be very good for your health. Few single sources contain both types of fiber, except flax seeds and some vegetables and fruit.

10.3.2
Why is Fiber so Important for Your Hormone Health?

Absorption:

Fiber forms a gelatinous barrier between your food and your intestinal wall, greatly slowing down the rate of absorption of glucose, fructose, and fat. This has the effect of substantially reducing the peak levels of these nutrients in your blood and your liver, and also greatly reducing the amount of insulin produced.

Satiety:

You eat a plate of pasta, and you're still hungry, why?

Putting food in your stomach does reduce your Ghrelin levels, which you might think would stop you feeling hungry. Unfortunately, you also require a little hormone that is produced at the end of the small intestine to tell you that you're satiated, which isn't produced for some time after you have eaten. So having plenty of fiber in your meal both slows down the emptying of your stomach, giving time for your Ghrelin levels to drop, but it also speeds up the rate of passage through your small intestine, which all help to tell you in time that you really do not want that second helping.

Detoxification:

Hormones and other compounds that are surplus to your body's requirements, particularly estrogen, are excreted in the bile, and if they are then bound up by fiber, will be eliminated out of your body. Similarly, cholesterol, which is used in your body to produce the bile acids that help you to absorb fats, binds to fiber preventing the cholesterol being reabsorbed and recycled and allowing it to be eliminated out of your body, which will help your body maintain optimal cholesterol levels. If there is insufficient fiber in your bowel both the cholesterol and estrogen will be reabsorbed from your colon, adding to your toxic load.

The same process applies to all the toxins that have been detoxified by your liver and excreted into the bile. Fiber is required to bind up this toxic waste so that it cannot be reabsorbed, and to allow it to be eliminated it from your body.

10.3.3
Prebiotics That Feed Your Microbiome

Prebiotics are special carbs which are not digested in your stomach or small intestine, so they become available as food for the microbiome in your colon.

There is good archaeological evidence that as a species we have always eaten useful amounts of foods containing prebiotics. Close to my home, the NZ cabbage tree contains useful amounts of inulin (a prebiotic) and the Maori, who touted it as a natural cure for colic, diarrhea, and other gut disorders, ate most parts of this tree regularly. Now that makes total sense, doesn't it?

The main prebiotics are:

Soluble Fiber – see above.

Resistant Starch

Some forms of starch are 'resistant' to digestion in your stomach and small intestine so they have similar effects to soluble fiber, in that they pass through into your colon to become the ideal food for your microbiome. They digest it into a short chain fat called butyrate, which is the preferred fuel for the cells that line your colon.

Butyrate also promotes gut wall integrity, dampens down inflammation in the gut wall, promotes insulin sensitivity, and helps you to feel full after a meal (satiety). Some people are even finding that they sleep better and feel calmer after eating resistant starch, which is not surprising given that the butyrate will be feeding the serotonin-producing bacteria in your gut.

Butyrate is so important for gut health that some health practitioners will supplement with butyrate while you are in the early stages of healing your gut. One of the best food sources of butyrate is butter from grass-fed cows (guess where the name came from).

Emerging research is suggesting that resistant starch may bind preferentially to some of the bugs responsible for SIBO and even the undesirable bacteria in your colon, to help you expel them out of your body. This effect is so powerful, that resistant starch is now included in the rehydration formula given to cholera patients.

The main natural sources of resistant starch are raw potato starch, green bananas (plantains – including the skins), and cassava starch, which you may be able to find in your health shop in the specialty flours section. Fortunately, a useful proportion of the starch in some starchy foods, like potatoes, rice, and legumes gets converted into resistant starch when the foods are cooked and then cooled. This starch will then feed your microbiome rather than giving you an insulin spike. Make a cold potato salad from steamed potatoes and don't throw out those surplus roast potatoes you couldn't manage, or the leftover rice from your Indian takeaways. Put them in the fridge and eat them warmed the next day. They are great for your gut.

> *"don't throw out those surplus roast potatoes you couldn't manage, or the leftover rice from your Indian takeaways."*

Inulin, oligofructose, and xylo-oligosaccharides

Inulin, oligofructose, and xylo-oligosaccharides are among a bunch of prebiotics with very forgettable names, but they are quite common in everyday vegetables, and they have similar beneficial effects on your microbiome as soluble fiber and resistant starch.

Those with the highest quantities are listed first:

- Chicory root
- Jerusalem artichoke
- Dandelion greens
- Garlic
- Leek
- Onions
- Asparagus
- Mushrooms

That list is all pretty delicious and they will all do nice things for your gut health because of their prebiotic action. However, if you are not used to eating lots of prebiotic foods, you may get a temporary surge in gas production. This is a sure sign that your health would benefit from eating more of these foods, not less.

10.3.4
Slow Carbs

The way your body responds to carbs that are not digested quickly, and so do not spike your blood sugar, is completely different from the way it responds to refined carbs (sometimes called white carbs or fast carbs). I call these 'slow carbs' and, in most situations, you can eat these relatively freely, unless you are trying to get into ketosis (See Chapter 11 Good Oils Make You Slim and Healthy).

Slow burning, non-starchy vegetables should be one of the basics of your diet, so make sure your plate is at least half full of vegetables such as broccoli, asparagus, chard, kale, spinach, silver beet, cabbage, lettuce, peas and Asian greens. Sea vegetables also come in this category and include wakame, nori, kelp, kombu, and many more. If you have never tried some of my suggestions, be adventurous, as all such vegetables are all extraordinarily high in beneficial minerals, protein, and other healing compounds.

The legume grains or pulses are also fiber rich, protein-rich, and nutrient-rich foods that tend to be underused unless you are vegetarian. While they have moderate amounts of carbs, these can only be digested slowly and so do not contribute to an excessive insulin spike. Try the red, blue, or regular lentils; chickpeas; green and yellow split peas; pinto, adzuki, black, navy, and other beans.

There are many brightly colored and delicious, not so sweet, fruit that are full of antioxidants and phytonutrients, and fall into this category of slow carbs, including the berry fruits - raspberry, strawberry, blueberry, blackberry, and some of the more brightly colored stone fruits such as apricots, black plums, and nectarines. Other slow fruits include tart apples, tamarillos, grapefruit and guava

Some other fruits naturally have a higher sugar content, so come in higher on the GI scale, and so should be eaten in moderation to avoid insulin issues. Fruits in this category include sweet red apples and pears, pineapple, cherries, mango, water and rock melons, ripe bananas and grapes.

I deliberately did not include soybeans in this list of slow carbs, as my view is that the only forms of soy that are safe for human consumption, in very limited amounts, are those that have been made by the traditional long fermentation process like miso, tempeh, natto and fermented tofu, soy sauce and soy milk.

Industrial, unfermented soy products like regular soymilk, infant formula, and meat substitutes are a very different story. Soy has the highest levels of 'troublemakers' of any seed, and while these are reduced by fermentation, soy still has high levels of phytoestrogens so can contribute to estrogen dominance.

To me, soymilk is a recipe for a women's health disaster as the phytates still present in it actively block the absorption of key nutrients such as iron, calcium, magnesium and zinc, and the high levels of phytoestrogens contribute to estrogen dominance.

CHAPTER 11

Good Oils Make You Slim and Healthy

"The best gift you can give yourself is a slim, beautiful, healthy belly"
Dr Mehmet Oz

11.1
Ketosis for Health

If you are carrying more belly fat than you like to have, you need to snack regularly to avoid low blood sugar, and you are unable to skip a meal, then you are a sugar burner (glucose-adapted). If that is not the way you want to be - welcome to the world of ketones, where eating MORE GOOD oils can make you slim and healthy.

Our bodies have evolved over roughly the last 2.5 million years to be hunter-gatherers, eating lots of fats from grass-fed animals and primarily burning body fat (being fat-adapted) as our energy source. Regularly having large amounts carbs in our diet (being glucose-adapted) only started a blink of an eye ago - in the last few thousand years as we started to move towards becoming farmers growing plentiful grain crops and, more recently, sugar.

Your body can only store limited amounts of glucose and glycogen, your blood the equivalent of 5 g of sugar and your muscles and liver about 600 g of glycogen – enough for about 90 min vigorous exercise. If you are only glucose-adapted, once these stores are burnt you start to feel hungry and tired. Your body will start to go into starvation mode and will start cannibalizing your precious muscle tissue to convert their protein into glucose and, at the same time, raise your cortisol levels – not good.

This happens because, when you are eating plentiful carbs, over time your genes have up-regulated all your body systems involved in glucose burning and fat storage. Unfortunately, this way of eating also causes your body to down-regulate all the gene systems required for accessing and burning fat for energy (you are glucose-adapted).

You will recall seeing in Figure 10.1, that the

Nutritional ketosis should not be confused with the serious condition - ketoacidosis. Ketoacidosis can develop in people with diabetes who are not able to produce enough insulin. Without enough insulin, your body starts to break down fat, producing a rapid build up of acidic ketones in the bloodstream, which can lead to diabetic ketoacidosis if untreated.

intake of fat had a minimal effect on raising your blood sugar and on insulin production (remember that insulin is your fat storage hormone). This happens because your body burns fat in a very different way from the way it burns glucose.

The fatty acids from your diet or your fat stores are either transformed by your liver into water-soluble fats called ketones, which are then burned by your mitochondria. Alternatively, your fatty acids can also be burned directly for energy by the mitochondria in your cells. Either way, there is less inflammation-inducing oxidation generated by burning fat than there is from burning glucose. Having a plentiful ketone supply also stimulates your body and brain to grow more mitochondria, which translates to you having higher energy levels and better brain function.

Ketones can happily cross the blood-brain barrier and make a very effective fuel for your brain. Recent studies have shown that your brain works about 70% MORE EFFICIENTLY when it is burning ketones instead of glucose (that's probably contrary to what you have been led to believe). Recent research using brain scans has shown that some areas of a brain damaged by Alzheimer's do not function at all on glucose. Yet when such a brain gets fed with ketones, some of these areas can light up and become active again, which is why good fats like coconut oil are really important for optimum brain function and preventing or reversing Alzheimer's.

Ketones also increase the levels of glutathione in your brain – your body's most powerful antioxidant. These two factors can translate into less brain fog, lowered risk for dementia and Alzheimer's, improved sleep and improved brain health overall.

A small proportion of the fatty acids can also be transformed, by the liver, into the glucose which is needed to fuel the red blood cells (some do not contain mitochondria, so they do need glucose for fuel). This means that your body has ZERO absolute requirements for carbs from your diet at all – there are no Essential Carbs!

As long as you eat dinner in the early evening and don't snack during the evening, then you naturally go into a mild state of ketosis (fat-burning) overnight and if you have a high fat, low carb, moderate protein ketogenic diet style breakfast, your body will continue to burn fat as the preferred fuel. However, if you have a sugary cereal or bagel for breakfast, your body immediately switches back into glucose-burning mode.

If you continue to eat a high fat, low carb, moderate protein diet, your body transitions quite quickly into a state called nutritional ketosis, where burning fat becomes your body's preferred fuel. You will also find your insulin levels drop, food stops being a focus for you, you can skip a meal without being bothered, and your mental focus improves.

You may even start to crave higher fat levels in your meals – CONGRATULATIONS - you are now fat-adapted, which means your genes involved in burning fat have now become up-regulated and your life will never be quite the same. Becoming fat-adapted can take anywhere between a couple of days to a couple of weeks, the key factors governing the time this takes being how severely you restrict your carb intake and how healthy your liver is.

While the beneficial effects of nutritional ketosis on your belly fat levels are obviously important, there is a rapidly growing body of evidence that the anti-inflammatory effects of nutritional ketosis are supporting a wide range of health benefits. The ketogenic diet was originally developed to help people with epilepsy, but there is now evidence of benefits for a wide range of mental conditions including autism, depression, Alzheimer's and Parkinson's – conditions for which there are no other very effective treatments. Nutritional ketosis is often viewed as a diet promoting fat loss, which it does, but it should also be viewed as a brain energizing diet.

Other conditions that have also been shown to respond to you being in nutritional ketosis include some of the biggies like heart disease, diabetes, PCOS, acne and even cancer. Cancer cells have an absolute requirement for sugar to survive and thrive, so using nutritional ketosis is rapidly becoming an important part of controlling cancer cell growth. Many people also find that over time they can reduce or even eliminate the drugs they need to take and so reducing their toxic load.

11.2
But That's Not What I've Been Told

Shouldn't I be avoiding fats?

Shouldn't I be avoiding cholesterol?

Don't fats make you fat?

Aren't saturated fats bad for me?

These beliefs beg the question, why is there so much confusion around fats and oils? It doesn't help that 'fat' can be an offensive term, as nobody wants to be called 'fat'. This has made it very easy for Big Media to demonize dietary 'fat' as being artery-clogging poison and to promote foods rich in bad carbs like sugar and refined flours.

As I explained in Chapter 8 The Hormonal Reasons Why Diets Don't Work, most of the confusion started with the publication in 1977 of the report 'Dietary Goals for the United States'. The key recommendations from this report were that people should increase carb consumption; reduce their overall fat consumption, particularly saturated fat, while increasing their intake of polyunsaturated oils. The report did also recommend a reduction in the consumption of cholesterol, sugar, and salt.

This report was followed by the 1992 Food Guide Pyramid, which recommended that fats and oils should be used sparingly. It had carbs at the base of the pyramid and recommended that the biggest proportion of your diet should come from the bread, cereal, rice, and pasta group – in other words, high levels of carbs and high levels of gluten. Enter the insanity of the 'low fat' craze.

The whole idea that for your health's sake you should eat more carbs and less fat is scientifically just plain wrong. When you actually look at the research the data supports the idea that if you eat good fats, you get slim and reverse heart disease and type II diabetes, while preventing dementia, cancer, and many other disease processes. The reality is that, within reason, the higher the PROPORTION of good fats in your diet, the more belly fat you lose and the better your brain and body functions.

The reality is that, within reason, the higher the PROPORTION of good fats in your diet, the more belly fat you lose and the better your body functions.

Since the publication of the two reports mentioned above, there has been a massive deterioration in the health of people in the USA and around the world. These reports are what triggered the beginning of the epidemics of obesity, diabetes, dementia, and related chronic conditions, which are still going on now.

Yet a recent research review has shown that the demonization of saturated fats was NOT EVEN SUPPORTED by the research data that was available to the Congressional Panel in 1977 when they came up with 'Dietary Goals for the United States' report – the power of the Big Three in action.

A recent research review has shown that the demonization of saturated fats was not even supported by the research data.

There have also been several reviews of studies done over the last 40 years about the health consequences of eating saturated fats, which have all shown that a higher intake of saturated fats is not associated with increased risk of heart disease, stroke, diabetes, or even death from any causes. A recent large Norwegian study concluded that "people who eat a lot of saturated fat are less likely to suffer from heart problems and, instead, have much healthier biomarkers, such as improved blood pressure, cholesterol, insulin and blood sugar levels".

This is contrary to the prevailing dietary advice you will get from most sources, which are manifestly not based on what the research data shows!

You could speculate for hours as to why this is so, but the important point you need to know is that saturated fats are NOT actively bad for you. As a group they are neutral to mildly beneficial fats. As you will see later, some plant sourced saturated fats like coconut oil are very beneficial for your brain function and health.

The idea that you should increase your intake of polyunsaturated oils is also clearly not supported by the research. (See below).

Fortunately, food policymakers are finally starting to catch up with the science, and in 2015 the United States Dietary Guidelines Advisory Committee removed previous recommendations to limit the amount of fat you eat after realizing that it doesn't make us fat or sick!!! They also got rid of the recommendations to limit the amount of cholesterol in your diet.

I'm sure you will find that much of what I've said so far is outside what you've been led to believe, but here's what the real science demonstrates.

11.3
Fat structure

Very quickly and simply, a fat molecule is a long chain of C (carbon) atoms with, in most cases, a hydrogen atom on each side of the carbon, another hydrogen atom at one end, and a fancy bit at the other end of the chain. See Figure 11.1

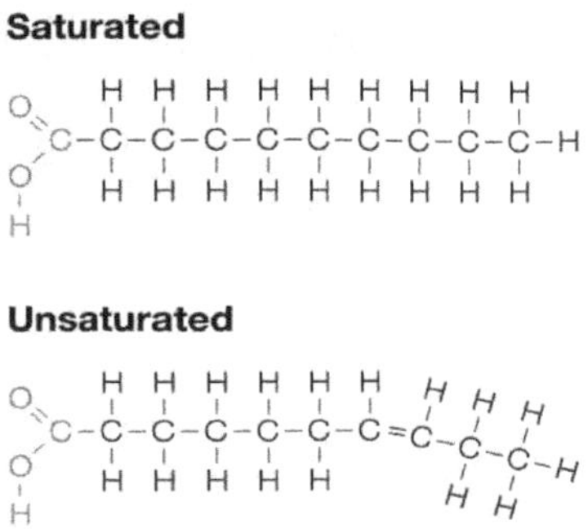

Figure 11.1 The structure of a C10 fat molecule

11.4
Saturated Fat

For a fat molecule to be called saturated, all the positions where a hydrogen atom could potentially be present are full up (hence 'saturated'). The shorter the length of the carbon chain, the more liquid they are at room or body temperature and the more easily they are digested. Saturated fats can be classified as either SCT (short chain triglycerides - C4 to C6), MCT (medium-chain - C8 to C12) or LCT (long chain - C14 to C18).

These classifications are important in that, the longer the fat molecule, the more energy is required to digest it. Both the SCT and the MCT are either burnt directly for energy (if you are fat-adapted) or absorbed into the liver and converted into ketones, so can provide very quick energy for your body and, more importantly, your brain. This characteristic means that MCTs from coconut oil are widely used for feeding people in crisis, such as in emergency rooms, and used by athletes for quick energy. They should also be the preferred fats for those who have had their gallbladder removed because they do not need bile for digestion.

The LCTs, which are at high levels in most vegetable oils and animal fats, need to be broken down by enzymes from your pancreas before your body can use them, so is a much slower and more involved digestion process.

Most animal fats have a reasonably high proportion of saturated fats. For instance, butter and grass-fed beef fat are around 50 - 60% saturated fat. Most vegetable oils contain very little saturated fat, the notable exceptions being coconut oil and palm kernel oil.

11.5
Unsaturated Oils

If a plant creates an oil that has two hydrogen atoms absent from the oil molecule, it is classified as 'unsaturated'. A double bond is formed between the two carbons – See Figure 11.1.

The double bond has two important effects: firstly, it puts a kink in the oil molecule, which changes how it fits into your cell membranes. Secondly, it is much less stable, so an unsaturated oil is much more readily damaged by light, oxygen or heat.

Omega-9 (ω-9) molecules have one double bond at C9 (counting from the right-hand end in Figure 11.1), so the parent Omega-9 is called oleic acid, and they are called mono-unsaturated oils. Oils rich in Omega-9 can be

VERY health promoting, but are not an Essential Fatty Acid (EFA), because our bodies can make Omega-9 from other oils if there is not enough in our food. Oils such as olive, avocado and macadamia oils are the best sources of Omega-9.

Omega-7 (ω-7) molecules are quite similar to Omega-9, in that they also have one double bond at C7 and your body does have the ability to make them. The parent Omega-7 molecule is called palmitoleic acid. Recent research has shown that Omega-7 can counter the risk factors responsible for 'metabolic syndrome', such as insulin sensitivity and inflammation, so can usefully contribute to belly fat loss.

Good food sources of Omega-7 include macadamia nuts, grass fed butter and cheese, eggs, olive and avocado oils.

Because of their single double bond, all the monounsaturated oils like Omega-9 and Omega-7 are five times more reactive than saturated fats, but they can be used for relatively low-temperature cooking.

Omega-6 (ω-6) molecules have two double bonds, starting at C6 so the parent Omega-6 is called linoleic acid (LA) and they are often called polyunsaturated oils. They are classified as an EFA, because your body cannot make them from other oils, so they must be obtained from your diet for you to be healthy – i.e. Essential.

Most readily available vegetable oils are high in Omega-6, so sources include canola, corn, cottonseed, grapeseed, hemp, palm oil, peanut, rice bran, safflower, soya bean and sunflower.

Because they have two double bonds, polyunsaturated oils are 25 times more reactive than saturated oils so they are easily damaged when used in cooking. Unfortunately, such oils are very cheap, so they are very widely used in processed food and for deep-frying, and this is a major reason why people are not thriving.

CLA (Conjugated linoleic acid) is formed when the double bonds are shifted to starting at C9 instead of C6 and sometimes they contain a natural trans bond. Natural CLA is found in the fat of cows, goats and sheep and if they are grass fed animals, their CLA content is up to 10 times higher than if they were grain fed. The CLA you can buy as supplements are made from chemically altered Omega-6 oils, with the double bonds starting at C10, so they do not have the same health benefits.

Studies have shown useful health benefits from you eating CLA containing foods from grass-fed animals, including loss of belly fat, lower risk of heart disease, diabetes and cancer. These results are NOT achieved when people take CLA supplements – nature knows best, so eat more grass-fed butter.

Omega-3 (ω-3) molecules have three double bonds, starting at C3, so the parent Omega-3 is called alpha-linolenic acid (ALA) and should really be called a super-unsaturated oil, but most authors mistakenly lump them in with Omega-6 as a polyunsaturated oil. ALA is also an EFA – which means it must be obtained from your diet for you to be healthy – i.e. Essential.

Good sources of the primary Omega-3 include flax seed, chia, and perilla seed oils, while walnut and hemp also include useful amounts of Omega-3.

Because super-unsaturated Omega-3 oils contain three double bonds, they are 125 times more reactive than saturated oils like coconut, so they are very easily damaged by light, oxygen and heat - in that order. They should NEVER be packaged in anything but completely lightproof containers (brown, green or violet glass is not good enough) and never used in cooking, although they can be added to your food as a tasty garnish at serving.

11.6
Your Omega-6/Omega-3 Balance

Your genes evolved on a diet that had roughly equal amounts of the two EFAs (i.e. a 1:1 ratio of Omega-6 to Omega-3), and yet your genes have only changed by a minuscule amount over the last 10,000 years.

The 1977 report 'Dietary Goals for the United States' recommended increasing the intake of Omega-6 oils, which gave the fledgling vegetable oil industry (aka Big Food) the green light to produce huge amounts of refined Omega-6 oils, which are now widely used in processed foods and dominate the supermarket shelves in their clear plastic bottles.

The effect of this explosion in Omega-6 oil consumption has meant that most people have somewhere between 10 and 30 times more Omega-6 in their body than they have Omega-3, i.e. a 10-30:1 ratio. This is a VERY long way from the historic 1:1 ratio. The health consequences of this imbalance are profound, and are summed up in the proceedings of a scientific conference on the subject: Omega–6/Omega–3 Essential Fatty Acid Ratio: The Scientific Evidence.

"A higher Omega-6/Omega-3 ratio is associated with increased risk for coronary heart disease, colorectal cancer, asthma, osteoporosis, arthritis, and neurodegenerative diseases, and various aspects of mental illness, violent behavior, and deficient cognition in both children and the elderly." Simopoulos & Cleland 2003

You might well be asking, "How could such a change in your Omega- 6/Omega-3 ratio affect so many serious conditions?"

There are three key factors involved:

- The 500 million new cells you produce each day use whatever EFAs or oils are available to make their membranes, which are critical to cellular function. For example, the primary Omega-3, ALA is a part of the oxygen transport system into your cells. Having enough Omega-3 is important for your energy levels, and most people get a lift in energy when they first start using Omega-3 oils in the right way, which is to emulsify them with a high sulfur amino acid protein such as you find in yoghurt, cottage cheese, sunflower or hemp seeds.

- Your body is capable of converting the primary EFAs to make the secondary EFAs needed to control inflammation and for healthy brain function. However this conversion is often down-regulated because of the Omega-6/Omega-3 imbalance. If you are not getting enough primary Omega-3 in your diet, then your body will struggle to produce enough of the secondary Omega-3s needed by your brain. You could address this by either upping your intake of oils rich in primary Omega-3s like flax or chia seed oils or by supplementing with blackcurrant or the right hemp seed oils or krill oil, which all contain preformed secondary Omega-3s.

- Your body also uses the secondary EFAs as a precursor for the prostaglandins and other eicosanoids, which respond ultra-fast to input from your environment. They work almost instantaneously at the cellular level in response to changes in your environment and hormonal system. They are involved in nearly all body processes, but particularly inflammation, so it's almost unbelievably important to have them in balance.

Unfortunately, the drug companies do not take a holistic view of prostaglandins, so drugs blocking prostaglandin synthesis are quite common, including the anti-inflammatory drugs aspirin, ibuprofen, naproxen, rofecoxib and celecoxib. Not surprisingly such drugs have a wide range of nasty side effects, are the leading cause of drug toxicity and are one of the leading causes of drug-induced death.

The eicosanoids made from the secondary Omega-6, GLA (found in evening primrose, borage, blackcurrant and some hemp seed oils) are anti-inflammatory and act as an important trigger for a wide range of changes in your body in response to adrenaline, infections or toxins and pregnancy.

The eicosanoids made from the secondary Omega-3s (see above), enhance the effects of those made from GLA and your body uses them to reverse the effects of an adrenaline rush. They are powerfully anti-inflammatory.

There is another set of eicosanoids made from the secondary Omega-6 called AA, which you get in modest amounts from meat and egg yolks. However your body will readily make AA from either the primary Omega-6 (LA) or GLA, so the main driver for the amount of AA in your body is the amount of Omega-6 oils you have in your diet. They are powerfully inflammatory and so actively oppose the good ones made from GLA and the secondary Omega-3s.

As you can see the various eicosanoids are designed to balance each other, and the main driver of the amount of each of these you have in your body is the balance of Omega-6 and Omega-3 in your body. Like so many other things in your body, it's all about the balance folks.

The widespread changes in our Omega-6/Omega-3 ratio have come about both because of an absolute decrease in the amount of Omega-3 available in our food supply. But also, a relative decrease, compared to the increasing abundance of Omega-6. This is because Omega-3 oils are highly unstable unless handled very carefully so, to achieve better shelf stability, food manufacturers actively avoid Omega-3 oils. Omega-3 oils are also more expensive than Omega-6 oils, giving another reason for food manufacturers to actively avoid them.

To correct this major Omega-6/Omega-3 imbalance in your body, three things need to happen:

- Substantially REDUCE your intake of refined Omega-6 oils by switching to healthier cooking oils containing saturated fats (such as coconut oil or butter) or Omega-9 oils (such as olive or avocado oils).

- Substantially REDUCE your intake of junk foods and processed foods containing refined polyunsaturated oils – the Omega-6 oils.

- Substantially INCREASE your intake of undamaged Omega-3 oils like unrefined flax or chia seed oil, which will also provide you with some undamaged Omega-6.

11.7
Healthy Oils You Should Eat Lots More

	SCT	MCT	LCT	Oleic ω-9	Omega -7	CLA	LA ω-6	ALA ω-3
Coconut	0.5	60	31	7		0.2	2	
'Grass Fed' Butter	7	9	55	23	1	3	1	1
Butter	6	7	57	25	1	0.4	3	0.4
Beef Fat		0.1	43	38	1	5	9	4
Olive Oil			14	74	1		11	1
Macadamia Oil			13	64	19		2	1
Avocado Oil			13	70	3		14	1
Safflower Oil			6	15			79	0.1
Flax Seed Oil			9	14			15	61
Chia Seed Oil			11	7	1		21	59

Table 11.1 What's in the good oils (%)

11.7.1
Butter and Cheese

Because of the whole saturated oil misinformation campaign outlined above, butter and cheese have had a bad rap for the last 40 years or so which has been heavily reinforced by advertising from the margarine industry (Big Food). The information given below refers directly to butter, but depending on the type, cheese has roughly one-third fat which of course shares all the characteristics of butterfat. However, read 11.9.3 Processed Cheese before you go nuts on eating cheese.

The butter made from milk from grass-fed cows, such as we are fortunate enough to have access to in New Zealand, has the following characteristics:

- It contains around 65% saturated fat and 16% is from the easily digestible SCT and MCTs.

- Very importantly, it contains around 7% of the SCTs, which are an ideal food for the cells lining your gut wall and your microbiome, so eating grass-fed butter strongly promotes gut health. For more detailed information see butyrate under section 10.3.3 Prebiotics that Feed your Microbiome.

- Grass-fed butter contains around 23% of the healthy Omega-9 oils, 1.4% Omega-6 and 1% Omega-3, which gives it a healthy 1.4:1 ratio of Omega-6: Omega-3.

  Such butter compares very favorably with the butter from more intensive farming systems where the cows are fed lots of oilseed residues and other concentrates containing Omega-6, which gives the resulting butter an Omega-6/Omega-3 ratio of between 7 and 10:1.

- Grass-fed butter also contains usefully higher concentrations of vitamin A, vitamin D, and vitamin K2 (important for calcium metabolism), and also the fatty acids CLA and Omega-7, which have been shown to help with belly fat loss and cancer prevention.

- Grass-fed butter also contains usefully higher concentrations of several important antioxidants, including Glutathione (2x more), vitamin A (5x more) and Vitamin E (2x more).

- It tastes delicious both as a spread and when used as a safe cooking fat for dishes such as stir-fries and pan-frying (especially with a little bit of olive oil added).

- When it is gently heated to form ghee, all the milk solids such as casein and lactose are removed. These are usually the bits that can cause dairy intolerance, making ghee safe for nearly everyone to eat. It also has a higher smoke point, which makes it one of the best cooking oils you could ever use.

(My family often accuses me of having more butter than bread – totally untrue).

As I have noted above, the delicious yellow butter, rich in Vitamin A, that we get from grass-fed cows is a totally different product from most of the butter in most other countries. This tends to be a pale, insipid butter made from cows fed on concentrates and (in the USA) injected with an rBGH (recombinant bovine growth hormone) derived from gene technology. How your butter is produced really matters.

"Don't blame the butter for what the bread did!" - Prof Grant Schofield.

11.7.2
Coconut Oil

Coconut oil, like butter, has had a bad rap for the last 40 years or so, but more recently it is being recognized for being the superfood it is.

The bad rap was completely undeserved, for the following reasons:

- It is the richest source (61%) of SCT and MCTs, which are absorbed directly into your liver and converted into ketones, which provide you with both quick energy and food for your brain.

- It contains around 46% lauric acid (a MCT) making it one of the best fuels for your brain.

- When your liver and brain are producing ketones, they also produce more glutathione, your body's master antioxidant.

- Your body can convert lauric acid into monolaurin, a compound that can destroy fat coated viruses such as shingles herpes, measles, and influenza, some bacteria and protozoa such as Giardia.

- It only contains about 7% Omega-9 and less than 2% Omega-6, which makes it a very stable oil and difficult to damage with heat. This makes coconut oil a very healthy cooking oil.

Thus, coconut oil is both an excellent brain food and an excellent cooking oil. Some people do not like the coconut flavor but you can get refined, deodorized coconut oil, which has no smell or taste. Because it's nearly all saturated fat, the damage caused by refining is not as serious as it is with Omega-6 oils.

You can also get MCTs, extracted from coconut oil as an oil or powder, which gives a more rapid boost in blood ketone levels and is widely used by bodybuilders and athletes as fuel while they are building lean muscle mass. Using some MCT oil as a supplement can aid your transition into becoming fat-adapted, but you CAN'T just eat a high carb diet and use some MCTs and expect to become fat-adapted – but yes you will get a temporary boost in your blood ketones and brain function. New on the market are pre-formed ketone supplements, which can give you an even faster temporary boost in your blood ketones and brain function.

In my view, the place for these is only as a temporary boost if you are starting to experience 'keto flu' or need a quick energy or brain boost when you would usually reach for that sugary snack. When you are fat-adapted you do not usually get the brain boost from MCT or ketone supplements, because you are already running on ketones. The concentrated MCT 8's and 10's and preformed ketones now on the market are very highly processed and refined, and thus I do not regard them as real food. Treat MCTs with caution when you first start using them as larger amounts can cause loose bowels.

Quality palm kernel oil is not as widely available as coconut oil but shares many of the nutritional features of coconut oil. However, its production system usually causes massive environmental damage (unless it is Certified Organic). If you don't like the coconut/palm flavor, you could always use a combination of butter and olive oil for your cooking.

11.7.3
Olive, Macadamia and Avocado Oils

Extra virgin olive, macadamia and avocado oils are all rich sources of the Omega-9 oils, which are consumed in high amounts as part of the very health promoting Mediterranean style diet.

It's important to note that because of the ready availability of freshly pressed extra virgin olive oil, this is the main oil consumed around the Mediterranean region and a key part of the very healthy Mediterranean Diet. It is only this undamaged olive oil, rich in phytonutrients, that has been shown to have health benefits.

There are no such health benefits associated with refined (in other words damaged) Omega-9 oils. This includes the refined olive oils (which are sold as virgin or 'lite' olive oil), hi-oleic sunflower or safflower oils, peanut oil, or rice bran oil. The quality of your oils really matters.

Olive and avocado fruits contain about 15 – 20% oil, macadamia nuts about 75% oil, along with lots of wonderful antioxidants and dietary fiber and taste delicious. All of these are wonderful additions to your diet.

11.7.4
Safflower Oil

I give safflower oil as an example of an Omega-6 oil which, if it is NOT refined, has a delicious buttery taste so makes a great base for your salad dressings. Unrefined safflower oil is also a very useful source of Vitamin E; 40 ml would provide about half your daily requirement of vitamin E.

Most people get way more Omega-6 in their diet than your body needs, so I'm not recommending you use lots of safflower oil. However, once you have corrected your Omega-6: Omega-3 imbalance you will need to include some unrefined Omega-6 in your diet, and safflower is my favorite.

There is a very wide range of very cheap and very nasty Omega-6 polyunsaturated oils sold in supermarkets and widely used in processed foods. These include canola, corn, cottonseed, grapeseed, hemp, palm oil, peanut, rice bran, safflower, soybean and sunflower oils. These are almost always sold as refined oils packaged in clear plastic. They are bad for your health if used as a salad oil and, as they are relatively easily damaged by heat, they are even worse for you if you use them as cooking oil (See 11.9.1 Refined Vegetable Oils). This does mean that the only health promoting oils you can buy in many supermarkets is extra virgin olive, avocado and coconut oils.

11.7.5
Flaxseed Oil

Flax seed, chia seed, and perilla seed oils are the only oils that contain more Omega-3 than they do Omega-6, and thus are capable of reducing your Omega-6/Omega-3 ratio.

Hemp seed and walnut oils often get called Omega-3 oils. However, they both contain more Omega-6 then they do Omega-3 so while they can be useful sources of Omega-3, they are not capable of improving your body's Omega-6/Omega-3 ratio.

Because all Omega-3 oils contain three double bonds they are extremely unstable, and they need to be processed with great care to taste good and be functionally useful in your body. If they don't taste good and have a bitter aftertaste, then they are damaged and will not actively support your body towards health. If your Omega-3 oils are not packaged in anything but completely lightproof containers, such as a safe black plastic or glass, they will taste bitter. BROWN, DARK GREEN OR VIOLET GLASS DO NOT BLOCK ENOUGH LIGHT TO PROTECT SUCH OILS.

"any color so long as it is black" Henry Ford

Ideally your flax seed oil should have a delicious, mild buttery/nutty flavor with no bitterness, strong or burnt flavor. Unfortunately, very few manufacturers around the world take the necessary care to produce such oil, so most flax seed oil on the market tastes pretty foul. It doesn't have to be that way. I am proud to be one of those few manufacturers who produce high quality, good tasting, flax seed, chia seed and hemp seed oils, made with health in mind.

One of the key roles in your body for the primary Omega-3 – ALA, is oxygen transport across cell membranes. If you emulsify flax seed oil with milk protein, you form a new water-soluble compound - a lipoprotein. This compound bypasses the normal oil metabolism and is absorbed directly into your bloodstream, and thus into your cell membranes, as the key component in oxygenating all your body's cells and maintaining the integrity of your cell membranes.

In a practical sense you can achieve this by having a flavored blend of cottage cheese (or quark) and flax seed oil (the Budwig recipe). There is no evidence to support the very common idea that for you to get better cell oxygenation it only works if you use cottage cheese or quark, as recommended by Dr Budwig in the 1950s (a very long time ago). Depending on your food preferences you can use any source of milk protein, egg protein, sunflower seeds or hemp hearts, which are all rich sources of the sulfur-containing amino acids vital to forming the key lipoprotein.

For most people, organic whole fat yoghurt is relatively easy to source and makes a delicious flavored smoothie with flax seed oil. When you take flax seed oil in an emulsion with any protein rich in sulfur-containing amino acids, most people will experience a lift in energy shortly afterwards because of the better oxygenation of their cells.

Because cancer cells do not thrive in a high oxygen environment, this combination of flax seed oil and milk protein is widely used as an important part of many protocols to heal from cancer, i.e. The Budwig Protocol.

11.7.6
Nuts and Seeds

Nuts and seeds are a wonderful way of getting more high-quality oil in your diet, along with plenty of protein, fiber and many beneficial phytonutrients like antioxidants, vitamins and minerals. If possible, source fresh raw nuts so the oils are not damaged by age.

Because of their good balance of nutrients, nuts and seeds are a great addition to your diet to help keep you in fat burning mode. One little trick that can help control your appetite before lunch or dinner is to eat a handful of nuts about 20 minutes before your meal. Doing this will reduce your Ghrelin production, which gives your body a chance to tell you that maybe it doesn't really need that huge lunch you intended to have before you ate the nuts.

Chia, flaxseed and hemp seeds and walnuts are useful sources of Omega-3. Hemp, pumpkin, sesame and sunflower seeds and walnuts are useful sources of Omega-6. Almonds, brazil, cashew, macadamia and pecan nuts and pumpkin and sesame seeds are all useful sources of Omega-9. Peanuts also contain useful amounts of Omega-9 oils but because they are not true nuts and grow underground, they are often contaminated with toxic fungus, so they can be pretty hard on your liver and are the 'nuts' most likely to cause allergies.

A really delicious way to get more good oils and protein into your diet is to branch out a bit and try a few different nut butters, other than the standard peanut butter. I sometimes make my own nut butter, and my personal favorite is ABC (Almond, Brazil and Cashew).

11.7.7
Dark Chocolate

Dark chocolate, with a cocoa content of at least 72% or greater, includes only oils from cocoa beans in a relatively undamaged form - these are the healthy saturated and Omega-9 oils. In contrast, other chocolates usually include a wide range of heavily processed and damaged vegetable oils, which are used to mimic the more expensive cacao oils and they also contain a substantial amount of sugar.

Depending on the cacao content, good dark chocolate usually contains more fat than sugar, which does give a more bitter flavor. Having a couple of squares of dark chocolate can satisfy that craving for something decadent without having a serious impact on your blood sugar levels. Because it is made from the whole bean, dark chocolate also contains useful amounts of dietary fiber and substantial levels of powerful antioxidants and some critical minerals, and has been shown to be heart healthy.

That made your day, didn't it?

11.8
Flax vs. Fish or Krill for Omega-3

Most authors advocate the idea that an Omega-3 supplement is one of the most important things you can do for your health and will advise you to get your Omega-3 from fish or krill oil. They suggest that your body is incapable of producing sufficient of the secondary Omega-3s EPA and DHA from the ALA in vegetable oils.

Such advice ignores the large volume of published research which shows that in healthy adults the conversion of ALA to EPA is usually in the order of 5 to 10%, and that the conversion to DHA is around 2 to 5%. In fact rates as high as 15 to 20% conversion to DHA from flax seed oil have been measured in young women of childbearing age and in preterm infants – presumably, an evolutionary trait designed to foster healthy brain growth in the fetus.

I recommend you consume around 0.5 oz of flax seed oil daily, which is the amount you need to form healthy cell membranes in the 500 million new cells you make each day. If you follow this recommendation your body is very capable of making the relatively small amounts of EPA and DHA it requires. When you consider that humans evolved in Eastern Africa, on a diet rich in green plant foods and grass-fed meat, (all good sources of ALA) and well away from the oily, EPA and DHA-rich cold-water fish, this should not be surprising.

That said - modern living in the form of stress, alcohol, high intake of damaged Omega-6 oils and metabolic syndrome can down-regulate the genes responsible for the first step in the conversion process of ALA to EPA and DHA, and LA to GLA and AA. There is a simple workaround to this issue that can be achieved by using secondary Omega-3s and Omega-6s from blackcurrant, hemp and evening primrose oil, or using a combination of krill oil and flax seed oil for the first couple of months of supplementing your Omega-3 levels. I am proud to be one of those few manufacturers who produce high quality, good tasting vegetarian oil blends containing the correct balance of both primary and secondary Omega-3s and Omega-6s made with health in mind – these help to make you feel better quickly.

Once your body has been treated to a regular intake of high-quality Omega-3 and Omega-6 oils, the genes responsible for making the enzymes necessary for the conversion to the secondary Omega-3 and Omega-6s, usually become up-regulated as your health improves, so taking these more expensive oil blends becomes unnecessary.

Another important point, missed by most authors, is that EPA contains five double bonds and DHA six double bonds, which makes them thousands of times more reactive than saturated oils. This fact means that getting undamaged fish and krill oil is nigh on impossible, especially as most fish and krill oils are encapsulated in clear gel capsules and not packaged in lightproof containers, so this light damaged oil will not be contributing to your health in an optimum way. Fish oils are not harvested from a sustainable resource and many are usually contaminated with potentially toxic heavy metals and pesticides. The industry is aware of this problem so such oils are very heavily processed to remove some of the toxins, leading to significant levels of damaged Omega-3s, meaning they do not contribute to optimum health.

Also, as I have already discussed in Section 11.6 Your Omega-6/Omega-3 Balance, our bodies need to have roughly equal amounts of Omega-3 and Omega-6 to have optimally healthy cell membranes. If you are taking a gram or two of fish or krill oil in capsules daily, this is going to do little to change this major imbalance which is very likely present in your body.

For your health's sake, you really should get lots more ALA Omega-3 in your diet.

11.9
Unhealthy Fats you Should Actively Avoid

11.9.1
Refined vegetable Oils

Most vegetable oil is produced in very large, high-tech factories, and is not produced with your health in mind.

The seeds or fruits are either cooked to break down the cell structure before pressing at very high temperatures and pressures, or the oil is extracted by using a synthetic solvent. Because of the damage caused by these extreme extraction methods, the oil then has to be refined to make it edible. The refining process involves adding strong alkalis, which not only removes many of the damaged molecules, but also all the natural antioxidants present in the oil. It is then dosed with strong acid to neutralize the alkali and deodorized by injecting very high-temperature steam through the oil (at up to 500°C). It then has synthetic chemicals added to protect against oxidation and crystallizing in the bottle.

Light is an extremely damaging factor for all oils and you should NEVER purchase any oil packaged in clear plastic or glass.

Unfortunately, the labeling of oils is not well regulated, so many oils which call themselves cold-pressed are not really so. It is likely to mean that the seed hasn't been cooked, but it is likely still pressed at very high temperatures and refined at high temperatures, which means that they will contain damaged EFA molecules, probably including trans-fats, and their electrical charge will be altered.

THERE IS ONE INFALLIBLE TEST THAT WILL TELL YOU WHETHER YOUR OIL IS REFINED OR NOT. If the oil tastes and smells of the seed or nut from which it was extracted, then it will be good for your health. No matter what the label says, if it is bland and tasteless and has no odor, use it for oiling your chopping boards, cricket bat or deck.

Most fats occur in the triglyceride form, with three fat chains linked together by a glycerol molecule. Such fats are electrically neutral and so they are insoluble in water. In unrefined oils, there is a small but important proportion of phospholipids which have two fat chains linked together by a phosphate

An Experiment with Margarine

I know some people are likely to struggle with this one, but for the reasons outlined above, all margarine is bad for your body and your brain.

For instance, children who ate margarine regularly scored significantly lower on intelligence tests than their peers. I know this is not what you get from the adverts or even from the Heart Foundation but, for your health's sake, you need to AVOID ALL MARGARINE, including those made with 'healthy oils', like refined olive oil.

If you are still not convinced, try this little experiment. Take a lump of butter and a lump of margarine and put them on a plate, somewhere accessible, but out of the sun.

A mouse in my house took three days to find them and eat all the butter.

When I threw the olive oil margarine out three months later, it was still sitting there, totally inert. The mouse wouldn't eat it; insects hadn't touched it; and no fungus had grown on it. Apparently, birds will not eat it either.

In other words, MARGARINE IS NOT FOOD. There are no enzymes in nature (or in your body) to digest it, so now you know the damage it does to your body, why would you eat it?

group. These are electrically charged and water-soluble which gives them a critical role in forming healthy cell membranes. The refining process both removes these important phospholipids and also causes the formation of a number of damaged fat molecules, including trans-fats.

We are electrical beings. Our body uses electrical potential to function so the electrical charge carried by undamaged EFAs is critical for the healthy functioning of your cell membranes. Your cell's nucleus is positively charged and the outer membrane negatively charged. Oils that have been refined do not carry an electrical charge and so are, to all intents and purposes dead, not life supporting, and should not be taken into your body.

It's a really good idea to start becoming an oil connoisseur and care about how your oil tastes. If it tastes of nothing it will provide some energy, but it's not good for you. Likewise, if it has any off flavors, particularly a bitter aftertaste that lingers, then the oil has been damaged during processing and will not be contributing to your health. As you might expect, the more unsaturated the oil, the more it is susceptible to processing damage. There are many flax seed oils (and fish oils) on the market which are really not fit for human consumption.

Fortunately, we are starting to see some gourmet oils coming onto the market, which have not been refined, so taste good and can be used to add new and delicious flavor notes to your food. I produce some of them.

11.9.2
Trans-fats and Margarine

You have probably heard that trans-fats are not great for your health, but what are they?

Trans-fats are a type of unsaturated fats that are rare in nature but are readily formed by the industrial processes used in the production of margarine, snack food, packaged baked goods, and fast food. The hydrogenation process makes liquid vegetable oil more solid by creating a synthetic saturated fat. Refined vegetable oil is treated at high temperatures, and pressures in the presence of a metal catalyst (nickel or aluminum) and hydrogen is pumped in to break the double bonds.

Trans-fats have been shown to be seriously damaging to your health, in particular promoting heart disease, inflammation, mental problems, insulin resistance and risk of diabetes.

Research has shown that the refining and hydrogenation processes damage fat molecules in a largely random fashion, so there are many unidentifiable, and probably toxic, new 'fat' molecules created. The high temperatures and pressures involved in refining vegetable oils, and the hydrogenation process, leave very few undamaged EFA molecules, and some of these will have been converted into trans-fats (which are easy to identify).

Damaged fats can sit on enzyme receptor sites in your cells and block access of real undamaged fats to the enzymes and, in the process creating a functional EFA deficiency.

Because of the adverse publicity trans-fats have generated, margarine manufacturers have devised a new way of producing hydrogenated fats that do not contain trans-fats (interesterified). However, such margarine still contains other damaged fat molecules, and the health consequences of eating such margarine have been shown to be just as bad as those containing trans-fats.

The key issue is that, if you want to be healthy, you need to avoid consuming damaged fats. Doing this can be quite difficult because they are so cheap and convenient for food manufacturers to use, that the use of hydrogenated vegetable oils is widespread in processed food. Unfortunately, the labels on junk foods and processed vegetable oils cannot necessarily be trusted, so you really need to avoid such foods if you want to be well.

Since your body uses whatever fats are in your bloodstream to make the cell walls of the 500 million of new cells it makes daily, eating ANY bad fats like margarine or refined oils is going to negatively affect many bodily processes.

11.9.3
Processed Cheese

Processed cheeses are another of those foods that have been highly modified to make it quick and easy to use and have a very long shelf life. Their processing involves taking all the reject cheese, which does not meet specifications, and cooking it with one or more of the following to get the required balance: whey protein, emulsifiers, milk, vegetable oils, salt, preservatives and food coloring - many of these ingredients have unpronounceable names and don't belong in real foods. The proteins and fats are damaged by the cooking process which, combined with the preservatives used, gives a very long shelf life, but also makes it very difficult for your body to digest.

Not a good source of either fat or protein, so do not include processed cheese in your diet - in many countries such 'food' is not allowed to be labeled as cheese.

CHAPTER 12

Detoxing Your Body

"The primary driver of chronic disease in the industrialised world is now environmental toxins"

Joe Pizzorno, ND.

There is increasing awareness that what we have done to our environment by way of pollution from industrial chemicals and processes, we have also done to our bodies. Our detox systems are very robust but they are simply not equipped to deal with the sheer volume of toxic heavy metals and synthetic chemicals (many of them suspected carcinogens) that we are routinely exposed to in our food, home environment, air, water, medicines, personal care products and our soil. This is one of the key reasons why that the older you get, the more difficult it can be to maintain good health, because these toxins will accumulate in your body if you do not take active steps to support your detox systems.

12.1
What Causes Cancer?

There are now many studies that have tried to sort out the relative importance of genetics and environmental factors in the incidence of cancer. These have involved the use of identical twins or adopted children and, the BAD news is, that such studies suggest that the influence of genetics on cancer is only moderate.

This doesn't surprise me, for two important reasons.

Firstly, once scientists had the tools to unravel our DNA or genetic code, there was a huge amount of excitement and hope that many conditions that seemed to have a genetic component would be able to be cured. The problem is that once they crunch the numbers, all they can say is that a particular SNP (piece of genetic code) or gene "is associated" with a particular condition. The association is purely a mathematical probability, with absolutely no proof of cause and effect.

In 2000, when the Human Genome Project first presented data to the world, it looked like 97% of your DNA had no apparent function – "appears to be junk DNA". Follow-up studies are now suggesting that we have an idea of the function of somewhere between 9 and 80% of your DNA, but we are a very long way from saying that if you have a particular gene, you WILL get a particular condition.

Secondly, we know already that what you eat and how you live can have a huge impact on the way your genes express themselves (the way information from a gene is used to make RNA or protein for use in cell functioning). We now have branches of research called Epigenetics and Nutrigenomics, which are studying the effects of foods on your gene expression, so your food is 'information' to your genes. This science is still in its relative infancy, but there is a hope that at some stage we may be able to understand your personal nutritional needs well enough to help you choose the right diet for you.

So having your breasts removed because a DNA scan shows that you have a gene that is associated with an increased risk of breast cancer doesn't seem like a great idea. Surely it would be better to change the way you eat and live to become healthier, so life will be more fun?

Since the influence of genetics on cancer is only moderate, then the GOOD news is that your environmental exposure to toxins and the way you eat are the major causes of cancer. Fortunately, such exposure can be under your control, should you so choose.

12.2
What are These Toxins?

I suspect that your attitude to industrial chemicals is probably a bit like mine used to be – if the chemical has been approved for use and there is no warning label on it, then it must have been tested and found to be safe – surely?

Sorry, that's not the way it is at all. Regulators like the FDA (Food and Drug Administration) and EPA (Environmental Protection Agency) in the USA seem to start with the assumption that new chemicals are 'safe' until proven otherwise. Consequently, in our modern world, we live in a virtual soup of around 80-100,000 synthetic chemicals, many of which have not been tested adequately for safety (certainly not how they interact with each other) and how they might impact on your body, and their use is largely unregulated.

Unfortunately, it gets worse than this. A chemical like BPA (Bisphenol A), which is the highest volume chemical produced worldwide, is used for can linings and on most EFTPOS receipts. Yet it has been shown to be a powerful xenoestrogen and thyroid disruptor. However, the industry has been given several years to find an alternative and to phase out the toxic chemical – while you continue to be exposed. Even worse - BPS, the increasingly widespread replacement for BPA, has already been shown to be just as bad and there are rumblings of plans to ban it – BUT more years of exposure for you.

It's very easy to become a bit ostrich-like about this problem, thinking that there's nothing you can do about it, the problem is just too big, or 'it can't be that bad'. So how bad is it?

It is impacting on your health, whether you like it or not - so it's very bad!

A 1990 study to look at the causes behind what the Doctor put on the death certificate, showed that the primary drivers of chronic disease in the industrialized world were nutritional deficiencies or excesses and lifestyle choices such as smoking – so these factors were the choices you made. A similar, much more recent study showed that while nutritional deficiencies or excesses and lifestyle choices such as smoking were still important, the primary driver of chronic disease is now the environmental toxins which we are routinely exposed to whether we like it or not. Unless you actively avoid them.

It's a global problem. It's estimated that 20% of the pollution along the West Coast of the USA comes from China.

For example, you would like to think that your placenta would protect a baby from exposure to toxins. However, in recent years, several tests on the blood from the umbilical cord of new-born babies has shown levels of contamination from well over 200 synthetic chemicals, including pesticides, flame retardants, dioxins, mercury and lead.

One of the most recent studies has even found BPA in umbilical cord blood. BPA is an endocrine disruptor known to affect a baby's brain at levels as low as 0.23 parts per billion, which is a very minute amount.

Some of the toxic heavy metals widespread in our personal environment include:

Mercury – found in tooth fillings, vaccines and top of the food chain fish like tuna or farmed fish.

Nickel – found in all junk food because of its use as an oil hydrogenation catalyst.

Lead – widespread in soil from its historical use in fuel additives and paint.

Aluminum – from drink cans, municipal water, vaccines and ALL underarm deodorants.

Cadmium – from dust in the air and the widely applied phosphate fertilizers.

Arsenic – from air and water (10% of USA public water supplies are contaminated), some chicken meat and rice. Widely used as a wood preservative.

Cesium - the most dangerous substance released in nuclear disasters like Fukushima.

All of these heavy metals, in various ways, disrupt mitochondrial function – the little energy factories in your cells. So a key effect of heavy metal toxicity is that you feel tired for no apparent reason. Recent international research has shown that Arsenic, Mercury and Cadmium are particularly damaging to your mitochondria and they, along with Aluminum, are all clearly associated with increased risk of Alzheimer's.

All pharmaceutical drugs should also be regarded as potentially toxic to you as all drugs have side effects, of varying severity, which affects some users. Some widely used drugs have also been shown to increase your risk of developing chronic conditions. For instance, PPI's (widely prescribed for acid reflux) have been linked to a 44% increase in the risk of developing dementia or Alzheimer's, and a 16% increase in the risk of developing heart disease (and double the risk of dying from a heart disease event).

Similarly, there is no evidence that statin use decreases mortality in women and the FDA now requires a label warning that using statins may increase your risk of diabetes, liver damage, memory loss and confusion and muscle weakness. Don't forget that many women report lowered libido when they are using hormonal contraception.

I hope you are starting to appreciate that in our modern world it is impossible to avoid many of these toxins getting into our bodies, so the reality is they are accumulating in your body unless you are consciously taking steps to get rid of them. This means that, for the sake of your health, you need to focus on better ways of getting them out.

12.3
The 'Pancake' Theory

You might well ask, "how come I'm not aware of the impact of these toxins?" As I have said before, everyone is different and so how toxins affect you and how well you can detoxify a particular toxin is a very individual thing. Your body wants you to be well and has an amazing inbuilt ability to absorb toxins and detoxify them – some people better than others.

Many years ago, one of my sons had quite severe asthma for a few years, and during his second emergency trip to the hospital I had a very interesting conversation with his doctor. I was struggling to understand why sometimes a food would trigger an asthma attack, but next time he ate the same food he wouldn't necessarily get asthma. Most of the time it felt as if it was a different trigger each time he got asthma, which was very confusing for us all and made managing his condition very difficult.

She explained the situation like this: your body's immune system can be likened to a stack of pancakes. Each of the stressors your body is exposed to represents a pancake. For your particular immune system, your stack of pancakes might include - intolerance to gluten; the mercury from your amalgam fillings; a low-grade threadworm infection; sensitivity to GMO soybeans; the anger you are holding on to from an incident at work; and the preservative in your skin care cream.

How many pancakes you can eat before you're full is different for everyone and depends on how big they are. Similarly, the number of stress pancakes your immune system can handle at any one time without becoming overloaded is different. In the same way, what YOUR body's immune system regards as a pancake can be very different from another person's.

For my son's asthma, at that time his immune system could handle a stack of, say, four pancakes before it became overloaded and triggered him into an asthma attack. However, the fifth pancake that appeared to trigger the attack could be different every time. One day he could eat an apple no problem, the next day an apple could trigger an asthma attack. It depended on whether the apple was pancake three or pancake five. Fortunately, as he grew up, his immune system grew stronger and able to handle more pancakes, so asthma is no longer a problem for him.

In the same way your ability to handle toxins differs from other people, both in your particular ability to handle some different toxins, and what your body regards as a toxin. One of my key objectives of this book is to help you identify what your body thinks of as a toxic pancake and how to get rid of, or reduce the size of, some pancakes so that your immune system doesn't get overloaded and negatively impact on your wellness.

12.4
Avoidance

Now that you have some awareness of the problem of toxicity in your environment, there are some simple steps that you can take in your home to minimize your exposure:

- As much as you can, choose to buy organic foods and products from free-range, grass-fed animals. This will minimize your exposure to pesticides and supply you with more nutrient-dense food.

- Washing fruit and vegetables can reduce some pesticide residues, but doesn't remove the residues from inside.

- Eat real foods made from produce typically found around the outside shelves of a grocery store and avoid the central aisles loaded with processed, pre-packaged foods. You will thus avoid synthetic food additives with names you can't pronounce and, contamination from the packaging used. You will also avoid many of the toxins produced by processing at high temperatures, etc., which is often part of the manufacturing of processed foods.

- Avoid food packaged with plastic wrap and canned foods, as these are both sources of potent xenoestrogens and endocrine-disrupting chemicals. Always use a plate to cover food being heated in a microwave, not plastic wrap.

- Use only household cleaning products made with natural ingredients (names you can pronounce) and perfumed with essential oils, rather than cleaning products with petrochemical solvents and synthetic perfumes.

- Do not use insect sprays in your house or have your house 'spider proofed' with very persistent insecticides. Insecticides are designed to kill primitive animals, and you are an animal, so these are generally the most toxic pesticides for humans.

- Use only personal care products made with natural ingredients. The regulation around the use of chemicals in personal care products is even less stringent than the regulations around food additives. Your skin does not provide an effective barrier against absorbing chemicals; so if you wouldn't eat your cosmetics, don't put them on your skin.

- Find out about your tap water. It is likely that someone has tested your local supply. If it is contaminated, you should install an appropriate water filter to clean it up – including your shower water.

- Replace your Teflon-coated non-stick cookware with stainless steel, ceramic, glass, or cast iron cookware. The gases given off by Teflon-coated cookware at temperatures as low as 200° C. will kill birds and do seriously nasty things to you. Recent research is suggesting there is no 'safe' level of exposure – it's in the same league as asbestos and lead.

  A great alternative for a non-stick fry pan is to use a cast-iron pan seasoned with fat. After serving, while the pan is still hot, run the pan under a cold tap and everything just rinses off. You have to re-season the pan with fat again if you use soap to clean.

  The other no-no to do with Teflon is microwaveable popcorn – most of such products use Teflon to line the plastic bag so that it doesn't stick, which gives you a significant dose of Teflon when you eat the popcorn.

- When you redecorate your home look for green, toxin-free alternatives to regular paint and vinyl floor coverings. Cork tiles make a wonderful finish on your kitchen floor. They are easy on the feet and most things bounce if you drop them.

- Carpets are loaded with fire retardants, insecticides, and other neurotoxins, and also trap environmental toxins, so carpets are not great, especially if you have a crawling baby in the house. Throw rugs are a much better alternative if you wash them thoroughly before you use them.

- The EWG (Environmental Working Group) website has some great consumer guides on how to find healthy food, cleaning products, personal care products, etc.   www.ITookCharge.nz/Environmental Working Group

*"if you wouldn't eat your cosmetics,
don't put them on your skin."*

12.5
Detoxification

Your body evolved its detoxification pathways a very long time ago; well before our recent exposure to synthetic chemicals. This means that if you really want to be well, you will need to actively support your body to detoxify on a regular basis.

This is required because your own liver, bowel, kidneys, lungs, brain, and skin detox systems are almost certainly overloaded and need your active support.

My recommended detox program for your body takes about nine days and involves making a point of consuming some things and avoiding others (See Chapter 16 Your 'Rapid Reset' Plan).

Ways in which you can support your body to detox include:

12.5.1
Bowel Movements

The primary detox pathway for chemicals that are not naturally water-soluble is from the liver, via the gallbladder, into the bowel and thus out of your body. The fundamental requirement for this pathway to work efficiently for you is to have a minimum of one to two bowel movements EVERY DAY, which probably requires you to eat at least 30 – 50 g of fiber per day (you are likely only eating 5 – 15 g per day).

To safely increase your fiber intake you need to take it slowly, otherwise it will just make the problem worse. If this is a problem for you, to get things moving, I recommend doing a course of colonic irrigation which will remove the impacted toxic sludge from the past and allow your bowel muscles to start working again.

Consistency does matter, so your stool should be neither too hard nor too soft. You might find it helpful to do a quick search for a 'Bristol stool chart', which is widely used by health professionals to help evaluate the health of your gut.

There are many potential explanations for loose bowels, but they can be an indicator of an internal parasite infection. If you have a health issue for which there is no other explanation, parasites are highly likely to be involved. Internal parasites are not just a Third World problem and estimates of infection rates in developed countries range from 35 to 95%, which is a pretty scary thought – do not ignore this possibility.

12.5.2
Eat Fiber

Having an adequate intake of dietary fiber is fundamental to achieving regular bowel movements. The fermentable fiber, often referred to as soluble fiber, absorbs large amounts of water and provides bulk, which is really important to help stabilize the rate at which nutrients are absorbed into your body. Fermentable fibers are present in vegetables, nuts, legumes, fruits and flax seed, and they are vitally important for maintaining a healthy microbiome in your gut.

The less-fermentable fiber, often referred to as insoluble fiber, provides a matrix for absorbing toxins and allowing them to be carried out of your body in your stool, and enhances fecal bulk. Such fiber is found in many vegetables, nuts, seeds, flax seeds and whole grains.

Because there is such strong evidence that increasing dietary fiber intake can reduce the incidence of heart disease, stroke, colon cancer, and diabetes, you should be aiming to eat a minimum of 30 g per day – preferably lots more. However, most people are not even eating half of that so it may require you to start taking some form of fiber supplement to help you have more regular bowel movements.

Liver Stressors

The most likely liver stressors that you will need to minimize or eliminate to achieve the body detox you desire include:

Alcohol – because your liver has difficulty breaking down alcohol, and it causes an inflammatory response, you must completely abstain from alcohol during my recommended nine-day 'Rapid Reset' program. See Chapter 16 Your 'Rapid Reset' Plan.

You're likely to find that such abstinence increases your feelings of well-being and so you may well become motivated to reserve alcohol for special treats or have several alcohol-free days per week. Doing this will also reduce your risk of getting breast cancer.

Sugar in any form – All sugars, but particularly fruit juice, contain a high proportion of fructose that can only be broken down by your liver. Thus, like alcohol, sugar causes an inflammatory response in the liver.

Since sugar is even more addictive than drugs like morphine, eliminating sugar during your nine-day 'Rapid Reset' program can be a challenge for some but, if you proceed as recommended, any cravings will only be short term.

Damaged fats – Any refined or hydrogenated oil or margarine will contain molecules that your liver does not have the enzymes needed to convert them into fuel for your body. Such damaged fats also severely disrupt your mitochondria. Trans-fats are just the tip of the iceberg. Many such fats are widely used in processed food, so you need to eliminate all such foods during your nine-day 'Rapid Reset' program. Eat 'Good Fats' instead.

Excessive protein – Your body does not have a mechanism for storing excess protein. If you eat more protein than your body needs, your liver has to transform it into sugar by a complicated process called gluconeogenesis. This stresses not only your liver but also your kidneys, which have to deal with the excretion of the extra uric acid and calcium (kidney stones anyone?). The resulting sugar either gets burnt for energy or is stored as fat; you need to loosely monitor your protein intake to make sure you get enough, but not too much.

12.5.3
Support Your Liver

It is estimated that around 75% of the body's detoxification activity happens in the liver, so it is really important that you support this process. Many fat-soluble toxins can readily move into cells and cause damage, so supporting your liver in removing these toxins should be the focus of any detoxification protocol.

Water-soluble toxins are usually not quite such an issue for your body because your cell membranes have pretty effective mechanisms in place to minimize their access to your cells (as long as you eat healthy fats), and your kidneys and skin are usually effective pathways to eliminate these.

There are three phases to the liver detoxification process:

Phase 1 – enzymatic transformation

This is where a group of

liver enzymes transform fat-soluble toxins into water-soluble compounds. Unfortunately, some of the resulting compounds can be even more toxic than the original chemical, so it's important that you don't attempt to detoxify too rapidly, otherwise you are likely to overload the rest of the detox system.

Foods that support Phase 1 in a good way include brassicas (such as broccoli or kale), sesame seeds, turmeric, berry fruit, citrus and green tea. It's important to note that drinking caffeine, smoking, and alcohol consumption all impact Phase 1 in a negative way. These need to be avoided while undergoing your detox protocol so that you avoid potentially overloading Phase 2.

Phase 2 – enzymatic attachment

This is where the second group of liver enzymes modify the products from Phase 1 to make them more water-soluble and less toxic. Having adequate antioxidant activity from vegetables and fruits is really important to help Phase 2 proceed efficiently. Brassicas, garlic and turmeric are also potent supporters of Phase 2 activity.

Phase 3 – transport

Water-soluble compounds require specific transporters to move them into and out of cells, including moving the products of Phase 2 out into the bile (from the liver), or into the urine and intestine for elimination. Brassicas, such as broccoli or kale, and apples are among foods that support this process.

Are you getting the idea that you need to eat lots of brassicas and turmeric to support your detox pathways? Eating lots of foods with vibrant colors will greatly increase your intake of the vital antioxidants. Eating lots of garlic and onions is also important as they supply organic sulfur, which helps you to eliminate heavy metals like lead and arsenic.

You can spend a lot of money on a detox formula, but a very powerful detox support drink you can quickly make at home is:

1 litre water (1 quart)

1 whole lemon (flesh and peel)

1 tbsp. fresh ginger root (or 1/2 tsp ginger powder)

1 tbsp. diatomaceous earth

Blend all these into a yummy drink with a high-speed blender and enjoy the benefits.

You could also add things like a bit of fresh turmeric, a few dandelion leaves (out of your garden) or other greens.

"Doing a coffee enema sounds such a hassle, is it really worth it?" I hear you ask?

I used to have reasonably severe prostrate issues which were sending me to the bathroom several times a night which, I can assure you, is no fun. Having tried a number of different approaches, with only limited success, I realized I needed to detoxify my body from the PCB's (very powerful xenoestrogens) I was exposed to as a child, so I decided to try the effect of coffee enemas.

Now, three years on, I no longer have ANY issues with my prostate and I feel a lot healthier than I have felt for many years. I attribute my recent use of coffee enemas as being one of the key reasons why I can say that, at 72, I feel 99% well and love my life.

Chlorella is particularly helpful for supporting heavy metal detox, as are the natural minerals diatomaceous earth and zeolite.

If your detoxification system becomes overloaded, particularly in phase 2, your body will park toxins into your fat cells rather than leaving them floating around. This can have rather unpleasant consequences if you start to burn belly fat, as the stored toxins will then be released back into your system. This means that you have to be really careful to support your liver while you're losing fat.

Your liver does not have an infinite capacity to handle food, drink and toxins, which means that you need to avoid consuming large amounts of food and drink which are known to stress your liver's ability to detox.

12.5.4
Coffee Enema

While the idea of this might sound a little gross at first, please don't dismiss it out of hand. Coffee enemas are a very powerful way of detoxing, so you will need to put more effort into the other methods I have suggested if you choose not to do this. After initial research with rats, coffee enemas started being used during WWII as a very effective method of pain reduction for injured members of the armed forces when drug supplies ran short.

The effect of coffee used as an enema is COMPLETELY different from drinking a cup of coffee. Coffee is very rich in antioxidants so, with a coffee enema, most of the caffeine and antioxidants present in the coffee are absorbed from the colon and taken directly to the liver, via the portal vein, where they greatly enhance Phase 2 and Phase 3 detoxification.

The use of a coffee enema is one of the most powerful ways of supporting glutathione production, your body's major antioxidant produced within the liver, which powerfully supports the whole detox process. The coffee enema enhances the production of glutathione, providing very powerful support for Phase 2 detoxification. The caffeine also relaxes the bile ducts to enhance the flow of toxins out of the liver into the bowel for eventual elimination, so supports Phase 3. Of course, it can also help promote a bowel movement.

Very little of the caffeine goes into the general blood circulation, so even people who are intolerant of caffeine can usually tolerate a small coffee enema.

Ideally you need to use freshly ground organic coffee, which is prepared using about one tablespoon of ground coffee per cup of filtered or spring water. Bring gently to the boil, simmer for 20 minutes and then allow it to cool to body temperature. Do test it with your finger first!

Most practitioners recommend inserting quite large amounts of coffee into your rectum, from 2 – 3 cups or even up to a liter and doing 2 – 3 enemas per week. Such a large amount means that you have to lie still for 15 to 20 minutes, and focus so you can retain the coffee.

I don't choose to make time to do this; I take a little and often approach by using amounts as small as 80 – 100 mls, most days. This is an amount I find I can retain relatively easily and still get on with my day. The other advantage of using such a small amount is that it easily fits into an enema bulb or syringe, which eliminates the need for messy enema bags or buckets.

I recommend you play with how strong the coffee is, how much you use, and when it best fits into your day (ideally first thing) to find what amount you can easily retain so YOU CAN DO IT EASILY, DAILY. I also make up several days' worth of coffee at once, which helps to make it much more doable within my routine.

12.5.5
Support Your Kidneys

The key function of your kidneys is to filter water-soluble toxins from your blood. The best way you can support this is to drink plenty of water to keep your kidneys active and flushed.

How much water should you drink a day?

There is no one answer to this question because it depends on the state of your health, how active you are, and what the temperatures are. As you move into becoming 'fat-adapted' you will need to up your water and salt intake, as running on fat as your primary fuel requires more water than running on glucose. If you are losing weight, you will need to drink a lot more water because, as part of the fat loss process, your fat cells will be dumping lots of stored toxins into your blood and into your kidneys.

When should you drink water?

You breathe out about a liter of water overnight, so drinking several glasses of water when you first get up is very important. Having a warm drink of water, with half a lemon in it, first thing in the morning is great for your gut in several ways and can often help to get your bowel moving.

Any water you drink at meal times dilutes the stomach acid which is vital for digesting proteins, so drinking while you are eating is linked to problems like acid reflux and gut health issues. Drink your water well before or well after your meals.

If you don't drink sufficient water you are at risk of developing kidney stones. Being only mildly dehydrated will also have an impact on your brain function and energy levels. There is some evidence that drinking water can temporarily boost your metabolic rate, and so drinking about 500 mls of water half an hour before a meal can reduce the amount you eat and contribute to fat loss. Sometimes that hungry feeling you get is - just your need for some water so, if you feel hungry, your first response should be to have a drink of water and then see if you really are hungry – that's a win-win way to behave.

Probably the best way to check on your hydration level is as simple as 'do you feel thirsty?' For most people the thirst mechanism in your brain is very effective at telling you when to drink.

If you are not one of these lucky ones, the other thing you can do to monitor your hydration levels is to check the color of your urine. If it's nearly clear and has no odor, you are well hydrated, but possibly drinking too much so that you're leaching minerals out of your body. The darker the color and the more aromatic your urine, the more dehydrated you are. You need to aim for consistently having light yellow colored urine.

Of course, your water needs to be free of contaminants such as chemicals, and taste good. Unfortunately, much of the water from your tap or a bottle doesn't meet this standard. You might want to look at a filtration system that selectively removes contaminants, but not the naturally occurring minerals.

I am lucky enough to have beautiful spring water at my house, but I'm still not great at drinking enough. I do make an effort to drink quite a lot of water when I first get up in the morning to make sure I rehydrate after the night. I also find putting a squeeze of lemon juice in my water bottle is a great incentive for me to drink more regularly.

12.5.6
Your Skin Detox Pathway

Sweating is a powerful way of eliminating toxins from your body, but few people sweat enough on a regular basis. Unfortunately, many of us sit at our desks all day in air-conditioned environments, so our skins can accumulate toxins, with little chance to eliminate them by sweating.

Saunas

Several studies have looked at using infrared saunas in the treatment of chronic health problems and found good evidence of benefits. Conditions studied include high blood pressure, congestive heart failure, heavy metal toxicity, rheumatoid arthritis, Alzheimer's and dementia.

Far-infrared saunas are more effective than traditional hot rock saunas, steam rooms, or hot tubs at detoxing your body. This is because this particular form of infrared radiation can penetrate more deeply into your body without overheating you so badly. Thus, most people find they can tolerate dry heat, infrared saunas for much longer than moist heat, and dry heat also enhances the amount of sweat you can lose in a session.

You can enhance the effect of a dry heat sauna's ability to remove heavy metals (such as mercury, lead, and cadmium) by having a high dose of vitamin C, either orally or intravenously, before a sauna session. This can enhance the excretion of mercury, in particular, by mobilizing mercury bound within your cells and facilitating direct excretion from your skin, which avoids the potentially toxic effects of mercury on your kidneys. Vitamin C can also stimulate the uptake of heavy metals by your liver for excretion via the gut, further sparing the kidneys.

Of course, the beauty of this is that by the sauna promoting improved blood flow to your skin, you can end up with clearer, softer and healthier looking skin. Saunas can also help with relieving aches and pains, and by promoting relaxation, help to reduce your stress levels. Another win-win option.

Epsom Salts Bath

Some of the same effects can be achieved by soaking in a nice warm bath, particularly if you add a cup of Epsom salts, ½ cup of Bentonite clay and maybe a little ascorbic acid and baking soda, and a few drops of relaxing Essential oil such as Rose or Lavender.

Importantly, an Epsom salts bath enhances the magnesium and sulfate levels in your body which are both important for liver health. To enhance this process, having an Epsom salts bath is a time when it is advisable to use soap during your bath to remove any fat-soluble toxins that get excreted into the oily layer on your skin and to allow the minerals into your body.

You can further enhance the experience by playing some mood music and lighting a few candles, and this is certainly a good way to destress at the end of the day. The whole experience can dramatically lower your levels of stress hormones.

12.5.7
Your Tongue Detox Pathway

In the ancient Ayurvedic (Indian) medical system, scraping your tongue is seen as a very effective way to cleanse your mouth cavity. Ayurveda regards your mouth as one of the main gateways between your mind/body and your environment.

When we sleep, our body is busy removing toxins by depositing them onto the surface of our tongue. If you don't scrape away these toxins, they get reabsorbed by your body which can lead to health issues.

Scraping your tongue first thing in the morning removes any build-up of toxins and bacterial film to give you fresh breath, and that gives you that snoggable quality which is such fun. Scraping works much better than a toothbrush to achieve this.

Scraping also helps with your ability to taste your food, which helps make what you eat more satisfying, so you will probably eat less, and it may reduce the need for adding sugar, salt, or excessive spice to make it taste better.

In Ayurvedic tradition "tongue scrapers should be made of gold, silver, copper, tin or brass, and should be non-sharp and curved so as not to injure the tongue". Stainless steel tongue scrapers are widely available, but I find a rounded, stainless steel soup spoon is easy to find and works really well.

Scrape your tongue gently from back to front for several strokes. You will probably want to rinse the spoon of the residue from the first few strokes. If you feel your gag reflex you have scraped too hard or too far back – just be gentle. Having said that, in the Yogic tradition they encourage you to gag, which clears some mucus from your 'monkey glands' in your throat that apparently accumulate toxins overnight.

12.5.8
Fasting

Fasting is 'choosing to forego food for a period as part of cleansing or healing routine' and, before modern medicine, it was one of the few options available – and it is wonderfully effective. The way people fast varies enormously, including the duration, and what you eat or drink during the fast.

Fasting can be a very powerful way to help detox your body, because it allows your whole digestive system to rest so that the energy you normally use to process food can be used to detox your body. It also means that the products of your digestion are not bombarding your liver so your liver can use all its resources for detoxification.

Recent research has also shown that fasting helps to boost your immune system by kick-starting the production of new white blood cells and HGH (Human Growth Hormone). After about one to three days of a water only fast your body has greatly enhanced stem cell production, which allows it to grow healthy new tissues. This is why fasting can be such a powerful healing tool. After only 24 hours of fasting your leptin levels start to normalize, and your gut has enhanced stem cell production and healing.

For many people, fasting allows them to experience some relief from conditions as diverse as allergies, arthritis and skin and gut disorders. Extended water fasting has also been used by people to successfully heal from a wide range of very serious conditions including cancer and Parkinson's disease – a good option to explore if you are short of money for your treatment.

Deliberately going into a fast takes some determination and courage – 'how will I cope without food'. Because of this, most people find that once they fast they have improved mental clarity and focus so that they feel lighter, more energetic and feel really good about themselves. Everybody's experience of fasting will be different so there are no hard and fast rules about how to do it.

Some of the considerations you need to think about are as follows:

How Long?

Mini (or Intermittent) fast - A daily (or most days) fast of just 12 – 16 hours is a wonderfully effective way to support your detox systems and brain function. It also boosts your production of HGH, which promotes muscle growth and longevity.

To achieve this, all you have to do is to have your evening meal reasonably early and not eat breakfast till a bit later than usual, with no snacks in between – easy really! As I have already mentioned, this will put you into a mild state of ketosis and enhances your transition into becoming fat-adapted, and it helps you feel light and joyful. Because I am already 'fat-adapted' I do not feel any hunger pangs when I do this, so most days my breakfast has morphed into brunch.

24 – 60 hour fast – This can be a good place to start if you have never fasted before, as it will help to give you a feeling for how your body reacts to a fast.

Some argue that you shouldn't fast for any longer than this because your body has an ongoing need for protein and nutrients to build new cells. If you're not fat-adapted, then your body may start to break down muscle protein to provide the sugar it thinks it needs as fuel. This is not a good place to be because it can be quite hard to rebuild muscle mass, and having plenty of muscle increases your metabolic rate and helps you to look and feel good. Once you are fat-adapted there is emerging evidence that 12 - 24 hour fasting can give superior athletic performance and even enhanced muscle building.

Once you are fat-adapted then the stimulation of your production of HGH, which happens when you fast, and your inherent ability to recycle nutrients, is sufficient for you to preserve your muscle mass. This means that long fasts can be profoundly healing for pretty nasty conditions like cancer.

For many people I think that this is plenty long enough for most purposes, and you can certainly feel great after such a fast. My thoughts are, having played with longer periods myself (mainly out of curiosity), is that you should have a really good reason to go for longer and think about getting some professional support if you do so.

The only way you can find out how your body reacts is to do it with an open mind, because it will take some courage to stick with it.

7 or 10 day fast - Some people use this as a seasonal or annual maintenance detox. Unless you are fat-adapted, very experienced at fasting and know how your body reacts to the fast, then it's a good idea to have some professional supervision when you are fasting for longer periods like this.

What to eat or drink during a fast?

Dry fasting - A dry fast is the most extreme type of fasting, where you forego all food and water for short periods. Such a fast is usually done for spiritual reasons, and I do not recommend you do this for detoxing, as you can overload both the liver and kidneys if you are not taking in any fluid.

Water fast - A water fast involves drinking plenty of water or herbal teas while you're fasting. My thoughts are that because just drinking water deprives your body of the nutrients required to help drive the detox pathways, it's probably not the optimum way of detoxing. However, a water fast IS the optimum way of allowing your body to heal from serious conditions. Again – it depends on how your body reacts and why you are choosing to fast.

Bone broth fast - A bone broth fast is the most stress-free way of fasting, particularly for your first time. You can make bone broth by simmering meat bones, preferably with some vegetables and vinegar added, for 24 – 48 hours. Such bone broth contains plenty of minerals, in a form very easily utilized by your body, and useful amounts of antioxidants. More importantly, it also contains useful amounts of protein, particularly in the form of collagen which is very healing, particularly for your gut, but also your skin, cartilage and bones. There are now some great commercial organic products on the market.

Having your bone broth hot is very comforting for your empty stomach, and can enhance your feelings of well-being during a fast.

Juice fast - While doing a juice fast is a very popular way of fasting because you don't get so hungry, I do not recommend a juice fast as an optimum way to detox. This is because juices, particularly fruit juices, all contain a high proportion of fructose which stresses your liver to utilize it, reducing the efficiency of your liver detox. My thoughts are that a bone broth fast produces a more effective detox. A freshly prepared vegetable juice made from carrots, green vegetables and maybe a green apple can work as a much better option than fruit if your body is very fragile and you are trying to help it heal from conditions like cancer.

My experiences - Having played with various types and length of fast, I have personally settled on doing a daily mini-fast of 12 - 16 hours – well most days. Now that I am fat-adapted, I just do not get hungry until mid-late morning. Very occasionally, I will do a one-day bone broth fast, which also works well for me. When I did longer fasts, I used to experience detox headaches for the first day or so, and feel really fantastic when I broke my fast. After using the other detox methods that I have discussed in this chapter, I now find that during a long fast I don't get any headaches and don't feel much different: I feel fantastic all the time. I aim to do a one-day fast about once a season, but it has to fit in with the rest of my life.

12.6
Sleep

Having an adequate sleep is ABSOLUTELY FUNDAMENTAL to the health of your body, brain and your libido. Your body and brain require 7 - 9 hours of sleep per day to allow it to repair, rebuild, and detoxify. You cycle through various stages of sleep repeatedly during the night, the normal pattern being five cycles of somewhere between 80 - 200 minutes each. The average cycle is about 90 minutes long, so five of these takes 7.5 hours, but some people may need as much as 10 hours (120 X 5).

During the earliest cycles you tend to spend more time in the stages of sleep that enhance physical repair, while the last cycle tends to spend more time in REM (Rapid Eye Movement) sleep, which enhances your mental repair. If you go to sleep one to two hours later than usual, this will likely cut out your fifth cycle, and you are likely to wake up to a very foggy brain.

The fluid system in your brain is akin to your lymphatic system which turns over slowly, only around 3 - 4 times per day. When you are asleep the glial cells in your brain contract, which greatly increases the rate of brain fluid flow to assist with the flushing of metabolic waste and toxins from your brain during the night.

You should aim to wake up feeling rested, rejuvenated and rearing to get into your day. If you don't feel this way, then you need to take some serious steps to improve your sleep pattern and treat getting enough sleep as the high priority it needs to be if you're going to achieve wellness.

"Studies show that over time, people who are getting six hours of sleep, instead of seven or eight, begin to feel that they've adapted to that sleep deprivation - they've gotten used to it. But if you look at how they actually do on tests of mental alertness and performance, they continue to go downhill. So there's a point in sleep deprivation when we lose touch with how impaired we are." Philip Gehrman PhD, CBSM (University of Pennsylvania Sleep Center)

Brain imaging studies have found that a sleep -deprived brain looks very similar to a depressed brain.

To help you get better restorative sleep, some factors to consider include:

12.6.1
Bedtime?

We now know that the old adage that one hour's sleep before midnight is worth two hours after has very sound physiological reasons. As I discussed in Chapter 8 The Hormonal Reasons Why Diets Don't Work, leptin is the hormone that co-ordinates the pattern of hormone release during the night to enhance your body's repair processes. The drop in leptin levels, which happens if you don't get to bed early enough, seriously disrupts your body's repair processes and can tell you that you need to raid the fridge and then it will store anything you eat as fat.

Working out your ideal bedtime greatly increases the chances that you'll get both the quantity and quality of sleep that your body needs. The main factor to consider is, when do you need to get up, which is usually determined by your lifestyle, your children, or your dog.

Say, for instance, you need to wake at 6 a.m. to get your day started. If your sleep cycle is the average 90 minutes long, then you will need 7.5 hours of sleep and need to go to bed at 10:30 p.m. Your ideal should be to wake up naturally 5 - 10 minutes before you need to get up, so if you are regularly being woken up by your alarm, then you need to try shifting your bedtime 15 minutes earlier and see how that goes.

If not feeling refreshed when you wake up in the morning is an issue for you, another factor to consider is that your body responds very well to consistency when it comes to sleep. So, going to bed at the same time and getting up at the same time (or at least waking up at the same time) should be one of your goals. That Sunday morning sleep in may not be such a great idea for you, so try being as regular as possible for a couple of weeks to see if things improve.

12.6.2
Melatonin

Your body's daily rhythm means that you start to make the hormone melatonin once it gets dark. Melatonin is not essential for sleep, but you will sleep a lot better if you have normal levels of melatonin. ANY exposure to light during your body's biological night reduces melatonin production and release.

Your circadian rhythm is only capable of being reset by about an hour forward or two hours back each day, which explains why we get 'travel jet lag' and can also have difficulty coping with shift work. The reason why it's easier to travel west than it is to go east, is that it seems to be easier for your body to shift your clock back by delaying the release of melatonin than it is to move it forward. You can also give yourself 'social jet lag' by partying late every night for a three-day weekend, which can make Tuesday morning not much fun. In fact some of the symptoms of a hangover may just be the result of your disrupted daily rhythms.

Not all light is equal, and the blue light that is part of normal sunlight is really important to help you stay alert and enhance your mood during the day. The problem is that most modern electronic devices and light bulbs also produce large amounts of blue light, which makes your brain think it's daytime when you use them at night.

It turns out that it's relatively simple to avoid blue light by using amber colored glasses or sunglasses, which effectively block the blue light from telling your brain that you should be awake. Studies have shown that using blue-blocking glasses during the evening allows you to produce as much melatonin as if it were dark, which can translate into major improvements in sleep quality and mood. If you don't want to use amber glasses you could use a red or orange reading lamp, or candlelight during the evening, which don't emit much blue light.

Another method is to use a program called F.lux on your computer or device, or engage 'Night Shift'. Both automatically adjust the color and brightness of your screen to your time zone, so that when it's dark outside the program blocks some of the blue light coming from your screen, giving it a faint orange color – these are not as effective as blue-blocking glasses.

It's also important to expose yourself to plenty of direct sunlight as much as possible during the day. Our positive relationship with the sun has evolved over a very long time, so the correct advice is 'avoid **sunburn**', not 'avoid **sunlight**'. It is particularly important to get outside, even briefly, as soon as you can after rising. Early exposure to sunlight destroys any remaining melatonin and bumps up your serotonin level, which helps you feel great during the day. This early morning sunlight exposure is also important for normalizing leptin levels in your body.

It is very important that when you're sleeping, you keep your bedroom as completely dark as you can make it. You may even want to invest in blackout curtains, or use a sleep mask.

You may also want to consider taking a melatonin supplement to help you sleep. Some cherries contain plant-based melatonin (phytomelatonin), which is more effective than synthetic melatonin for promoting sleep (and dark cherries also contain powerful antioxidants). Quality tart and sweet cherry juice concentrates contain standardized amounts of melatonin, and they can be taken just before bed to assist you sleeping.

Try taking around 30 µg of phytomelatonin (or 0.5 – 1 mg synthetic melatonin), which is likely to work for most people, to assist you getting into a restful, restorative sleep. Melatonin can also help with jet lag after a long flight. If melatonin doesn't work for you (it does for nearly everyone), try taking 50 - 100 mg of 5-HTP - a natural form of the amino acid tryptophan, the precursor to melatonin – this is likely to help.

12.6.3
Cortisol

Your cortisol level fluctuates in response to your circadian rhythm. Ideally it drops during the evening to reach its lowest point about midnight and starts to rise again between two and four a.m. This increase during the very early morning is a part of what wakes you up ready for your day, and your cortisol should peak about an hour after you get out of bed, which is why the morning tends to be your most productive part of the day.

If you get to bed late, then your cortisol levels will still start to rise, two to three hours after you go to sleep as part of the awakening cycle, which severely restricts the amount of deep, restorative sleep you achieve.

What this all means is that your body's hormonal system is designed to function optimally when you get to bed and go to sleep no later than 10 - 11 p.m. I know this might seem like an impossible task for you, but if you take on board and use some of the strategies discussed in Chapter 14 Detoxing Your Mind, this will become a whole lot easier.

12.6.4
Alcohol

Aside from your hormones, one of the more common causes of waking up tired is the use of alcohol the night before. Although alcohol does tend to make people fall asleep quite quickly, the reality is that alcohol disrupts the REM sleep phase which is when most of the repair and rejuvenation happens in your brain. Try to have several alcohol-free days per week.

If you feel that alcohol might be part of your sleep issues try giving up alcohol for a month. You might be quite shocked at how much better you sleep, and how much more energy you have as a result.

12.6.5
Building Blocks For Sleep

Nutrient deficiencies such as magnesium, potassium, calcium, and the vitamins D and K are relatively common, and all these nutrients work together synergistically to support your wellness and particularly your sleep.

Your liver is particularly susceptible to the influence of the inflammatory eicosanoids produced from Omega-6 oils, so restoring the Omega-6/Omega-3 balance is really important for liver function and sleep.

You will also find my recommendations outlined in Chapter 14 Detoxing Your Mind, will do a lot to support you to maintain healthy sleep patterns.

12.6.6
Prepare Your Bedroom for Sleep

As I have already discussed, it is vital to eliminate light from your bedroom to allow you to have a restful sleep. If you need to use light to help you get to the bathroom in the night, you might want to think about installing a low- intensity salt lamp (or an orange/red light bulb) beside your bed that you can use in the night to see without damaging your melatonin levels.

Keep your bedroom quite cool as studies have shown that the optimum temperature for sleep is between 16 and 21°C (60 to 70°F).

Minimize the presence of alarm clocks etc. close to your body as, for some people, the EMFs (electromagnetic fields) from devices can disrupt your production of melatonin. It's a great idea to turn your Wi-Fi off at night and to put your phone into airplane mode, to reduce your nighttime EMF exposure. Some people who are very sensitive to EMFs even go so far as to install a kill switch beside the bed to cut off all power to their house as they sleep, which can be very effective for enhancing their sleep quality.

12.6.7
Go with the Flow

Getting enough sleep is really essential for good health, so it's important that if you feel sleepy you listen to your body and get some extra sleep – learn to nap.

There should be no shame in feeling that you need to sleep in the afternoon. For me, if I have had a run of bad sleeps, an afternoon siesta at the weekend acts as a reset to get me back into sleeping well again.

If you do go for a nap, I suggest you don't initially put a timer on. Your body might just need a power nap of around 20 minutes - NASA has shown that a nap like this improved astronaut performance by 34% and alertness by 54%. For some people, having longer than this disrupts their usual night-time sleep cycle, while others may need 2 - 3 hours. Listen to your body and learn what suits you best.

CHAPTER 13

Move Your Body

"Exercise is the closest thing modern science has found to a wonder drug. Exercise does not just make your body stronger, but it actually works its magic to protect and preserve brain function."

David Perlmutter, MD

There is little doubt that most of us in this modern world could do with getting some more exercise, which would make a major contribution to our health and well-being.

Not surprisingly, your HGH (Human Growth Hormone) levels are at their highest when you are a child and growing rapidly, and they normally decline after puberty and as you age. However, maintaining high levels of HGH can do very nice things to your rate of aging, and the way you exercise can have a powerful impact on your production of HGH – it's not just about doing more, it's also about doing it better.

The second factor that best predicts the rate your body ages at, is the length of the telomeres or caps that protect the end of your chromosomes from fraying (like the little aglets on the end of your shoelaces).

If preserving your youthful vigor, looks, libido and strength is important to you, then naturally enhancing your HGH levels and the length of your telomeres are the two best ways of helping you feel and look younger. The steps I outline in Chapter 16 Your 'Rapid Reset' Plan, have been shown to enhance your production of HGH and the length of your telomeres, but the way you exercise can also have a powerful positive effect on your rate of aging.

Exercise also has a powerful impact on your brain function by stimulating the production of BDNF (Brain-Derived Neurotrophic Factor), which is heavily involved in maintaining your memory, your ability to learn and your happiness. Exercise has been shown to be more effective at enhancing your mood and reducing depression than any antidepressant drug.

However, as I have already pointed out in Section 7.5.8 Exercise and Progesterone, it doesn't take an awful lot of exercise to mess with your cortisol levels and your sex hormones, in a way that can accelerate your rate of aging. You are the only one who can judge where your sweet spot is so that you get enough activity to get the powerful benefits of exercise, but you don't overdo it.

To figure out what you need to change about the way you move (or don't move) requires you to get very honest with yourself about what your goals are and what feels good for you.

Let's face it, if you sign yourself up for a season at a Cross Fit Gym and, after a few sessions you find that the high-intensity workout just doesn't do it for you. It doesn't make your body feel good, and everyone else seems to be able to do it so much better than you. Are you going to be able to keep this up in the long-term, just for your health's sake? I don't think so.

If you can find something you love doing that gets your body moving some more, then go with that, because that is the exercise you will be able to keep up in the long-term, which is the important thing. So here are some thoughts which may help you to find the movement that works for you.

13.1
Dance

Does moving your body to the sound of music appeal to you? Then find some form of dance class that you can do locally that feels like fun to you. Maybe it's the high-intensity Jazzercise or Zumba Fitness classes where you can get high on the rhythm, build some muscle and increase flexibility.

Maybe it's a partner dance such as Tango, Salsa or Ceroc that appeals to you that you can have fun with your partner, or go out and meet somebody new.

Or maybe it's just dancing at home to your favorite music at the end of your day, which becomes your meditation and your way of getting in touch with your feminine side.

13.2
Swimming

Does swimming come naturally to you or are you like me, and sink if you stop moving? Swimming provides a very complete workout for your body by using every muscle and both firming and shaping your body without putting any stress on your joints. The other lovely quality of water is that it is so much denser than air, that every little movement becomes like a resistance workout for your whole body, so you get results faster.

Even better, because the water is cold, it sucks the warmth out of you so that you burn more fuel during swimming than any other exercise, just to maintain your core temperature. Michael Phelps (multiple Olympic gold medal swimmer) ate 12,000 calories a day when he was in training (the average man eats 2,500 calories per day). Granted he normally trained 3 – 4 hours a day, but it was the loss of body heat to the water that meant he had to eat so much to maintain his body weight.

13.3
Walking

Walking is another wonderful activity, especially if you can do it out in nature. Power walking on a treadmill with music blasting in your ears is going to have a completely different effect on your body and mind from going walking in nature, being grateful for the sights, smells and sounds, and breathing in some new additions to your microbiome from the air around you.

It is easy to turn such a walk into a walking meditation that does wonders for your state of mind, and the exposure to sunlight will enhance the amount of vitamin D your body produces. Or maybe it's an opportunity for you to get together with, and bond with, somebody from your tribe and chat about what's going on in your life – also very important for your stress levels.

13.4
Cycling

Like walking, cycling is another wonderful activity, especially if you can do it out in nature rather than in a gym.

Your knee is one of the most complicated joints in your body so, not surprisingly, many people end up with knee issues – especially runners. Cycling regularly is a very effective way of building up the muscles and ligaments that hold your knee together because it's a flowing exercise without any jarring impact.

After a knee injury in the mountains, 40 years ago, I had an ongoing weakness which caused me problems for several years. I then moved to a city and started biking to work most days, for only a couple of years, but I have not had any knee issues since then.

13.5
Burst Training

If one of your objectives in life is to gain lean muscle mass, then Burst Training is one of the best ways to achieve this and massively boost your HGH levels at the same time.

Burst Training also goes by several names, such as Tabata's or HIIT (High-Intensity Interval Training). To get started with Burst Training you need to find something you love doing, that gets your body moving very vigorously, then go with that, again because that is the exercise that you will be able to keep up in the long-term.

At its most basic, Burst Training consists of you doing an activity that will get you COMPLETELY breathless after 20 - 30 seconds of hard effort.

It really doesn't matter what the exercise is; it can be anything from using gym equipment like an elliptical trainer or weights, skipping or sprinting up stairs or a hill in the sunshine, sprinting on a bike, or sprinting in the pool. Whatever appeals to you is great.

After the first breathless phase, what happens next depends on how long you want to spend doing this activity. If your recovery periods are 90 seconds (a common choice), the whole process will only take 20 minutes. Professor Tabata only allowed 10 seconds recovery, so the whole process took less than four minutes.

Extensive research has shown that such an intense activity trains and enhances your body far more effectively than long, slower workouts (often referred to as Cardio) and it greatly boosts your HGH production and the length of your telomeres. Only four minutes of Tabata's can get you better fitness gains than an entire hour of running on the treadmill. But, if you do it properly, it should be really, really hard work. Your choice!

If you decide to give it a go, you ideally need to design your program so that you can repeat each burst eight times and still function afterwards (even though you may feel you might die). Your recovery period in between bursts can be as short as 10 seconds or as long as 90 seconds - your choice; the only stipulation is that you have to keep moving gently in between bursts.

Warm up gently first. As you might imagine, you will need to start this activity fairly slowly to ease your body into it. This might look like you doing only one or two full bursts and the rest at a much slower pace. You should only do this once, or a maximum twice, per week as your muscles will need recovery time if you do this properly. You will also need to eat more protein than you have been used to, just to feed your muscle growth and more flax seed oil than you have been used to, just to prevent damaging inflammation and fuel your muscle recovery.

As you might have gathered from the way I have written this section I did have a few goes at burst training, but I quickly decided that taking some care about the way I eat, and detoxing my body and mind, is my preferred pathway to boosting my HGH levels and lengthening my telomeres so that I can live a long and joyful life. Having said that I do get enough exercise to remain fit enough to do a hard days skiing, or do acrobalance with my sons without feeling dead the next day.

Your overall wellness will benefit if you incorporate more frequent movement into your life. Your brain is particularly sensitive to the benefits of exercise, but it benefits most from you doing something that lifts your heart rate, perhaps by going for a walk around the block or preferably in a park or as natural environment as possible, or some Tai Chi before breakfast or at lunchtime. Or you could simply put a reminder on your phone or computer for you to take a walk to the water cooler every hour.

WHATEVER WORKS FOR YOU, AS LONG AS YOU DO IT.

CHAPTER 14

Detoxing Your Mind

"Live today. Not yesterday. Not tomorrow. Just today. Inhabit your moments. Don't rent them out to tomorrow."

Jerry Spinelli

You will find this chapter rather more subjective than anything I have written so far. At the same time, I would like you to take on board the idea that this is the most important chapter in the book. I say this because even if you detox your body and change the way you eat, you will find that in time you will revert to the way you were if, at the same time, you do not detox your mind – it is that important. This is likely one of the key reasons why all the other things you have tried in the past have not worked for you in the long term.

Because the way your mind works is the sum of all your personal experiences, this means that choosing the best way of detoxing your mind is going to be a very personal decision based on what resonates with you right now. It's much less science-based. Having said that, there is a lot of research being done which demonstrates the very beneficial effects that detoxing your mind in various ways has on your overall wellness.

I have been on my own journey to detox my mind for about 25 years. This chapter is about the resources that I have come across, that I have investigated and/or used. You may not find what you're looking for in my suggestions. I hope you at least take on the idea that detoxing your mind is really important if you want to be well and live the life of your dreams, so that it motivates you to search for a way that does work for you.

As you have seen, your stress hormones adrenaline and cortisol can severely disrupt all the other hormone systems in your body and push you into 'tend and befriend' mode. So widespread is this disruption that you CANNOT hope to get all your other hormone systems in balance if you do not find a way to de-stress.

Your body is not able to distinguish between traffic jams, your boss yelling at you, or a wolf chasing you. The key thing for you to recognize is that, while some of your stress levels come from physical causes, like a driver pushing into your traffic lane without signaling. However the vast majority of stressors in your life come from your emotional response to people and happenings in your life and the mind talk your ego creates as a result.

These are the stressors in your mind which, if they are not detoxed or cleared, have an amazing ability to fester in your mind over time. To me there are two components to the process of detoxing your mind.

Relaxation Response. This is using your inbuilt relaxation response to reset your stress hormones, by using short-term stress relief techniques. For example, you could try breathing, meditation, prayer, mindfulness techniques, being grateful, yoga, tai chi, massage or soak in a hot bath. These can assist your body to actively move out of stress response and into the relaxation response and you should use them every day. Research at Harvard has shown that using such techniques can have a major positive impact on your life.

"May the Force be with you." Master Yoda

Mind Mastery. Achieving this is the second aspect of mind detox, and to me it is equally important. It's learning to be the master of your mind in a way that allows you to clear yourself of ego-driven mind-talk about your past and your fears for the future. For most people, this mind-talk contributes significantly to the levels of distress they experience. When you start to achieve mind mastery and spend more time in the present, you'll find you start to create the life of your dreams.

"The force is an energy field created by all living things. It surrounds us and penetrates us; it binds the galaxy together." Obi-Wan Kenobi

I find it a bit bizarre, in a world where quantum physicists such as Einstein and Bohm are celebrated for their insights into the nature of our universe, yet many people still struggle to understand the role of energy in our everyday lives and our health. The concepts of quantum physics tell us that there are no separate parts to anything and that everything and everyone is connected to everything and everyone else; we are not separate. Equally, pretending that what is going on in your mind does not affect your body does not reflect the science.

Quantum physics also tell us that matter isn't really made of energy, but simply is energy – that includes you!

Your own life force, or energy, is centered in your mind, and scientists from Princeton have now established that our minds and our intent can alter the outcome of external events with no physical intervention.

So we really can, and do, shape our own reality with our conscious intent. That's what the movie 'The Secret' was all about – how The Law of

Attraction (probably more accurately called The Law of Creation) works, WHETHER YOU BELIEVE IN IT OR NOT.

14.1
Relaxation Response

As I have discussed, failing to de-stress greatly disrupts the smooth running of all your hormone systems and your body as a whole. Any stressful event or thought that causes the release of the stress hormones, adrenaline and cortisol, puts you into the 'tend and befriend' mode where you will find it a struggle to take care of yourself, rather than everyone else.

Initiating the relaxation response is the key to getting your body out of the stress hormone mode, but how to achieve this is different for everybody. For most people, blobbing in front of a TV set does NOT, by itself, tell your body that it does not need to be in stress mode. To get your hormones back in balance, you probably need to guide your body into the relaxation response actively.

In this chapter I am aiming to help you find some tools that you can use, depending on what suits you best, at this time in your life. It will likely change over time.

14.1.1
Belly - Breathing

The simplest way to tell your body that you are 'safe' and it does not need to be in stress mode is to breathe into your belly consciously. Doing this may feel quite strange because most people tend to breathe into the top half of their lungs with relatively shallow, rapid breaths. Doing so is a toned down version of what you do when you're panting or stressed.

Please take a moment to shut your eyes. Place your left hand on your heart and your right hand on your belly. Take several moderately deep breaths ensuring that your right hand on your belly moves and your left-hand doesn't. This simple act sends a very powerful signal to your brain that you are 'safe' and that you do not need to produce any more stress hormones. Use it as often as you need to help you to calm down and move your body out of stress mode.

Once you have done this a few times and it no longer feels strange to breathe in this way, you will find that you can belly breathe without having to put your hand on your belly. You will then find you are able to use belly

Mind hack your 'day.'

Try ending your 'day' when you arrive home from work in the evening – which means starting 'tomorrow' in the evening.

Give yourself 10 – 20 minutes as soon as you arrive home to initiate your relaxation response. This will start a virtuous cycle by clearing any rubbish in your head from your day, which will drastically improve your relationship with your family during the evening, which will help you to get to sleep at the right time for you, and which will make the rest of your 'day' so much more productive.

I'm sure your ego is saying that you don't have time for this in your life? Yet you will find that when you have properly relaxed your evening will go so much more smoothly that you will get more done. You effectively create MORE time.

breathing, even in public, whenever you feel stressed or overwhelmed.

The more you use this technique, the better you become at being conscious of your stress levels. With some practice, you will be able to tune in to consciously reduce the levels of the destructive stress hormones running around in your body.

14.1.2
Sleep

Restful sleep is a state when your body and mind are in deep rest and relaxation. Going to sleep does not necessarily mean that your body goes into the relaxation response, so you will have a much better sleep if you make sure you engage the relaxation response BEFORE you try to sleep.

I have already discussed sleep in Chapter 12.6 Sleep, so I will merely reiterate that getting adequate deep and restful sleep is absolutely essential. It's a very powerful way to restore and repair your mind and body. If you're feeling tired and brain-fogged and that it would feel really nice to have a cat nap, you should do your level best to honor that feeling and create a way that you can have a 20-minute power-nap. Ask a friend or your partner if they can look after the children for half an hour.

Your body telling you that you need sleep is not something you should feel ashamed of or ignore. I know your ego (and your partner?) will be reeling off a list of all the things you need to do, you can't possibly afford the time to sleep right now.

However, the wonderful thing is that having a nap is NEVER time wasted. You will find when you have rested, that your work goes so much more efficiently that you will actually get more done. You effectively create MORE time.

Listen to your body and love yourself enough to honor its need for rest and repair.

"...Your body telling you that it wants to sleep is not something you should feel ashamed of or ignore."

14.1.3
Initiating the Relaxation Response

The relaxation response is when you are in an altered state, where your mind is still awake, but body and mind are in deep relaxation. It is the opposite of the stress response, or 'Tend and Befriend'.

Watching television or browsing Facebook do NOT initiate the relaxation response; so you need to find a technique that works for you to consciously attain this state.

Relaxation response, meditation and prayer are, to me, terms that are effectively the same, which may be not how they are commonly understood. Some people may respond negatively to the idea of meditating, perhaps for religious reasons. Studies at Harvard University have shown that your body initiates exactly the same relaxation response as you can get from meditation with a 'mantra' by using ANY repeated phrase. You could use a phrase that has some religious significance to you, if that works for you.

Many studies have shown that the relaxation response provides deeper rest and repair to your body than sleep. This could be because there is increased harmony between the different parts of your brain during the relaxation response, which is not seen in either the wakeful state or in a deep sleep. One study of cancer patients who started meditating showed that within only eight weeks their gene expression had made positive changes – so you don't have to be your genes.

You achieving the relaxation response is so important for reducing your ego's mind talk, and your wellbeing, that I have given you more resources at www.ITookCharge/RelaxationResponse In there I talk about how to use the latest technology to make it really easy, as well as some of the more traditional approaches.

14.1.4
Is Meditation Right for You?

You may find that conventional meditation doesn't feel right for you. It may even feel like a form of torture to be sitting still and focusing on your breath or listening to audio tracks. It is possible that you may be subconsciously avoiding meditation because you don't really want to connect with the real you underneath all your ego's b***s*** mind talk. Your ego may feel quite threatened by you starting a process to take back the control of your mind because it involves that scary thing called change.

Another potential reason why you may find meditation difficult is that some women, when they are in their feminine energy, may not feel comfortable sitting still. You may feel it is more in your nature to move and flow. So, while a man – or a woman who spends much time in her masculine energy – may be comfortable with sitting in silence to meditate, this may not be right for you at all.

In many spiritual traditions, the feminine form of meditation was as sacred dance – any form of dance or ritual movement, done with the intention to connect with your divine feminine. In other words, anything goes. What sacred dance means to you is entirely your choice.

It might be useful, especially initially, to keep it a bit light-hearted. Create a playlist of music you only sing along to in the shower or feel a bit silly admitting you enjoy to other people. Really try to let yourself go and dance like no one is watching and, if you can manage it, do it in front of a full-length mirror.

Walking in nature can also be turned into a walking meditation if you choose to focus on your time for walking as a precious luxury, when you can engage all your senses rather than as something you have to do to get your daily exercise. Scan the horizon which exercises and relaxes the powerful muscles in your eyes; notice the colors of the leaves on the trees and the way they rustle in the wind; the color and scent of flowers you pass; and feel your stress levels drop as you relax into the moment. This process is a world away from treating your walk as a 'must do to lose some belly fat or get you fit', whilst striding along with music blasting into your ears.

14.1.5
Get an Oxytocin Fix

As I explained in Chapter 3 It's Not You; It's Your Hormones, increasing your levels of oxytocin can work very powerfully to create feelings of love, bonding, calmness and connection, as oxytocin directly counteracts the effects of cortisol. If your cortisol levels are high, they can contribute directly to feelings of loneliness, depression, burnout or rapid aging.

High cortisol/low oxytocin can also mean that you may struggle with your relationships because it feels easier to detach, disconnect, and walk away. This can potentially be very dangerous for your intimate relationships. But it can also mean because you don't have the energy to connect with friends and don't want to interact with people, you could get into a downward spiral that could potentially end with depression. For women, in particular, interacting with your 'tribe' can be a very important way of lifting your mood and feeling good about your life – 'befriend'.

Because cortisol and oxytocin directly oppose each other, an important way to lower your stress hormone levels is to work on ways of increasing your oxytocin levels. Some of the simple ways to increase your oxytocin levels are to play with your child or your partner, laugh a lot, or just give something of yourself to someone else.

Playing or cuddling with a soft, strokeable pet like a cat or dog is also a way to increase your oxytocin levels. Not surprisingly, many studies have shown that you heal faster if you have a pet in your life. You're likely to have lower blood pressure, less risk of heart disease, and reduced anxiety and feelings of depression from your interaction with a cuddly pet.

A very powerful way to de-stress yourself is to find someone close to you and share with them a genuine 'oxytocin hug' – a hug lasting around 20 seconds or so. Your body is programmed from birth to respond to skin contact with the production of oxytocin. The more skin in contact and the longer the contact is for, the more oxytocin you will produce.

Kissing is also important, as your lips are packed with 100 times more nerve endings than your fingertips, so a real snog with your partner can have a wonderful effect on destressing you at the end of your day (or any other time).

If you don't find you have any time in your day to destress in any other way, then sliding naked into bed and spooning your naked partner, or snuggling your young child who is causing such chaos in your life, will do wonderful things to melt away your feelings of stress and rebalance your hormone levels.

Getting your oxytocin fix in non-sexual ways, as I have suggested above, is also important for supporting your libido. The wonderful thing about having a fired-up libido is that this is likely to lead to lovemaking, either with a partner or yourself and then, for women, oxytocin and dopamine (your pleasure hormone) are the two hormones that spike really high when you orgasm. According to several sources, multiple orgasms, (ideally at least three) gives you pretty much a complete hormonal reset.

If you don't have a partner or you want to masturbate, then consciously think about it as making love to yourself. Maybe try a hot bath by candlelight, enhanced by your favorite essential oil (cinnamon, clary sage, fennel geranium, jasmine, neroli, rose, ylang-ylang are some of the suggested oils that may promote sexual energy or libido). Maybe play some sensuous music. Take time to revel in the whole experience with lots of stroking yourself all over to enhance your oxytocin levels, which will enhance the intensity of your orgasms. Above all, play with what feels good and enjoy yourself.

14.1.6
Massage

To receive, or even give a massage is another powerful way of getting an oxytocin fix. While you may find that some forms of massage feel better to you than others, it's pretty hard to go wrong with a massage. Just the act of having somebody using their hands on your skin and your muscles feels pretty delicious.

Certain forms of massage are designed to achieve some therapeutic effect, to work through some form of muscle issues or tight spots you might be experiencing. Some of these can be quite intense, verging on the painful, such as deep tissue or sports massage. Relaxation massage is more focused on the feel-good aspect, but a good therapist will still find those muscle knots and help alleviate them.

Massage therapy improves your circulation, enhancing the delivery of oxygen and nutrients to your muscles and helping to remove waste products. It also induces the relaxation response, lowering your heart and breathing rate, your blood pressure and enhancing your immune system.

Swapping massages with your partner can be a wonderful win-win situation.

14.1.7
Yoga, Tai Chi, Qigong

All of these exercise systems are based on ancient Eastern teachings designed to help you enhance the energy flow in your body, move and stretch your muscles and joints and to assist you to connect with your breathing. Very importantly, they also are very powerful techniques for getting your body and mind out of 'stress' mode and into 'rest and digest' mode. There are other similar techniques, but these are the three that I have tried.

My personal favorite is yoga because I have had back issues off and on for many years and I find the poses taught in the class in my local town are great for maintaining flexibility and is a very effective preventative system for not having back issues. I have tried doing yoga at home, but I find it very easy to put it off to tomorrow. I also really enjoy the energy of a class where everyone is there for the same purpose - to enhance their well-being.

14.2
Mind Mastery

"The problem with our ego is that it is made up of only past experiences, and we are allowing it to use our past to create our present and our future" - Andy Shaw

If you are like most people, your ego, or mind talk, or little self, or the nutter in your head – whatever you want to call it (I am going to refer to it as your ego) is very active in your head generating conflict. It occupies a lot of mental energy and mind space with criticisms, insults and degrading thoughts of yourself and your actions or, even more destructive, by judging other people.

The problem is that you've been having this conversation with yourself for so long that you now think that your ego is you – it's not. It's just a third party renting space in your head which, more often than not, sabotages you at the turning points in your life. The ones when you could have allowed greatness into your life, but you don't follow through with the commitments you made to yourself.

If you let it, your ego will come up with all these reasons from the past as to why it would be dangerous to change, or it will take you into fear of the future and all these 'what if' scenarios of what might happen if you were to change. So, the role of the ego is to keep you 'safe', based on your past experiences. The unfortunate side-effect of this is that it also keeps you small, by trying to keep you from taking the risk of trying something new. Doing something new will inevitably expand your life – maybe not always in the way you hoped, but it does anyway.

The best way to silence your ego is to be fully present in the moment, right NOW. I hope this chapter can give you some techniques to help you to master your ego, to allow you to look at the world in a more positive light, and to start to create your own reality.

Let's start the journey towards getting the mastery of your mind, so you have it on your side to help create the life of your dreams.

14.2.1
Your Ego

"Am I in control of my mind, or is it in control of me" - Andy Shaw

If you don't like the way your life is right now, then you haven't been making conscious choices to direct it. You have just been going along with the choices your ego has made for you, as I was – harsh, but true.

I believe that the vast majority of the cells in my brain and body want me to be happy, healthy and successful. However, like most people, a tiny proportion of cells somewhere in my left-brain are highly skilled in creating stories and thought patterns that can really derail me feeling good about myself and, at the same time, make it really hard to make some real changes in my life. Your ego is very clever at coming up with mind-talk that tells you, "You're not good enough," or, "You shouldn't have done that," or, "What will people think of you?" It can and does add a significant amount of stress into your life.

Typically, your storyteller ego centers on events that have occurred in the past, or about what might occur in the future. While it can be useful sometimes, warning you to make changes with caution, this mind-talk is more often a waste of time and energy. It can be very emotionally draining, and a block to you making the tangible progress you'd like to see in your life. Although a fairly extreme way of looking at it, many people may feel as if they are at war with their brain as to who has mastery over it: your ego or you.

As I discussed in Chapter 2 How Your Brain Works, we now know that when you are growing up your mind is like a sponge. Until you are about six or seven you are not really capable of passing judgment on what you hear, so you tend to believe everything told to you. This means that it is a very rare individual who arrives in adulthood without some form of false beliefs along the lines of, "I'm not lovable", "I'm not enough", "I'm not good enough", or, "I don't deserve this".

Another factor highlighted by recent research started in the USA, is the significant influence of ACE's (Adverse Childhood Experiences) on your long- term health. The ongoing research has highlighted a stunning link between childhood trauma and the chronic diseases people develop as adults, as well as social and emotional problems. The ACE's included in the studies range from personal experiences such as physical abuse or emotional neglect, to the behavior of other family members, such as a parent who's an alcoholic or the victim of domestic violence, to the disappearance of a parent through divorce, death, abandonment or being imprisoned.

Of great concern is that they found that the toxic stress from such childhood trauma was very common, affecting two-thirds of children from employed, white, middle-class, educated people. The higher the number of ACE's in your past, the higher your risk of health, social and emotional problems, yet most people usually experienced more than one type of ACE. If you want to check out your ACE score, go to www.ITookCharge.nz/ACE

You might think that it should be relatively easy to get past such experiences and mind-talk as you get into adult life, but the reality is that your mind heals in a very different way from your body. Your physical body has an amazing ability to heal itself as long as you feed it the right building blocks and help it detoxify. For your mind, while you absolutely can heal from any event from your past, it can be a long and slow process to find the right way for YOU to detoxify and get rid of your pain from the past and your negative self- beliefs. This is definitely not a 'one size fits all' process.

"I can't express anger. I grow a tumor instead". Woody Allen

Many people choose to not even try, going through their lives almost on autopilot, leaving most of their choices to their ego. In fact, where you are in your life is the sum of all the choices you have made so far. There is no point in blaming somebody else for where your life is now, because the reality is you chose it – every bit of it. Probably a lot of your choices were unconscious, but you have possibly also made some conscious choices that helped to keep you small because it was less challenging that way.

Did you have an emotional response to that idea? Anger maybe? Or disbelief? If so, that was your ego reacting to the idea that you might be going to change something, with uncertain or challenging outcomes. Just observe your response and feel what is really true for you and the emotional response will dissolve.

"Reality is negotiable." Albert Einstein

Depending on how you tackle it, mastering your mind can take a lot of effort and potentially take a very long time but, believe me, if you haven't already done it, it's worth it.

It involves you choosing to own the power you have to bring your mind into the present. Make a conscious decision to stop worrying about what has happened in the past or what might happen in the future, and to move deliberately towards your goals. Since nothing stands still, your choices are either moving you towards where you want to be or carrying you away from your dream life.

It also involves you taking full, unconditional responsibility for everything that happens in your life. No more blaming or judging other people for what has happened or saying "it's not my fault". This process is not going to be easy for you, but the rewards for you taking on that responsibility are huge.

14.2.2
How to Gain Mind Mastery

The first step in getting out of negative thought-loops, or ego talk, is actually to recognize that you're hooked into these loops. For some of us, being conscious of what our brain is saying to us comes more naturally. For others it's a real challenge to observe what our brain is doing.

So what do I mean by being conscious? It is estimated that your brain is processing around 16 trillion bits of information per second, but the average person is only aware of about 2,000, so there is an awful lot of stuff going on in your brain that you are normally unaware of. What you are aware of is usually only the bits that your ego thinks are important or threatening, based on past experiences. However, ideally one of your objectives in this process would be to become more aware of what is going on in your brain – more conscious.

I'm sure you've all heard about the power of positive thinking, but it's not easy to think positively for the majority of the time. Possibly a more useful way to look at it, is to try to develop awareness of the negative thoughts that are running loops in your head and try to eliminate these. If you can achieve this, by systematically paying attention to your negative thought patterns and not allowing them to continue, then you are automatically thinking more positively.

I found once I became conscious of my thought-loops, I could also become aware of how they made my body feel. Did I feel anxious, fearful, or angry? If they didn't make me feel positive, then I learned I only have to wait 90 seconds for the chemistry of that emotional response to dissipate so I can take control.

This is where you can start to use techniques such as talking to your ego and saying, "Thank you for sharing, but I'm not interested in thinking about that right now." Or, "I choose not to think about tomorrow, I choose to go to sleep". Are you present right now? Just by asking yourself that question you flick yourself into the NOW.

I now know that it only took 90 seconds for the biochemistry of emotions in my brain to capture me, and then the biochemistry was gone. So, if something made me angry, I was unconsciously choosing to stay with the anger rather than letting it go as soon as my biochemistry changed. So when you have a row with someone you love and notice yourself staying angry with them; ask yourself "why am I choosing to stay angry with someone I love?" I have found that simple question to be a real relationship changer.

There are, of course, multiple ways to achieve the intended result. You just have to find a way that suits you and helps you to take control of your mind talk.

I have found that paying attention to my mind-talk is vitally important for my mental well-being. Making the decision that internally abusing myself is not an acceptable behavior was a major step towards finding a deep inner peace. The most powerful technique that I have found to help me achieve this and move towards the life of my dreams has been the process of learning to 'Debug My Mind'.

14.2.3
Debug Your Mind

The movie 'The Secret' was centered on how to use 'The Law of Attraction' to create the life of your dreams, particularly financial dreams. It has been watched by over 200 million people and has spawned a thriving industry around teaching personal development to help you literally create your own life. I have personally read quite a few interpretations of this idea.

Unfortunately, the success rate achieved by the students of most of these teachers is abysmally low. According to recent Credit Suisse data, the number of people who achieve a net worth of over US$1 million is still just 0.7% of the world's population. The majority of people who start down the personal development route have achieving wealth as one of their major goals, so why aren't we suddenly seeing an abundance of millionaires?

According to the author, Andy Shaw, most teachers in this space are really clever and have the right mind-set to achieve success for themselves, but haven't figured out how to teach other people to achieve the right mind-set. You may well be thinking that that's not true because some people do succeed; yes they do, but not many. You probably also don't want that to be true, because that may mean that the nagging thought in the back of your mind that you personally can never become successful might also be true.

That was certainly the situation for me, having tried several different approaches over the years. I then came across Andy Shaw, who believes he has created the system to reliably teach you how to achieve the required success mind-set, which comes as a recently produced two book series called Creating a Bug-Free Mind and Using a Bug-Free Mind.

In these books Shaw likens your mind to a computer that has been contaminated by junk or bugs, to the point where it starts to run really slowly or even freezes up, so you need to do a reset so that it will run smoothly again. Similarly, your mind accumulates 'bugs' such as limiting self- beliefs, judgments, misunderstandings, assumptions and other beliefs about the way things are to you.

The most pervasive junk is your memories from the past. This is where your ego spends most of its time because it seems 'safe' because it's been there before. Your ego is not capable of logical thought, so it relies totally on experiences from the past. If, in a given situation in the past, you did something and got a certain result, as far as your ego knows the same response will have the same result in a future situation. To your ego, that's safety because it 'knows' what will happen. There is no need to take the risk of doing something new, because 'dragons might live there'.

Unfortunately, this also means that your attempts to change the way you think and to change your life have a strong tendency to be sabotaged by your ego, which seeks to keep you in the past, where you are 'safe'. This is the force that keeps you small or stuck in an unhappy relationship or an unfulfilling job because it's too 'risky' to break out and follow your dreams.

Being in control of your mind means being able to live in the present and accept WHAT IS - being able to forgive, not judging, knowing how to let go of feelings of worry and powerlessness, and much, much more.

My way of using Andy's books has been to read a page or two at a time, usually just before I go to bed, and then reread the next day to really allow the lessons to sink in. A fascinating part of the process for me has been that, if I have had a challenge in my day, I always seem to be reading a section that evening, that's relevant to my challenge. It helps me to take that particular bug out of my mind and look at life differently.

Does it work? It has for me.

14.2.4
Consolidate the Positive

This is self-directed neuroplasticity. You are rewiring your brain for joy, pleasure, and happiness.

The neuropsychologist Rick Hanson, author of the book Hardwiring Happiness, taught me about how our brains tend to operate as though we have 'Velcro' for the bad, and 'Teflon' for the good experiences in life. His research suggests that this negativity bias means your brain reacts more intensely to bad news, compared to how it responds to good news.

If you take this idea into your relationships, this means that to develop strong, long-lasting relationships that thrive, you need to have a ratio of five times more positive interactions than negative interactions. This could well be a major reason why research suggests that only about 30% of couples are considered semi-happy or better.

Dr Hanson suggests that the most effective way is to 'take in the good', noticing something good that happens and taking three simple steps to turn it into a lasting emotional memory.

1.   Notice a positive experience.

This activates a positive mental state. Choose a positive experience that happened recently and consider it fully. Perhaps it was a physical pleasure like inhaling the scent of roses on a walk, or an emotional pleasure like feeling close to someone who matters to you.

2.   Enrich it.

Next, install the positive experience in your mind. Get a feeling for how it affected you on a sensory level. Notice the associated feelings of wellness, sights, smells, and how it made you feel. Allow yourself to open to the feeling and let it fill your body, mind and spirit. As Dr Hanson recommends, find something fresh or novel in it. Recognize how it could nourish you, which then rewires your brain away from the bad aspects and toward what is good for you.

3.   Absorb it.

Let the positive feelings from this experience seep into you, providing soothing and calmness, filling you with gratitude and positive emotions. Create the feeling of being on your own side and let it sink into you. Let the good become part of you. Surrender to it — not in a passive manner, but in a way that serves your highest good.

This is self-directed neuroplasticity. You are rewiring your brain for joy, pleasure and happiness. You could try to start making these ideas into a habit by consciously practicing them daily for the next three days. If you can find the inspiration to continue for three weeks, by then it will be a habit.

14.2.5
The Importance of Now

Time is the most pervasive illusion to the human psyche because there is actually only NOW; there is no yesterday and no tomorrow. If this seems a bit weird to you, think of a simple task and then try to do it tomorrow or half an hour ago. You can't, can you? You can only do it NOW, in the present! That is because there is only now, and you live only in the now, so your life is timeless.

It's important to realize that NOW is when you create your future, so if you are unhappy now, the chances are that you will create an unhappy future. Our life situation is as it is, as a result of time and the (usually) unconscious choices our ego has made along the way.

You might not realize that you have a choice about what you think, and even how you feel. I used to think I was a product of my brain. I had no idea that I had some say about how I responded to emotions surging through me.

Let's try a little test to see how good you are at staying present. Please think of a time in your life when you were really joyful for a few minutes, and life felt just perfect. Now the fun bit – focus your whole attention on that event, try and remember the scene like a movie playing in your mind, the sounds and smells, your feelings, making it as vivid as possible.

How long were you able to stay in that scene without any other thoughts intervening? The first time I tried this I managed about three or four seconds before my ego chipped in with a comment. A very effective way of enhancing your mind mastery is practice this exercise regularly until you can hold such a joyful memory for a good 15 seconds – preferably longer.

14.2.6
How Do I Spend More Time in Now?

The simplest way is just to ask yourself the question 'am I present', because as soon as you are conscious enough to think about being present, then you are.

When you are fully present you are just aware of your environment and what's going on around you, but you are not reacting to it in any way or analyzing anything. See how long you can go before you have your next thought.

Being present is where the magic happens. Your subconscious mind has space to come up with solutions to any issues or problems you may have in your life, without any reference to the past, or interruption or confusion coming from your ego's commentary on what you should do, based on the past.

A very powerful way to settle the mind is to pay attention to your breathing. The chances are that if your brain is awash with negative self-talk, then you will be feeling tense and edgy and taking fairly shallow breaths into your chest. This is where 14.1.1 Belly – Breathing, comes in again, for not only are you sending a very powerful signal to your limbic system that you are 'safe', but it also feels good because you are fully present in that moment. This is why many ways of initiating the relaxation response, like meditation, yoga and qigong all place a large emphasis on being aware of your breathing.

14.2.7
Make Now Count

Another powerful tool is to pay close attention to the sensory information coming into your body as you are doing things. Ask yourself, "How does it feel to be here, doing this?" Pay attention to really tasting the food you put in your mouth. Try to identify the flavors and see how well they are balanced, or would the hint of another spice in there make it even better next time you cook it?

Pay attention to the texture of your foods and how they feel in your mouth. If you are enjoying a particularly delicious creamy dessert, try sensuously feeding your partner a mouthful... or two... or three. Have fun with your food, and preferably share it with the people around you. It's really hard to engage in negative self-talk when you are having fun in the moment.

For many people, one of the quickest ways to shift your mood is through the use of smell. Light some incense, a smudge stick, or essential oil burner and let the smell of lavender, spices, sage, or rose lift you up out of your feelings of stress. When a random smell wafts past, hook into it, try to identify it and let it move you into the here and now.

Take a moment to look at the view in front of you. You can either look at the big picture and enjoy the whole expanse and marvel at the beauty of the world we live in, or become aware of the contours of individual objects, notice specific trees, focus on the cloud types, and identify the birds around by the different songs you're hearing.

Notice colors, the beauty of flowers that you walk by on the street, or the bright dash of color in the outfit of a passer-by. If you love the violet top of a woman passing by, just say so. It will give you both a lift in the day and bring you both to the present.

Close your eyes for a moment and try to identify three different sounds you can hear. Relax your mind and expand your perception so you can identify sounds both near and far. Listening to music you love is also a great way to bring yourself back to the here and now. Let the sound move you, not just emotionally but also physically. Just allow your body to sway, or dance, or play in response to the rhythm.

Put a reminder on your computer or phone for you to tune into the present every half hour during your day. Close your eyes and tune into where in your body you are holding tension. You can help release this tension by giving the muscles a brief squeeze or massage, systematically squeezing and releasing them, or try to visualize sending your breath to the area.

Our largest sensory organ is actually our skin, so you can bring yourself into being present by closing your eyes and just becoming aware of the temperature of the air, the texture of your clothing on your skin, the feel of glasses on your nose, or the brush of your hair on your shoulder.

There is no more powerful way to bring you back to present than the feeling of somebody else's skin. It was programmed into you at birth when your mother held you close to soothe your first cries. Stroking your partner brings a wonderful feeling of intimacy and can bring you totally into the moment. Similarly, giving or receiving a massage brings you into the moment, but is also a wonderful way to de-stress your body and help it to detoxify waste.

Many people use movement or exercise to become present. Yoga, tai chi, and other martial arts are wonderful tools for personal development, relaxation, and mental growth.

14.2.8
The Power of Your Energy

As I mentioned at the beginning of this chapter, the science of quantum physics first demonstrated that the power of our thoughts or intentions could move subatomic particles. There is now a wealth of research that shows that our thoughts can affect inanimate objects.

Similarly, there is now a wealth of research showing that sending your thoughts and intentions can make a real difference to the health of someone, no matter where they are in the world. It doesn't make a difference what modality you choose to use, be it prayer, sending Reiki, or shamanic distance healing - they all get the same results. (Lynne McTaggart explains this research further in her book The Intention Experiment).

There are many options for healing and balancing your personal energy, such as Reiki, homoeopathy, ortho-bionomy or acupuncture. Try them on yourself, or go to a practitioner trained in any of these modalities. These can have a very powerful effect on your body to help bring it back into balance. I am trained in and use Reiki and ortho-bionomy, so can attest to their powerful effect on people. They work to get your energy flowing to help get rid of those nagging aches and pains, which are often just places where energy is stuck in your body.

14.2.9
Your Intuitive Right Brain

"Many highly successful people acknowledge that their ability to trust their intuition and act on their instincts has been a very important component of their success."

There is a strange dichotomy in the Western world where we revere someone like Albert Einstein, who brought us quantum physics yet, at the same time, many of us believe that if you cannot smell something, taste it, hear it, see it, or touch it, then it doesn't really exist. All of these sensory experiences that we call 'real' come from the stimulation of our sensory receptors, which transmit energy to the brain which then creates our picture of the world. So what really is reality? If I were to look at your child, would I see the same person that you do? Of course not, so your 'reality' is different from my 'reality'! Neither experience is right nor wrong; they're just different.

It's important to acknowledge that we have a right brain, which is sensitive to the nuances of body language, subtle interpersonal energy dynamics and, very importantly, it is intuitive. To hear the intuitive wisdom of my right brain, I must sometimes consciously divert my attention from my chatty, story-telling left-brain. (You might find it helpful to help get this section into context, to go back and have another look at Chapter 2 How Your Brain Works)

There is no need to question WHY you are subconsciously attracted to some people or situations and are repelled by others. It's not helpful. The reality is, you are reading their energy field. So listen to that 'gut feeling' or that intuitive nudge from your right brain and trust your instincts. The more you use and trust your instincts, the better you become at interpreting these nudges. Many highly successful people acknowledge that their ability to trust their intuition and act on their instincts has been a very important component of their success.

"Intuition is always right in at least two important ways. It is always in response to something. It always has your best interests at heart"
Gavin de Becker

This relationship with energy is recognizable when we are engaged in many sporting activities, in which everything influences everything. If I am shooting with a bow and arrow, I don't just focus on the target's bulls-eye. I visualize the path between the arrow tip and the bulls-eye. But I don't just see myself at point A and the bulls-eye at point B, and analyze how much force I should pull with and exactly where to aim, which are all left-brain concepts. I focus on the fluidity of the process as a whole, using my right brain.

In fact, many top athletes now actively engage their right brain intuition to improve their performance by simply visualizing themselves successfully completing their task. We now know that this is just as effective as carrying out a physical rehearsal of the same task. You can even extend this to strengthening your muscles – visualizing yourself lifting a weight has been shown to have about half the impact on your muscle strength as actually lifting the weight, and can be done anywhere – who needs a gym membership?

A key word for your right brain is 'joy'. Your right brain is thrilled to be alive and in many ways has the outlook of a child, where the world is a wonderful place, and you are at one with the universe.

Another key word for your right brain is 'compassion'. It allows us to see a homeless or disabled person with an open heart; without pity, judgment, fear, disgust, or aggression. If I reach out to somebody with genuine compassion, I feel myself move into the 'right here, right now' with an open heart. If we are willing to be supportive of others, this helps us to accept support from the universe for ourselves.

Happiness is actually the natural state of your right-brain, and your birthright. At any point in time, you can make the choice to use any of the techniques I have just talked about, move into the here and now, and experience how wonderful this world is.

The saying goes that there are more connections in your brain than there are stars in the universe. I find it helpful to think of the circuits in my brain more like a network of highways. If I habitually turn 'left' at any given junction, I could well end up in a place of fear or anger. However, I am always able to make the choice to turn 'right' at that same junction, which is more likely to take me to a place of joy or happiness.

To help my brain learn to turn 'right' more often, I choose not to watch the TV news (in fact I don't watch television at all), nor watch scary movies, nor hang out with people whose habitual response is anger. Instead, I choose to hang out with people who are habitually happy and help me to feel joyful.

14.2.10
Resentment

"Resentment is like drinking poison and then hoping it will kill your enemies." Nelson Mandela

Resentment is the mental loop that we get into, about somebody whom we think has harmed us in some way by neglecting us, or doing something that was unnecessarily hurtful, thoughtless, or mean. Resentments can arise from very real events, for instance, resenting all men for the way some of them treat their women. Unfortunately, all too often, resentments are fueled by imaginary events where we feel that someone – say, a family member – should have done something more for us or loved us more.

The problem with ALL resentments, from whatever source, is that they become part of our personality because of our basic choice not to forgive, forget, and move on. Resentments allow someone we feel has wronged us to rent space in our mind. We tend to subconsciously want to hang onto our painful past, even though we may say we want to let it go. Perhaps this is because we believe that by hanging onto our resentment, we will achieve the justice we think we are due.

The reality is that, by clinging to our hurt and angry feelings about someone, we block our capacity to move on in our lives and deal with the wounds we have received, or think we have received. The second reality is that, at the same time as we hang on to and foster these negative emotions, the person we're resenting is probably not giving the situation a second thought. We are the ONLY ONES being kept down by our resentment.

The particular process I used may not work for you, but it's really important for your future state of mind, and your development towards your greatest potential, that you find some way of getting resentments out of your head.

My experience with resentment

I once went to a weekend personal growth workshop, where one of the issues we spent a lot of time on was understanding what resentment is and why resentments are so toxic to us. We then did a really interesting exercise, where we were asked to write down all of the people we resented in our lives. Then we were asked to go down that list and write the number of years we had held each resentment for.

My mother was top of my list, and I was about 55 at the time, so my 'resentment years' totaled over 200 (and that was not the highest number in the room!).

Over the next few weeks I spent a lot of time working to understand why I so resented my mother. I talked about it to quite a few people (including my mother, which didn't help at all) to the point I was getting really bored with the story. My problem was that I couldn't get the story out of my head as we weren't given any tools to use to let go of it at the workshop.

Then I came across this little process which sounded pretty 'woo woo', but I was at the point where this whole story was renting a lot of space in my head, and I was pretty desperate to get rid of it. So I decided to give it a go. The key to the process, apparently, was the idea that the 'divas of the forest' are always there to help humanity. I should tell my story OUT LOUD to a tree – preferably one with personal significance – and end it with an apology to the person I resented, for resenting them, then make a pact

with the tree that the story then became our secret.

I am lucky enough to have 15 ha of virgin native forest on my farm, so I went to the biggest tree in the forest – an 1100-year-old totara. I told my story out loud, and several new additions to the story popped out (I think because I was talking rather than just thinking). Then I apologized to my mother for resenting her all those years and made my pact with the tree that all this was our secret (which is why I can't give you any more gory details).

I know it sounds crazy, but this totally worked for me. I was then able to see my mother for who she was when I was born – a 40-year-old woman with new twins and three other children, just doing the best she could. This allowed me to truly love my mother but, even more importantly, I discovered that it had allowed me to start loving myself and get rid of the 'I'm not lovable' story out of my head as well.

Was my resentment against my mother the reality of how our relationship was, and of how much she loved me? Absolutely not. But I had been holding onto the family stories I grew up on believing they were true because, as a child, my mind was in the theta state of accepting everything as truth.

I have since applied this technique to a number of pretty nasty situations where I could easily have made myself very miserable resenting very real things people have 'done to me'. It has worked.

14.2.11
EFT or Tapping

EFT (Emotional Freedom Technique) is a weird sounding combination of the ancient Chinese technique of acupressure (tapping) and modern psychology, in the form of affirmations made while tapping. It was discovered in 1980 by Dr Callahan, a psychologist, and then refined and simplified by Gary Craig some ten years later.

The result was the development of a very simple tapping process that could be easily learned and used on yourself. Importantly, Gary created a community around EFT, allowing the technique to be learned, applied, and shared freely. Because of this, hundreds of thousands of people all over the world have used EFT to resolve emotional problems and physical conditions.

The technique has been well researched and has been shown to powerfully reduce any 'not safe' feelings induced by both physical and mental challenges, thus reducing the stress response from the limbic brain. EFT is now widely used by mainstream therapists and psychologists for a very diverse range of physical and emotional issues, but it is so simple that you can learn and apply it on yourself (or your family) for free.

The range of conditions people have used EFT for is huge, but some common ones include back pain, limiting beliefs, money issues, body image issues, fear of spiders and cravings. I have used it many times on myself, to great effect, so if you want to explore further, go to www.ITookCharge.nz/EFT and check it out.

The neat thing about Gary's gift of EFT to the world is that amazing things can happen. For instance, a group of volunteers crowdsourced to send a team to Rwanda to work with orphans who had been traumatized by seeing their parents murdered. EFT had a major impact on the lives of these children (and the volunteers), helping them to heal from PTSD and other effects of trauma.

14.3
Take a Media Holiday

In our modern world there is a very heavy emphasis in the print media, radio, and television on sensationalizing events such as mass murders, natural disasters, and political game-playing. This can very heavily feed into your brain's negativity bias to give you an extremely negative view of the world.

The reality is that there are many, many amazing things happening in the world every day. They just don't get reported in the mainstream media as often. We live in a world of amazing abundance, where technology has transformed our lives in the last 50 years or so.

About ten years ago I decided I didn't need the negative input into my life from the media, so I stopped watching television, particularly the TV news. This had such a positive effect on my mindset that I decided to stop buying newspapers as well. Even better! Do I miss them? To my surprise - not at all. I find it much easier to maintain a positive worldview and see that my life is full of joy.

If there is something important that happens in the world that I should know about, somebody will tell me, and if it's not important to me, then it doesn't matter. I now have a similar attitude to the social media, so only check up on my personal Facebook, etc. every few days.

You may find taking a media holiday really challenging, so I suggest you make a firm resolve to try it for a week initially and see how you feel at the end of that week. I suspect that you may like the way it feels so much that you want to extend it.

14.4
Gratitude

Practicing gratitude is an extremely effective way to counteract your brain's negativity bias, and many, many studies have demonstrated the effectiveness of gratitude in contributing to health, better performance in sports and at work, an improved sense of well-being, and faster healing after a trauma like surgery.

Because we inherently tend to focus on the negative – what is broken or lacking in our life – it can be quite difficult to feel grateful on a regular basis. This means that we actually have to find a way to focus attention on the gifts in our life on a regular basis so that it becomes a new way of looking at things and a new habit.

No matter what your life is like, you can always find things to be grateful for: maybe it's the big-scale things it's easy to overlook in daily life, like your intimate relationships or where you work or where you live.

If those things aren't so great right at the moment, then what about the small-scale things you can focus on. Like the legs that carry you around, hands that can manipulate objects, that last red leaf of autumn, the butterfly that passes you on your way down the street, the sun on your skin, the taste of chocolate...

Practicing gratitude is not about pretending that there is nothing wrong with your life, it's about readjusting your focus and attention so that you consciously give thanks for the good things in your life. Some practical ways to bring more gratitude into your life could include keeping a gratitude journal for a while. It's probably best if you write a list of the things you're thankful for on a daily basis for a start, to help develop your new habit. After a while you may find that just keeping the journal where you can see it on your way to bed, or first thing in the morning, can remind you to think gratefully.

When you are grumpy about something and feel like taking your feelings out on somebody else, try making a short gratitude list in your head while you take some deep breaths instead of muttering nasty things under your breath. You are likely to be amazed by how much better you feel towards those around you.

Make a game of finding the hidden positive in a challenging situation and be grateful for it.

Practice gratitude as part of your night-time routine and notice how doing so impacts on your feelings, your ability to get a good sleep, and on your life.

14.5
Community

"Without a sense of caring, there can be no sense of community."
Anthony J. D'Angelo

The study of the long living 'Blue Zone' communities around the world has reinforced the notion that the way, and who, you hang out with can have a profound effect on your life. People who have a strong sense of support from those around them have a more positive outlook on life.

"You need to associate with people that inspire you, people that challenge you to rise higher, people that make you better. Don't waste your valuable time with people that are not adding to your growth. Your destiny is too important." Joel Ostee

Make sure your community will enhance your life. Because your brain tends to feel comfortable running along familiar paths or highways, it's also important for you to challenge yourself by spending time with people who are like you want to become. If you hang out with people who have a positive, happy outlook on life, you are far more likely to develop a positive, happy outlook on life as well. Similarly, if you hang out with successful people, it is well recognized that you are much more likely to become successful yourself.

"You become like the five people you spend the most time with. Choose carefully." Jim Rohnn

14.6
Conclusion

"The most important trick to being happy is to realize that happiness is a choice that you make and a skill that you develop. You choose to be happy, and then you work at it. It's just like building muscles."
– Naval Ravikant

The secret to hooking into any of the peaceful states discussed in this chapter is to have the willingness to call a halt to the destructive loops of thought, worry, and self-talk that your ego uses to distract you from being in the present moment.

Some people choose not to hold onto passing feelings of happiness or joy because the familiarity of intense negative emotions like anger, frustration, or jealousy gives them the illusion of strength and power.

We were all born into this world with the capacity to be happy at any time, so start straight away to make conscious choices that bring you joy now, rather than waiting for the right time to feel happy. Does it really work to say to yourself, "When I get a new car, I will be happy," or, "When I retire from this boring job, I will be happy," or, "When I die, I will go to heaven and be happy"? Do you really believe this? Or is this your ego just trying to keep you 'safe' from the unknown? The only time you have is NOW, so choose to be happy now and it will help you to create more joy in each step you take toward the ever-elusive future.

Go forth and be present...LOL.

CHAPTER 15

Heal Deeper

"Optimal health is your birthright"

Amy Myers,MD

We live in very exciting but polarizing times. By now I have shown you that the rapidly emerging science is giving us a whole new understanding of relatively simple things we can do to heal our own bodies by making some different lifestyle choices. This same science is also showing us how we can substantially increase our longevity, while at the same time maintaining our wellness and quality of life.

Yet, at the same time, in New Zealand 88% of the loss of healthy years is coming from non-communicable diseases – the chronic physical and mental conditions, such as heart disease, stroke, cancer, diabetes, obesity, arthritis, mental illness, addiction and dementia. So while we may be living longer, only about 70 - 80% of that increase is in years of good health, which means that we are also spending a longer period in ill health.

Thus, many people are kind of just existing, with debilitating chronic conditions or have some form of FLC (Feel Like Crap) syndrome, so life is just hard work and not fun anymore. Unfortunately, many medical practitioners are not trained to know how to deal effectively with such chronic conditions. You may find yourself bouncing around from doctor to doctor not getting any real answers or relief and, more importantly, not being able to live your life to the full.

While many doctors can, in some cases, help you to become symptom-free I feel that to some extent, they can be missing a part of the big picture of how you can achieve wellness just because of their focus on your symptoms and how to get rid of the symptoms.

"The satiated man and the hungry man do not see the same thing when they look upon a loaf of bread." Rumi

It is fantastic that a growing number of Functional or Holistic Medicine practitioners around the world, are applying some of the emerging science I have discussed to heal people who have supposedly incurable, chronic conditions such as diabetes, autoimmune conditions, cancer and Alzheimer's – yes you did read that list correctly. The approaches that have been shown to work are always multifaceted – there are no pills or 'silver bullets' for such chronic conditions.

Such practitioners are trained to look for the cause of your problem rather than to merely treat the symptoms, so that after treatment, most people can live normal, happy and symptom-free lives, often without medication, just from making what seem to be relatively simple changes to their diet and lifestyles.

While such doctors are more likely to help you to become symptom-free (which is fantastic; no question), I feel that, to some extent they are still likely to be missing a part of how to help you achieve wellness because again, the focus remains on your symptoms.

If you are willing to shift your focus from controlling your symptoms to your achieving wellness, then there are two additional key concepts that I would like you to embrace on your journey towards wellness. Firstly, the Pancake Theory and, secondly, that Everything is Interconnected.

15.1
The Pancake Theory

I want to take the pancake analogy that I introduced in Chapter 1.8 A Woman's Rapid Reset for Body, Mind and Hormones and discussed further in Chapter 12.3 Detoxing Your Body, and stretch it a little further. Your body has an amazing ability to adjust to what's going on in your life and keep going. You may have a stack of eight or ten, but most probably thirteen, individual pancakes which are stressing your being and your immune system, and yet you may be barely aware that your body and mind are not functioning at peak performance.

I think we can all aim a lot higher than that and go for the 90-100% state of wellness. To me, this means minimizing the size of, or eliminating as many pancakes as possible, not just the ones which are causing you obvious symptoms. This is what I have done, and the things I achieve at the age of 72 attest to the fact that this is not hard to do.

So what might this look like in practice?

Let's say you went to a doctor with an ugly red rash on your chest that just wouldn't respond to any of the topical creams you had tried. In the course of your doctor taking your history, it emerged that you had some ongoing gut issues, including constipation, which suggested you had some leaky gut problems.

Your doctor put you on a regime of a gluten-free diet and probiotics to help heal your gut and a range of supplements, including vitamin C and fish oil, to dampen down your inflammatory response. This treatment seemed to work fine, eliminated several pancakes, the rash cleared up and the gut issues (though you'd never really thought of them as a problem in your life) went away. Great.

The only problem with this scenario is that, as is often the case, it doesn't include looking deeper into the reason why your body needed anti-inflammatory Omega-3 fish oil to heal the inflamed skin. What it really indicates is that your body has a high Omega-6/Omega-3 ratio, which has been widely shown to be an underlying factor in many chronic conditions.

This suggests either that you weren't getting enough primary Omega-3's in your diet, or that your body wasn't making enough of the anti-inflammatory secondary Omega-3's because you were using too many Omega-6 oils in your diet. Probably a bit of both.

A lack of awareness around the important science of balancing your Omega-6/Omega-3 ratio to avoid chronic conditions seems to be widespread. Yet, just by tweaking the treatment by replacing the fish oil with some flax seed oil daily you could eliminate another pancake or two, greatly reduce your risk of developing other chronic conditions, and also end up with your skin glowing with radiant health.

For another example, let's say you feel sluggish and cold all the time, and you recently started to gain weight even though nothing in your diet has changed. You go to your doctor who is switched on about thyroid issues (lucky you), so does all the right tests and discovers you have a sluggish thyroid. This is making you hypothyroid because your iodine intake is too low.

Your doctor puts you on the usual iodine supplement and, within a couple of weeks, your energy returns and the weight starts to slip off you effortlessly. Great.

The only problem with this scenario is that, as detailed in Chapter 6.8.2, your thyroid is designed to scavenge any available iodine for its own needs. This means that the supplement you are put on very likely does not supply sufficient iodine for your breast or brain health. Thus you remain at risk of developing breast cancer, a range of mental conditions or brain fog. It looks like you've eliminated a pancake but in reality, it's still there, so your pancake stack is just reduced in size.

Another way to look at the issue of just treating symptoms is to consider the amazing ability your body has to heal itself without your knowledge. By the time you actually notice any symptoms of an ailment and are motivated to fix them, your body has already been working really hard to minimize their impact. So, when you do finally start to notice symptoms, they just represent the tip of the iceberg. If you and your doctor just work at getting rid of your symptoms, there is inevitably a whole lot more of the iceberg hiding underneath that's not being dealt with.

15.2
Everything Is Interconnected

It's a fundamental principle of quantum physics and the universe that everything is interconnected. More particularly, I have been at pains to demonstrate throughout this book that your body's hormonal systems are all interconnected. For example, you can't be living in a stressed-out state without this affecting your body's sex, thyroid and metabolic hormone balance.

Similarly, you can't be living with ongoing negative self-talk coming from your ego, without it affecting your stress hormone levels, and therefore all your other hormones.

If you have a heart attack and the surgeon inserts a stent to alleviate the blocked blood vessel, does this mean that all the other blood vessels in your body are fine? Of course not. Having a heart attack means you are much more at risk of having a second heart attack or stroke. Even three years after a heart attack, your risk of having another heart attack or a stroke remains 2 - 3 times higher than your peers.

Similarly, if you are diagnosed with ANY autoimmune condition, your risk of developing a second autoimmune condition is five times higher than your peers.

You can't live in the modern world without having ongoing exposure to toxic heavy metals like mercury, nickel and lead, and endocrine disruptors that are affecting your hormonal balance. For example, every time you touch the receipt from an EFTPOS machine you are absorbing some BPA (or BPS) which, in some countries, has already been banned from use in food can linings because it is known to be a potent estrogen mimic.

What this really means for you is that if you develop ANY symptoms of being unwell, this is the tip of your iceberg showing and this is your body warning you that all is not right, and your stack of pancakes is getting too high. You would be wise to do something about it.

15.3
The Thirteen Most Common Pancakes

To summarize what you have learnt so far about things affecting your health:

1. Ongoing issues with self-destructive mind talk, which seeks to keep you in the past or worrying about the future, rather than living in the NOW.

You would be an unusual person in this modern world if this was not the case unless you are already taking serious measures to gain mastery of your own mind, rather than letting it run on autopilot, without you making conscious decisions.

2. Sufficient distress in your life to be causing your body some health issues from the elevated stress hormone levels.

You would be a very unusual person in this modern world if this were not the case unless you are already taking serious measures to de-stress yourself most days.

3. Issues with a stuttering thyroid, which will come from the impacts of toxins, stress and mineral deficiencies.

Your thyroid is the most sensitive part of your body to damage from environmental toxins and mineral deficiencies. Your stress hormones can also have an important negative impact on your thyroid function. Women are 5 - 8 times more likely than men to have thyroid problems.

4. Less than optimum amounts of all the minerals you need to be well.

This does not mean you will have overt deficiency symptoms, but unless you are regularly eating seafood and sea vegetables or supplementing with food-based minerals, you will have some suboptimal mineral levels in your body.

The widespread use of soluble fertilizers (which seldom contain trace elements) in our food production systems means that your food is not a complete source of all the minerals you need. Add to this the fact that many soils around the world are inherently deficient in key minerals like selenium, zinc, iodine and magnesium and you have a recipe for hormonal imbalance and a sluggish metabolism.

5. Some degree of estrogen-dominance, coming from your ongoing exposure to the xenoestrogens in our environment and food, which disrupt your hormone balance.

You will notice this as some symptoms of PMT leading up to your period or, if you are a little older, you are likely having hot flushes and other symptoms associated with menopause – this does not have to be that way.

Your exposure to xeno estrogens and other endocrine disruptors is impossible to avoid completely. If you are not taking steps to reduce your toxic load already, you would be wise to do so to help you to achieve wellness.

6. Some degree of insulin and/or leptin resistance and metabolic syndrome,

because of your intake of sugar and refined carbs.

Unless you are taking active steps to minimize your intake of sugar and refined carbohydrates, such as white rice or white flour, bread or pasta and cooked potatoes, then the blood sugar spike that comes from eating such foods will mess with your metabolic hormone balance.

7. Some degree of imbalance of your gut, mouth and skin microbiome and the leaky gut that goes with it, because of our widespread overuse of antibiotics, sanitizers and prescription drugs.

Your microbiome does NOT restore itself over time after you have taken a course of antibiotics. Rather, with every course of antibiotics you take, your microbiome gets less and less diverse and is therefore less able to help you maintain wellness. Again, you would be an unusual person in this modern world if this were not the case, unless you are already taking serious measures to nurture your microbiome by eating a diet containing plenty of prebiotic foods, rich in dietary fiber. You also need to be eating a range of probiotic fermented foods and using probiotic supplements.

8. Some degree of gluten intolerance.

The latest research has shown that EVERYONE has a negative response to gluten, which falls somewhere on a spectrum from a very brief opening of the tight junctions in your gut wall that you will not be aware of. At the other end of the spectrum is a full-blown autoimmune coeliac condition, where any exposure to gluten or gluten like molecules will give you major gut inflammation and other health issues. Because gluten is used so widely in everyday foods, processed foods and cosmetics, the more unwell you are, the more likely it is that gluten is contributing to the problem.

9. The EFA balance in your body is heavily laden towards Omega-6 dominance.

This makes you very vulnerable to developing chronic conditions because of the inflammatory imbalance that this causes, and likely also causes a functional Omega-3 deficiency. If you eat some processed food and are not actively supplementing with oils containing the primary Omega-3, like flax seed or chia seed oil, then this will be a given for you. Having a few capsules of fish or krill oil is not enough to correct this imbalance.

10. A degree of chemical toxicity, which is underlying some of your health issues.

A very recent study suggests that environmental toxins are now the primary driver of chronic ill health. Even new-born babies have been shown to have over 200 synthetic chemicals and heavy metals in their cord blood. This means that unless you are actively supporting your bodies detox systems, these toxins will be having a negative impact on your health.

There are so many hundreds of man-made chemicals and toxic heavy metals used in our food, food production systems, personal care products, tooth fillings, in building materials and furnishings and being released into our air and water, that it is inevitable that you have accumulated some of these toxins in your body.

Many of these will be fat-soluble and will have accumulated in fat cells around your body. If you start to lose weight these will be released back into your bloodstream and potentially overload your liver detox pathways, potentially making you more unwell. You will need to support your liver and kidneys to enhance their ability to detox your body.

11. A need to move your body a bit more to achieve the wonderful benefits that accrue from exercise.

Getting an optimum amount of the right kind of exercise impacts on the functioning of every part of your body, even parts that you would not suspect. So, for instance, this includes your oral health, brain health and gut health.

Alternatively, you may be at the other end of the spectrum where you exercise a little bit obsessively – and it doesn't take a whole lot of exercise to mess with your stress and sex hormone balance.

12. Some degree of sleep deprivation.

Unless you are minimizing your screen time in the evening or using blue blocking glasses, then your sleep quality will be suffering. Unless you are routinely getting 7 - 9 hours' sleep every night, then your brain and your body will not be able to do the detoxing and repairing required for you to be well. Even one night of poor sleep is sufficient to reduce your reaction time, make you cranky or emotional, your thinking slows down and your immune system starts to suffer.

13. Less than optimum amounts of all the vitamins and phytonutrients you need to be well.

Your less than optimum microbiome means that your bugs are not likely to be producing all the B vitamins, vitamin C and vitamin K that your body needs. You are almost certainly low in vitamin D unless you get plenty of sunlight exposure without the use of sunscreens or eating lots of fatty fish – this is a major. You are likely low in vitamin A unless you are eating plenty of brightly colored fruit and vegetables, grass-fed dairy products (yellow butter) or liver. You are almost certainly low in vitamin E unless you are using plenty of unrefined vegetable oils like olive and safflower, or eating plenty of nuts like almonds or hazelnuts, and sunflower seeds.

The widespread occurrence in people's lives of the thirteen pancakes listed above can lead to extreme frustration in your search for greater wellness to alleviate your symptoms. Of course, the size of each of these individual pancakes is going to vary a lot depending on your particular situation. Nevertheless, they typically all contribute to a level of CHRONIC INFLAMMATION.

The frustrating result of your pancake stack is that pretty much whichever practitioner you choose, and whatever they get you to do, will address at least one of these pancakes. Reducing this pancake may or may not give you some relief from your symptoms.

Most practitioners have a specialty area that they are most familiar with. Since chronic inflammation has such a wide range of symptoms, doctors are likely to find a possible cause that fits their specialty area and recommend specific tests to confirm their suspicion. If the test results come back positive you are put on a course of targeted treatment which will probably address some of your symptoms, but likely fails to address your broader health issues.

Such treatment may or may not alleviate some of your symptoms, depending on the nature of your remaining stack of pancakes. Does it leave you feeling totally well and totally loving your life? Highly unlikely. Such a process can easily lead to you going on a long and expensive search for the practitioner who is going to find the solution to all your problems. I'm sure many can attest that this process can go on for months, or even years, with little real progress in your state of wellness for all your time, expense and effort.

15.4
Chronic inflammation

We are all familiar with the inflammation that is your body's natural response to injury, an insect bite, or infection, which is an amazing and healthy process. If you cut yourself, your body feels the pain and immediately begins an inflammatory, immune and healing process that neutralises harmful bugs, cleans up any debris from the injury, and starts to heal the wound.

We tend to be less aware of the silent, chronic inflammation that is usually happening deep in our bodies and in our brain. It often does not cause any pain but is generating a constant supply of free radicals that start to overwhelm our antioxidant systems and damage our DNA, aging us and causing chronic diseases of every description. There is a growing consensus in medicine that every chronic disease has, at the heart of it, uncontrolled chronic inflammation – from Alzheimer's, autoimmune conditions, cancer, depression, diabetes, and heart disease, right through to the common cold.

One of the major sources of chronic inflammation is the food we eat, which tends to be high in pro-inflammatory ingredients such as sugar, white flour, damaged Omega-6 oils, and acid-forming foods like processed dairy, processed meat, and soft drinks. At the same time our diet is lacking in good oils, real food protein sources, and vegetables, which are all rich in antioxidants and other nutrients that help to prevent and control inflammation.

Low-grade infections such as gum disease (gingivitis), and internal parasites, also contribute to chronic inflammation. So do allergies, food sensitivities, and physical injuries that don't heal properly because of a pro-inflammatory diet. Fat cells, especially those around your belly, also produce large amounts of inflammatory chemicals.

Many environmental toxins are also inflammatory. Everyday chemicals such as cleaning products, perfume, air fresheners, glues, adhesives, latex, plastics, and synthetic fibers can all trigger an inflammatory response in many people. Pesticides, such as Roundup (glyphosate), and prescription drugs such as antibiotics, NSAIDs (painkillers), statins (heart disease), and proton pump inhibitors (acid reflux) can all disrupt your gut microbiome, causing a degree of leaky gut and leakage of undigested food molecules into your bloodstream. These promote food allergies and silent, chronic inflammation which develops over a long time, making it very hard to find a cause and effect relationship.

Chronic stress also causes your body to produce hormones that promote chronic inflammation. It could be stress from perceived physical or social threats, whether they are carried over from childhood or from your adult life. Because your brain regulates the way your body handles systemic inflammation, this means that social stressors such as conflict, isolation, and rejection, and perceived or anticipated threats that may never come to pass, can all promote inflammation in your body. High levels of cortisol from stress or excessive exercise also disrupt your gut microbiome in a way similar to the way toxins do.

Lack of enough restorative, healing sleep or insomnia can also cause your body to produce high levels of inflammatory chemicals.

Because we are electrical beings, the lack of grounding in our modern way of living disturbs our electrical field. We now know that we need to ground ourselves frequently by direct skin contact with the earth. Research has shown that such grounding has measurable effects on your inflammation levels, wound healing, pain levels and sleep. Some people are more sensitive to this than others, but take every opportunity you can to go barefoot on the ground. To get the best results you may even need to explore ways of grounding yourself while you are in bed by lying on some form of metallic tape connected to an earthed wire.

Inflammation is now being seen to be the common element in virtually all disease. By allowing chronic inflammation to continue we are aging ourselves prematurely, causing us to look old, feel tired or FLC, and be susceptible to every imaginable disease – so what to do? – Read on.

CHAPTER 16

Your 'Rapid Reset' Plan

"Once you make a decision, the universe conspires to make it happen."

Ralph Waldo Emmerson

16.1
Do It NOW

Controlling chronic inflammation takes a whole mind-body approach. Each of the three legs of your stool of wellness – what you eat, toxins in your body, and toxins in your mind – all contribute to your inflammatory state. The beautiful thing is that all three legs can be under your control - IF YOU SO CHOOSE. Knowing this gives you the power to choose to prevent and reverse inflammation, which then gives you the power to choose to control your state of aging and your degree of wellness. What a wonderful goal.

The other lovely thing about primarily targeting inflammation is that, with the right approach, this is something that can be reversed quite quickly so that you are likely to start to see results within a few days.

So are you ready to decide to commit to following my program for just nine days? That's just two weekends and one workweek, which I hope feels like a manageable chunk of time. By then you are likely to be starting to feel pretty wonderful and hopefully will feel motivated to continue for an additional two weeks, making three weeks in total.

Three weeks is long enough for your body to grow a completely new lining for your gut made from healthy building blocks. It is also enough time for you to have formed new habits around your lifestyle, which is what is required to cement these changes into your life so that you can start to look and feel youthful, energized, sexy, and loving life.

It's really important for your progress that you commit to addressing all three legs of your stool of wellness - See Section 1.7:

16.2
Detox Your Body

Please have another look at Chapter 12 Detoxing Your Body, to refresh your mind on the details and do these as a minimum.

a. Get your liver/bowel system working properly so that you have a minimum of one to two bowel movements every day. This will mean that you are supporting your liver to eliminate fat-soluble toxins. Monitor the texture of your stools.

b. Keep yourself hydrated with plenty of water so that your kidneys can eliminate the water-soluble toxins efficiently. This is crucial for any detox/weight loss program, as your body needs more water and salt while you are adjusting to being fat-adapted. Monitor the color of your pee.

c.   To start to detox your brain you need to get the 7 - 9 hours of sleep a night that your body needs to be able to rest and repair your physical body and mind.

d.   Put some movement into your day – it is fundamental to your good health, to reducing inflammation, and enhancing healing from a wide range of conditions as diverse as depression, gum disease, heart disease and Alzheimer's. There is good evidence that you cannot reverse the effects of 8-10 hours sitting at a desk during the day with a single visit to the gym or swimming pool.

e.   Enhance your body detox by eating the right food and supporting the process with tools like infrared saunas and coffee enemas.

16.3
Detox Your Mind

"Never stop holding yourself accountable for your own happiness. It's no one else's job to make you happy. Happiness really is an inside job, and when you base that happiness on other people or outside conditions, you're setting yourself up for misery." - Robert Kiyosaki

If you have excessive stress levels and high cortisol, you will NOT be able to get all your other hormones in balance, particularly the sex hormones that control your libido. Getting your stress and cortisol levels under control is a must. Please have another look at Chapter 14 Detoxing Your Mind to refresh you on what you need to do. It's important that you focus on both mind- detoxing areas:

Relaxation Response

These techniques are designed for you to use frequently, ideally on a daily basis, to help you to unwind from your day and prepare for a deep, restful sleep.

As a minimum, try to find a meditation technique that you enjoy. Explore the samples of the technology solutions available free on my website – www. ITookCharge.com/RelaxationResponse

Mind Mastery

To me, this is more about clearing the junk of your past from your mind, learning to stop worrying about the future, and starting to live NOW. As a minimum, bring some mindfulness and gratitude for the good bits in your life and find an effective way of clearing your resentments.

16.4
The Building Blocks

The eating program I have designed for you during the initial 'Rapid Reset' phase is essentially a high quality, low-carb diet of 'real' foods that your great grandmother would recognize (rather than 'fake' foods that come in a packet with an indefinite shelf life). It's designed to transition you into nutritional ketosis and to start to up-regulate your gene pathways for burning fat. Such a diet will not only supply your requirements for essential nutrients, but will also start to dampen down the inflammatory fire in your body, give it a chance to heal, and improve your brain function.

16.5
Low-Carb Reset Phase

By low-carb, I am talking about an intake of only 5 - 10% of your calories coming from carbohydrates, which translates to about 20 - 60 g per day. For those of you who really want to know the numbers, this means you will be getting about 65 - 75% of calories from good fats or oils, 20 - 25% from protein, and 5 - 10% from carbs, with no need for calorie restriction.

However, I would like you to forget about 'counting your macros' (protein, fat, carbs and fiber) and start listening to your body. Counting things can easily lead you into guilt and stress if you have 'too much'. The easy way to achieve the results you want is to eat lots of 'above-ground' vegetables, a moderate amount of protein at each meal, and lots of good oils and good fats.

One of the most common mistakes for people trying to get into nutritional ketosis is not eating

Metabolic Flexibility

Does the above statement seem hard to believe? On a recent Friday night my family requested 'fish and chips' for dinner. I ate two large pieces of fish (too much good protein), quite a lot of chips (bad carbs and bad fat) and a few antioxidants in the form of tomato sauce.

The next morning, I was still not hungry at 11.30 am but I had to go out for the afternoon, so I had my usual smoothie for 'brunch'. My body had just slipped back into fat-burning, and I felt great, with no ego nonsense about "should I be eating this way?", because I knew that was how my body would react. That's how having metabolic flexibility allows you to live.

enough fats. By cutting the carbs, you are trying to get most of your energy from fats, which means eating way more fat than you are used to. Forget your 'fat phobia' and use lots of butter and coconut oil in your cooking – it will taste delicious.

Because both fat and protein make you feel 'full' for much longer than carbs do, you are unlikely to feel like snacking between meals to 'keep you going'. If you do feel that need sometimes (and everyone does) then try the following suggestions, depending on where in the 'Rapid Reset' you are at:

- A teaspoon of coconut oil as liquid or powder.
- A knob of butter on a slice of cheese (my favorite).
- A small handful of nuts.

You may find people suggesting that low-carb diets are ineffective for achieving real health benefits, but you're likely to find their research covers much less extreme diets, where up to 40 or even 50% of calories are still coming from carbohydrates.

The way I am recommending you eat during the first nine days is pretty consistent with the ideas behind the Ketogenic, Paleo, Primal, GAPS and Wahl's fraternity, but with some important differences:

1. I focus on you rebuilding your microbiome and your gut lining to reduce this source of inflammation drastically.

2. I focus on you resetting your genes to allow you to become a fat-burner for the long-term.

3. I place a big emphasis on eating lots of above-ground vegetables to provide plenty of prebiotic fiber, vitamins, minerals and phytonutrients.

4. I want you to keep your protein intake in the low to moderate range. If you have more protein than your body needs, your liver has to process it into sugar to get rid of it.

Don't panic - eating this way is not necessarily the way you will want to eat for the rest of your life. The 'Rapid Reset' phase is designed to up-regulate your fat-burning genes so that you become fat-adapted. Once you enter this state your body becomes able to switch easily between burning fat or carbs, which gives you a huge amount of flexibility over what you choose to eat. You will want to continue eating a high-fat diet because it makes your mind and body feel so switched on and alive. But if there are no quality high-fat dishes on the menu, you can eat a higher carb meal no problem, you enjoy the carbs and then your body switches straight back to fat-burning mode - this is real METABOLIC FLEXIBILITY.

This effect means that after doing the initial 'Rapid Reset' phase, you are encouraged to reintroduce some of your favorite foods and see how the 'new you' reacts to them. Decide for yourself whether they are still for you. You may well find that they don't make you feel good anymore.

If you have had ongoing issues with any of your digestive organs, kidneys or heart, or you are pregnant or lactating, then you should talk to your doctor before implementing my recommendations. The principles are all sound, but you may need to take things a bit more gently than I am suggesting.

If acid reflux or heartburn is a major issue for you, this will make it very difficult to restore your gut health and your overall health. To help you sort this I have written a separate e-book on the subject www.ITookCharge. nz/AcidReflux . The book includes a section on simple 'do at home' tests you can use to find out WHY you have such an issue and what to do from there. I strongly recommend that you do not just continue to use antacids or proton pump inhibitors, as they have been widely shown to have nasty effects on your gut microbiome and hence your overall health.

You are probably better not to start this process if you are just coming up to your period. Since your fat cells both produce estrogen and can also store estrogen, you could well experience some hormonal weirdness as you start to break down stored fat, which may release some stored estrogen. This could look like mood swings, enhanced or decreased libido, or spotting which may occur while your hormones sort themselves out and come to a new balance. If you're in menopause you might get more hormonal weirdness – sorry!

16.6
How it Works

Eating a low-carb and high-fat diet of real food works, over time, to achieve the desired result of up-regulating your ability to be a fat burner by cutting out the sugar, processed and other bad carbs, and by limiting the fruit you eat to low GI berry fruit. Doing this helps to reset your metabolic hormones by lowering any insulin and leptin resistance you may have, and it minimizes the amount of the very damaging fructose in your diet.

You get some carbohydrates from the above-ground, non-starchy vegetables you are encouraged to eat lots of, like all the brassica family which includes broccoli, cauliflower, cabbage, kale, and Asian greens. Others to eat plenty of are spinach, chard, asparagus, and zucchini. Eating such vegetables automatically means you are getting lots of a wide range of different types of fiber, which we now know is necessary for a healthy, diverse microbiome.

It's also really great to choose lots of brightly colored vegetables, which are rich in antioxidants: red lettuce, purple cauliflower, purple sweet potatoes, bell peppers, and tomatoes. Basically, the more intense the color, the higher the levels of antioxidants and the more anti-inflammatory they are. Very importantly, they also promote the kind of healthy microbiome balance that we now know is associated with loss of belly fat.

I think it is fundamental to your journey towards wellness that you drastically increase your intake of vegetables. For instance, a recent Australian study showed that eating 5 - 7 serves of vegetables per day was a powerful way of reducing the effects of psychological stress in women.

Eating a low-carb diet of real food also makes it easy to increase the amounts of high-quality oil you are eating. This aids in your transition into becoming fat-adapted, and since ketones are anti-inflammatory, this powerfully helps to dampen down inflammation. Eating plenty of good fats, particularly the Omega-3 ALA, will also start to restore your balance of EFAs to a healthy 1:1 ratio which again, is powerfully anti-inflammatory.

Importantly, having a plentiful amount of oil in your meals increases the time your food stays in your stomach so you feel fuller for longer, you are less interested in snacking on carbs, and your total fuel intake spontaneously drops. Good fats also greatly reduce the size of your insulin and leptin response, compared to eating carbs or protein, so your metabolic hormones will quickly start to come into balance.

Eating plentiful good fats just makes you an all-round better person. Your body starts to burn fat, which is great for your belly fat and self-esteem. Your brain has a steady flow of energy that helps it to function more efficiently, so you feel energized and on top of things. Your food cravings go away, so you become a nicer person to be around, so your relationships improve, so it's not hard to feel happy and full of joy.

The most fattening and addictive foods to avoid are the dangerous duo of fast carbs from sugar and refined carbs containing, or cooked in, lots of damaged fats - you know - the ones you just can't stop eating. Think potato crisps, doughnuts, french fries, cheesecake, and cookies. I know they taste great but these are the sorts of foods that can go straight to your belly fat, increase inflammation, and do nasty things to your health.

"The most fattening and addictive foods to avoid are the dangerous duo of fast carbs, from sugar and refined carbs containing, or cooked in, lots of damaged oils."

Having a moderate amount of protein at each meal also helps to spontaneously drop your food intake because protein has roughly twice the effect on you feeling fuller for longer. Having enough protein and moving your body more during this phase also helps you to maintain, or even increase, muscle mass while you're losing belly fat. Increased muscle mass increases your resting energy burning, which helps you to feel warm and burn more fuel - just by living.

Maybe you need to increase the amount of protein you eat, this DOES NOT mean eating lots of meat. A piece of meat or fish, smaller than the size of your palm, once a day is plenty. Eating more than this is more than your body needs, so it will turn it into glucose, which you do not want. There are plenty of other healthy sources of protein like eggs or cheese and there are many delicious vegetables with useful levels of protein like green peas or beans, spinach, squash, mushrooms and asparagus.

The beauty of a low-carb diet is that it's pretty easy to follow. Pretty much everyone knows what 'carbs' are: bread, cookies, sweets, pasta, and potatoes. If it's either obviously sweet or obviously starchy, you know you should shun it during this 'Rapid Reset' phase.

It also works fast, so it's not unusual to lose useful amounts of belly fat in the first week (some of that will be water), have more energy and feel substantially better, which is great for your motivation to continue down this path. The best diet for you will always be the one you will stick to because you're excited about the way it makes you feel.

The other blessing of eating a low-carb meal is that the high-fat content makes it taste delicious. Just imagine yourself eating a fatty, grass-fed steak, fried in butter; some lightly steamed broccoli doused in butter; and a quick stir-fry of purple onion, garlic, capsicums, and zucchini cooked in coconut oil. Would that feel like being on a 'diet' to you? Yet a meal like that takes only 15 – 20 minutes to prepare (just drop the steak if you're vegan).

16.7
Start to Heal Yourself

It all starts with a nine-day plan. As indicated above, I recommend you consciously commit to the nine days because it's a manageable chunk of your life. If you can, imagine yourself doing this for just nine days, knowing that during this time you will likely see some major changes in the way you feel – does this feel good?

For this 'Rapid Reset' phase to work quickly some things just have to be eliminated COMPLETELY during the first nine days. Yes, I am suggesting 'cold turkey' here. Giving these up will not be as painful as your ego is telling you it will be. We are talking about starting the rest of your life here and your future wellness.

All of the substances on the following list have the potential to be addictive, so cutting just a bit out each day can be distressing, painful, and almost always ends in failure. The research shows very clearly that to get off any addictive substance reliably, gradual withdrawal simply DOES NOT WORK.

If you feel that you can't do this and that your life just won't be worth living for nine days without any of the substances on this list then, I'm sorry. I have obviously failed to convince you that your 'happiness, belly fat, and sexiness' and your long term health depends on it.

In that case, please pay it forward and pass this book on to a good friend who might benefit from it, and email me your receipt and bank details to david@ITookCharge.nz for a full refund - no explanation required.

Foods to eliminate for the first nine days (Phase 1):

1.   Coffee and all forms of caffeine - because of its effect on your stress hormones.

This also includes things like energy drinks, black tea, green tea and chocolate. Yes, even decaf coffee at this early stage because this still contains some caffeine and it can also be acid forming in your body.

You can choose a turmeric latte or there are lots of delicious herbal teas that are alternatives. It would be helpful to the 'Rapid Reset' process to choose herbs that support digestion and liver detox such as peppermint, ginger, chamomile, lemon balm and lemon verbena, or the roots of chicory, dandelion or burdock.

2.   Sugar in all its forms - because of its effect on your stress and metabolic hormones, liver, and dopamine.

This includes all fruit juice, honey, and all sugar substitutes including herbs like stevia and Luo Han Guo. I include the last two because sugar has two addictive elements: the blood-sugar rush itself, and also the sweet taste. It's hard for your body and mind to separate the two. Continuing to use sweet herbs during this 'Rapid Reset' phase is just going to make life more difficult for you in the long term. You will find that your taste buds quickly adapt to the lower levels of sweetness in your diet, so you will not miss it nearly as much as your ego thinks you will. See Section 16.5 for snack suggestions.

3.   Starch and gluten in all its forms - because of its effect on your gut and your stress, metabolic hormones and dopamine.

This includes wheat and all the other grains including rye, barley, oats, rice, corn, quinoa, amaranth, millet and sorghum. This is because of both the easily digestible starch content and also because of the presence of gluten or gluten-like storage proteins.

You should also avoid the starchy vegetables in all their forms, including potatoes, yams, corn, sweet potatoes and parsnips.

4.   Alcohol in all its forms - because it is a liver loader that will negatively impact on your livers ability to detox other chemicals during this crucial early stage.

This includes all the usual suspects such as wine, beer and spirits, but I also suggest you probably add kombucha to this list. Depending on how it's made, kombucha can contain significant amounts of alcohol, sugar, and caffeine.

5.   Dairy is not addictive like the first four but can often upset your digestive system so is likely to be important to eliminate, just for Phase 1.

Dairy contains proteins that can be a little bit like gluten, in that they are quite sticky and can be hard to digest for some people. This means that dairy may promote inflammation in your body. I include all liquid milk and butter, but not yoghurt, cheese (the fermentation modifies the protein and milk sugar (lactose) to more digestible forms) or ghee (because that has had all the protein and lactose removed, just leaving the good fats).

If you have access to raw, grass-fed or organic dairy products, then there is probably no need to eliminate these – quality matters. They are unlikely to pose a problem for your digestion because they contain many live enzymes, which help you to digest them more easily.

6.   Soya beans, in all its forms - because of the many anti-nutritional factors soy contains, making it very hard on your gut.

7.   Some people should also add eggs to this list - because like dairy, the albumin in the egg is a bit of a sticky protein.

If you are really struggling with an autoimmune condition or think you might have had an issue with eggs in the past, then eliminating eggs for this nine-day period would be a good thing to do. Most people will be fine with genuine free-range eggs where the wonderful health benefits you get from this top-quality food outweigh the small risk of being intolerant to them. Research has shown that the good fats, protein and cholesterol in eggs help protect your liver and heart, feed your brain and increase your resting metabolism, which both help you to lose belly fat and feel energized.

8.   Similarly, most people should add nuts to that list of foods to eliminate,

because peanuts are one of the foods more likely to cause allergic reactions.

Because peanuts are harvested from the earth, they often contain toxic chemicals from mold. If you are really struggling with an autoimmune condition, or think you might have had an issue with nuts in the past, then eliminating all nuts for this nine-day period would be a good thing to do.

For most, starting to eat lots more of the nuts from trees, such as walnuts, almonds, cashews, pine, and macadamia nuts, will give some more easy food options and provide lots of healthy good fats and proteins.

16.8
Before you start

If you have been a big consumer of processed foods you may have to do a pantry makeover to get rid of temptation. It will make your journey a whole lot easier if you can get the rest of your 'family' (including children) onto the same program – the power of community at work. Yes, the first few days may be a bit of hard work but, after that, you will all feel so much better.

Experience has shown that it is particularly important for a woman's body to be in an alkaline state while you are transitioning towards becoming fat-adapted. While you are preparing to do the 'Rapid Reset', to help alkalize your body for optimum results, you should increase your intake of:

Fresh vegetables and fruits, which are the most alkalinity promoting foods. Raw foods - Ideally try to consume a good portion of your produce raw.

Plant proteins – Nuts, seeds, mushrooms and beans (if you can tolerate them) are all good choices.

16.9
Reset - Phase 1.

My recommendation for Phase 1 is that you start on a day when you can allow yourself to take things a bit easy for a couple of days, so probably over a weekend.

Just to refresh - this initial step is designed to do seven important things, namely:

1. Get you off all caffeine, sugar, gluten, refined carbohydrates, soy products and alcohol in a way that minimizes any cravings you may experience.

2. Start to heal your digestive system and gut from damage caused by your diet, exposure to antibiotics and toxins.

3. Start to reset your leptin and insulin sensitivity which, once accomplished, will normalize your relationship with food.

4. Start to gently detox your body in a way that doesn't overload your detox systems.

5. Get you into moving your body more in ways that reduce stress and promote the production of HGH (Human Growth Hormone).

6. Start to experiment with ways of detoxing your mind to help you reduce your stress hormone levels.

7. Start to upregulate the important gene pathways that will convert you into becoming fat-adapted, and also allow you to be able to make the secondary Omega-3s and Omega-6s your body needs to reduce inflammation.

16.9.1
Your First Weekend - The Bone Broth Fast

Begin with a bone broth fast for two days, which means you do not eat any solid food, but you consume warmed bone broth several times a day, whenever you feel you might like something to eat – no restrictions on quantity. Bone broth is a stock made from the bones and connective tissue of animals, birds or fish, simmered with vegetables and a dash of vinegar (which helps to extract the minerals).

Bone broth contains useful amounts of protein including collagen, glycine, arginine; vitamins and minerals; electrolytes; and antioxidants like glucosamine. All these make bone broth the most powerful food you can have to start to heal your gut. Also, all this collagen does do nice things to your skin.

I suggest that it's pretty important for this first weekend for you to plan to severely restrict your social life as you may get some detox symptoms, potentially including headaches and bad breath. For those of you who are higher up the addictive scale, this first couple of days could be a bit hard work, as you may have cravings for some of the foods I have recommended you eliminate.

Some people may even experience something often called the 'carb flu' when they're coming off sugar and refined carbohydrates, which apparently feels pretty much like regular flu, with potential symptoms including headaches, hunger, short temper, anxiety, exhaustion, and brain fog. For a FREE workbook to help guide your 'Rapid Reset' go to www.ITookCharge/RRWorkbook

Vitamins from Food

Some authorities claim that all phytonutrients, like the antioxidants, are just vitamins waiting for a name – your body needs them.

What follows on from this idea is that real vitamins are not just simple, chemical compounds that can be manufactured in a factory. For example, the vitamin E family, as we currently know it, contains eight different molecular forms. This means that vitamins are families of nutrients that occur together in nature, and we don't necessarily understand how or why they work or interact.

Since the food from modern industrial agriculture tends to be quite low in minerals and vitamins, I encourage you to get as much of your food as possible from organic, or local farmers' market sources, or grow your own, which will be fresher and a better source of phytonutrients and bugs. When you choose supplements, try to source those that are derived from food, rather than being synthesized in a factory. Quality matters.

16.9.2
Your Phase 1 Reset Routine

1. When you first get up, if at all possible, go outside for at least a few minutes to get natural daylight in your eyes, to help reset your melatonin, leptin, cortisol and dopamine hormones.

2. Have a hot drink within about half an hour of rising. This tells your body there is no famine this morning so that it does not initiate a cortisol spike which would put your body into belly fat storage mode. Doing this is only important while you're still living in a glucose-adapted state, so will become less important as you transition into a fat-adapted state.

Ideally, have half a lemon squeezed into a mug of bone broth or hot water, or use a teaspoon of raw cider vinegar. Having such a mildly acid drink stimulates your digestive system and helps your body to start producing acid to aid in the digestion of food.

3. During the day, and as needed throughout the weekend, I suggest you drink as much warm bone broth as you want. Have servings around 200 - 400 mls (7 - 14oz) maybe five times a day. You could be drinking up to two liters per day, whatever feels good to you. The warm drink helps you to feel less hungry, and the protein content helps to stop your body starting to break down your muscles as fuel which could potentially happen during the early stages of becoming fat-adapted.

There are a few fundamentals of fasting that you need to be aware of:

•   Make sure you drink lots of pure water.

•   Don't try to exercise vigorously. Take it easy.

•   Simply listen to your body and act on what it tells you.

- Eat some easily digested food if you're feeling weak or very hungry - it's not a competition. Drink some more bone broth or eat an avocado or some berry fruit.

4. Have a high-quality bowel-detox supplement (See Appendix A.6), which includes plenty of dietary fiber to help get your bowel moving, and ingredients designed to heal the gut. You could add this to one of your early drinks of bone broth.

The primary detox pathway is from the liver, into the bowel, and hence out of your body. The fundamental requirement for this pathway to work is to be having a minimum of one to two bowel movements EVERY DAY. Use more of your supplement if required, to achieve this goal.

5. Sleep and daily rhythms. You need to aim to get the seven to nine hours of sleep your brain and body needs to repair, clean house and detox overnight and reset your hormones. If this is an issue for you, reread section 12.6 Sleep and get it sorted.

Ideally, you would also try a curfew on the use of visual technology after about 9.00pm (their high output of blue light disturbs your melatonin levels) and be asleep by 10.00pm. An alternative to this cut-off is to wear 'blue-blocking' (orange tinted) or sunglasses after sundown, which is likely to make you feel sleepy earlier than you might normally – it really does work.

The daily cycle of many of your hormones depends on your circadian rhythm which, for many people, is disturbed by the excessive use of technology at night and lack of time spent outside in full daylight. The most important time for you to spend time outside in natural daylight is first thing in the morning because this helps to normalize your leptin, dopamine and cortisol levels.

6. Mind Detox

"News is to the mind what sugar is to the body." - Rolf Dobelli

You might also want to consider that much of the content you see on the TV news, read in the newspapers or even on the Internet, is predominantly negative and, to a greater or lesser extent, is designed to keep you in fear. Because of this I gave them all up several years ago and, believe me, it is much easier to have a joyful outlook on life when you go on a media fast, and I have so much more time in my day. I have found that if you really need to know about something happening anywhere around the world, someone will tell you – it works.

During the evening or early morning, try listening to a meditation audio track to help reset your body's stress hormones. Samples of meditation aids are available on my website at www.ITookCharge.nz/RelaxationResponse for you to experiment with. Try to find something that works for you. Doing some form of meditation for at least 10 minutes per day, and preferably 20 minutes twice a day, should ideally become a non-negotiable for you so that it becomes a part of the rest of your life.

7. Sunday Night

By the end of the weekend you are probably going to be feeling pretty hungry; so you may well feel that going another night without real food is just not worth it. Don't be discouraged. If you've done a full 48 hours with just bone broth, well done - you're on your way to taking charge of your life again.

Try to manage another night without real food as it will make the transition into nutritional ketosis that much smoother. It does this by helping to up-regulate the genes responsible for you starting to easily power your body by burning fat as fuel instead of sugar, and resetting your metabolic hormones. Also, the longer you fast for, the more powerfully your body starts to heal.

Make sure YOU make the decision, not your Ego.

8. Listen to Your Body

It's really important that right throughout this process you start to take responsibility for monitoring your own progress by listening to your body. The messages your body will be giving you may be quite subtle, but they will be there, so please do not ignore them or pretend they are not real.

For instance, if your body is not coping well AT ANY STAGE with the increased fat intake, slow down and introduce more food from my 'good carbs' list. These are slow burning, minimizing your insulin response and will feed your microbiome in a healthy way.

It will be very helpful for you to start to understand how your body is working if you keep a daily journal of the food you have eaten, the state of your mood and the state of your poo. Review once a week and you will probably find that you can start to connect the dots of what works for YOU.

A simple and effective way to achieve this might be to use your phone to take a photo of your meal before you start eating, giving you instant recall of what you ate rather than you having to write it all down. You can then make some quick notes of how you feel after each meal. The combination of photos and notes, will allow you to track down patterns of foods that do or do not suit you – use technology to help you.

16.10
Reset Plan: Phase 2 – Day 3 to 9

I reiterate – an important goal of this exercise is to get you into a state of nutritional ketosis so that you start to become fat-adapted. This happens because your body will up-regulate the genes responsible for your fat-burning metabolic pathways. Once you have achieved this, your body will slip easily into a fat-burning mode whenever you want it to, rather than you trying to live the rest of your life in nutritional ketosis. This will give you the freedom to eat a high-fat diet most of the time, but also leave you not having to worry about what that delicious looking dessert on the menu will do to your new found wellness.

I don't believe most of us were designed to live in a permanent state of ketosis, as our ancestors most likely lived under conditions of feast or famine, depending on how successful the hunt was. Even the Inuit had a brief summer when they were able to access more carbohydrates in the form of plant foods and berries. That said, some people feel fantastic when they live in a state of semi-permanent nutritional ketosis.

16.10.1
What Can I Eat Now?

Well no processed or packaged food for sure. I also include processed foods with a 'paleo' or 'gluten-free' label in this ban, as many of them are of dubious quality.

So initially it's just real food that your great-grandmother would have recognized:

- Lots of non-starchy, above-ground vegetables, ideally fresh or frozen (but not canned because of the toxic can liner), and raw carrots.

- Extra-virgin coconut, olive, macadamia, flax seed and avocado oils, butter and fats from grass-fed or free-range animals.

- Mushrooms and other fungi.

- Free range eggs.

- Any grass-fed or free-range meat – not processed or smoked.

- Any wild caught fish or shellfish – not processed or smoked. Not farmed fish.

- Organ meat - especially the liver from organic animals, but heart and kidneys are great too.

- Cooked-and-cooled potatoes (think potato salad), raw potato starch, plantain, green banana and cassava flours (all good sources of resistant starch).

- Raw, organic dairy products, including hard cheeses.

- Coconut, flax, chia, pumpkin, almond and hemp flours.

- Any berry fruit. NO fruit juices.

- Herb teas.

- Fresh or dried whole herbs and spices (rich in antioxidants).

- Salt and pepper.

- Drink lots of water.

It's important to get as wide a variety of vegetables as possible; you should include at least something from the following three groups in your main meal of the day:

1. The brassica family – kale, broccoli, cabbage, cauliflower, brussels sprouts, bok choy and related vegetables (they contain a compound called sulforaphane, which has been shown to have potent anti-cancer and weight loss activity).

Also, onions, shallots, garlic, and leeks. These two groups are all rich in sulfur, so they enhance your body's ability to produce glutathione - your body's most important antioxidant.

2. Leafy greens - which basically mean that wide range of greens you can make a salad from, e.g. spinach, lettuce, sorrel, purslane, rocket, etc. There's a very wide range of leaves utilized in various cuisines around the world, and many of them have fascinating flavors.

Some of them, like spinach, chard and beet greens, also taste great when lightly steamed or sautéed in coconut oil or butter, with a hint of spice.

Many common weeds have delicious often unusual flavors, and make a great addition to salads if you can access them. Many of them are probably hiding in your garden. Try the leaves of watercress, purslane, dandelion, plantain, violet, sheep's burnett and sheep sorrel.

Although they don't strictly fit in this category, other green vegetables such as courgettes, asparagus, celery, artichokes, kohlrabi, zucchini, okra, peas, green beans, fennel and endive are all wonderful sources of phytonutrients and taste great.

3. Brightly colored vegetables – you know, those beautiful purple carrots, potatoes and sweet potatoes, red, yellow and orange capsicums, red beets,

purple and red tomatoes, and eggplants. All these wonderful colors represent highly active plant pigments that have a wide range of antioxidant and anti-inflammatory effects in your body, and they support your microbiome. Eat the rainbow.

Rather than give you a few strict recipes that you must stick to, I have chosen a couple of basic recipes, which are among my favorites, that are available on my website – www.ITookCharge.nz/Recipes

There are many hundreds of recipe ideas readily available on the web - just try searching 'low carb or keto recipes'. I recommend you check out the many websites with varied and wonderful low carb creations. Many of these (especially the desserts) you will look at and say, "That's low-carb???"

There is a lovely term for this approach to food that I came across on a visit to the USA, called 'recreational cooking'. 'Slow food' is a similar idea – food prepared with love and imagination that tastes fantastic and does wonderful things for your health.

If that's not you, and you choose not to spend a lot of time or thought on creating a varied diet, then I suggest you find a very limited number of recipes that suit you, shop only for these, and cook only these during this 'Rapid Reset' phase. Keep it really simple.

16.10.2
Your Phase 2 Reset Routine

I recommend your daily routine during the second phase of your 'Rapid Reset' looks something like this:

1. As early as possible, get yourself some exposure to natural daylight.

2. Have a hot lemon drink, ideally with a bone broth base, or collagen powder added.

3. Take a high-quality bowel detox supplement.

4. Breakfast.

It's important you eat a breakfast that has a good amount of high-quality protein, to provide the basic building blocks for your cells and to help your body to detox. It's also important to have plenty of the good fats, both to provide the building blocks for anti-inflammatory compounds and your cellular structure, but also to provide energy for your body in the form of ketones.

Your breakfast should have as few carbohydrates as possible since your body has been in mild to moderate ketosis (fat-burning mode) during the weekend and overnight. As a consequence, if you start your day without carbohydrates (think - no sugary cereal), then your body will tend to stay in the fat-burning mode for the rest of the day, enhancing your transition into nutritional ketosis.

There are many and varied ways to provide these requirements – just search 'keto breakfast recipes'. I personally find the quickest and simplest way to achieve this is to have a 'green smoothie' most mornings, with plenty of coconut cream as a ready source of ketones.

You can make such a smoothie both slightly sweet by the use of raw yoghurt, and fruity by the use of berry fruits, which are wonderfully rich in antioxidants, dietary fiber and relatively low in sugar. Alternatively, your smoothie can be made more savory by the use of a ripe avocado as the base, with some fresh herbs, like mint, or spices for flavor.

If you choose to make a cooked breakfast, a great base for this can be leftover vegetables from the night before, made into a quick frittata or fry-up. When you cook starchy vegetables like potatoes, it's a great idea to make sure you cook plenty, which can then be refrigerated overnight to convert them into resistant starch to feed your microbiome and warmed in a frying pan with plenty of coconut oil or butter and added to your breakfast or lunch. Or try an egg grilled in a half avocado topped with cheese.

If all else fails, grab a handful of your favorite tree nuts or a mouthful of nut butter as you rush out the door, or a piece of cheese and butter.

5. Mid-morning break.

With a slow burning breakfast, as suggested, you should not be hungry by mid-morning so restrict yourself to a hot drink of bone broth or herbal tea.

6. Pre-lunch.

About 20 minutes before you expect to eat lunch or dinner seems to be about the perfect time to set up your ghrelin and other appetite control hormones, so that any food cravings come under control. You are then more likely to be comfortable with eating less overall food at the upcoming meal. Eat a few of your favorite nuts like almonds or cashew nuts or, if you don't particularly like eating nuts have a good spoonful of nut butter (better if it's not peanut butter).

7. Lunch.

The same principles apply as with breakfast. Plenty of good fats, moderate amounts of protein, and minimal amounts of carbs, ideally all from vegetables or a salad.

If you're away from home during the day then lunch can be a bit trickier. It's an ideal opportunity to take some leftovers from the previous night's dinner and just warm them gently to preserve the resistant starch.

If you usually buy something for lunch, then a meat or fish salad is usually not too hard to find. You do need to be VERY careful not to get caught by hidden gluten in the form of croutons or thickeners in the salad dressing. You may need to ask for some olive oil and lemon juice to dress your salad.

Sushi or sashimi are possibilities because of the resistant starch in the pre-cooked rice. However this option is usually very low in fat and protein, so you may need to supplement with some nut butter or another good source of fat to keep you going.

8. Mid-afternoon break.

Again, with a slow-burning lunch, as suggested, containing plenty of good fats, protein, and fiber from vegetables, you should not be hungry at mid-afternoon break time. Again restrict yourself to a hot drink of bone broth, herbal tea or lots of water.

If, however, you are starting to crash, (and being tempted by that birthday cake bought by your best friend) try taking just a teaspoonful of coconut oil or a couple of teaspoons of your favorite nut butter. You are likely to be amazed at how quickly this works. It's almost instant. I highly recommend having both a jar of coconut oil and nut butter in your desk drawer for such emergencies.

9. Dinner.

Try and plan your day so you have time to prepare something delicious for dinner. Pretty much the same principles apply as with breakfast – plenty of good fats, with moderate amounts of protein.

However, this is the meal where you should try to ramp up the number of vegetables you eat, as getting a few extra good carbs at this time of day can actually help the whole process along. Having some good carbs (slow carbs) for dinner means that you are unlikely to get a blood-sugar trough in the middle of the night, which might stimulate the release of cortisol and make it difficult for you to stay asleep.

The simplest and most delicious way I know to achieve the sort of balance you need is to make a stir-fry with a piece of fatty meat the size of your palm, or a handful of mushrooms chopped up. Then throw in lots of chopped vegetables - as wide a range of types and colors as possible. Very lightly sauté your meat or mushrooms in plenty of coconut oil, or a combination of olive oil and butter, then add half a cup of water and your vegetables and cook lightly with a lid on the pan. Season with some umeboshi vinegar (a natural flavor enhancer) and herbs or spices. If the result is too much juice, just take the lid off for the last couple of minutes - Yummy.

Again, if you're eating out at a restaurant that produces 'real' food (not fast food), then a meat or fish salad is usually not too hard to find. The other simple solution is just to ask, "Can I just have more vegetables instead of .... (whatever starch is on offer i.e. rice, potatoes, pasta, and corn)". Probably Thai and Mexican are the easiest menus to work around, but low-carb eating is so common these days that most restaurants are happy to help.

Don't forget to check if there's any gluten hidden in the dressing or sauces.

It's important to eat dinner a good 3 - 4 hours before you go to bed, in other words, ideally no later than 6 - 7 pm, for two important reasons:

a)   It will make it easier for you to get off to sleep quickly when you get to bed.

b) It will be the beginning of your mini-fast, lasting 12 – 16 hours, which does very nice things to your metabolic hormones, particularly insulin and leptin. Such a mini fast will also ensure that you wake up in a state of mild ketosis, ready for another fat-burning day.

10. Give yourself a treat

It's okay to treat yourself to a couple of squares of chocolate containing 75%+ cacao mass (the higher the number, the better). Or maybe a quick dessert of some frozen berry fruit blended up with coconut cream or cream, a bit of flax seed oil and topped with a few shavings of dark chocolate.

Please try not to think of this whole process as deprivation. Rather, think of it as a new way of eating which tastes delicious because of the high

Omega-3 is Not Just Fish or Krill Oil

Having studied the science around the Omega-3s for nearly 27 years, I am acutely aware of the importance of including plenty of the primary Omega-3 (ALA) in your diet. It enhances your energy levels, puts a glow in your skin, and helps get rid of chronic inflammation.

Only by adding flax or chia seed good fats into your diet, can you get enough Omega-3 in your diet to start to bring your Omega-6/Omega-3 ratio into balance.

oil content, and is starting to make you feel like a new woman. The way this whole process works for you is very dependent on your mind-set.

16.10.3
Monitor Your Results

As I have suggested, you will likely find it very helpful to start a 'food, mood, poo' journal to note down how you're feeling after every meal and how your bowel is working.

Only by tuning into your body in this way can you start to pick up on the subtleties of how your body is responding to different foods, and thus learn what will serve you in the long term.

You may also find it helpful to apply to join our closed Facebook group – I Took Charge, where you can share your experiences with others on the same journey and ask any questions you like. This is monitored regularly and I will do my best to answer all your questions. By doing this you not only help yourself to learn what works for you, get inspiration and support, but you will also help others with their motivation and learning.

16.10.4
Everybody is Different

While it might seem that what I am recommending is very prescriptive, I only recommend this way of eating during the 'Rapid Reset' phase.

As I have said earlier, you are the only one who really knows what suits your body and makes you feel great, which is why it's important for you to become very aware of how you are feeling – it will also bring you into being present. No Doctor or author can do this for you.

Remember - "Do not believe anything I say, take only that which has the ring of truth for you." - Djwal Khul

16.11
Reset Plan: Phase 3 - Days 9 to 21

I will be very surprised if by Day 9 you are not starting to feel pretty good about yourself and starting to look at life in a very different way from the recent past. If you feel ready for it, then you could stop here – you will have already shrunk your stack of pancakes a lot.

If you are still struggling a bit, I encourage you not to give up; this may just be a slightly longer journey for you. In this case, you should carry on the way you have been eating until at least Day 21 and then re-evaluate. Most will have achieved nutritional ketosis by now but occasionally some people can take longer. However, please remember, it does take about 21 days to build a new gut lining and new habits – both are key objectives.

I also encourage you to go back to your food diary and see if there are any clues as to why you might be struggling.

Maybe you didn't handle eggs well and got a bit of a funny tummy every time you had eggs in your meal – in which case eliminate the eggs and otherwise carry on the way you have been eating until Day 21.

If you're in the first group and thriving, now is the time when you could start to reintroduce some of your favorite foods that you have been missing. Just introduce one at a time for three days and, if that goes well, try adding another favorite food for the next three days. If you can access quality, grass-fed dairy products that are rich in good fats, then I suggest you start with reintroducing some of these. Probably some butter is a good place to start. If that goes well, then try some full cream, natural and organic yoghurt (that has not been pasteurized after manufacture to prolong its shelf life. Yes – even some organic yoghurt makers do this).

By now you should be well on the way to being 'fat-adapted' and you may notice that if you have a low-fat meal for lunch, like a chicken salad or sushi, you may well crave fat at some stage during the afternoon. That's when your jars of coconut oil and nut butter can come to your rescue. Or you can make your own 'fat bombs' – there are some amazing recipes online.

Celebrate the fact that you are craving fat, not sugar – your body will be.

16.12
Onwards and Upwards

Eating this way is not necessarily the way you will want to eat for the rest of your life, so after doing this 'Rapid Reset' phase you are encouraged to reintroduce your favorite foods one at a time and see how the 'new you' reacts to them over three days. Decide for yourself whether they are still for you. You may very well find that they don't actually make you feel good anymore.

Once you have been through the 'Rapid Reset' phase and up-regulated the genes responsible for fat-burning, i.e. become fat-adapted, then you will have a lot more flexibility in the way you eat. You will find that your body can easily switch between fat-burning and glucose-burning, which gives you a high degree of flexibility about what you eat and what your body burns as fuel. It's important for your wellness that you vary the way you eat quite a lot – your body evolved to live this way and thrives on it.

For instance, many women converting to a high-fat diet discover that what food makes you feel the best changes throughout your cycle. You may find you need to eat a little more protein for a few days around ovulation, or need to eat a few more good carbs around the time of your period. If you have a carb craving, it is really important for you to remember to listen to your body and honor what it is telling you. If you are craving carbs, then have some more good carbs (or even not so good – maybe gluten free chocolate cake). Your body probably needs the extra insulin that you get from eating the carbs to help balance out your sex hormones.

The other great news is, now you are at a point where the occasional binge on the foods you feel like you're missing is important to help to make sure your body doesn't think it's going into a famine. This means that if you are out for a meal and there are no good low carb options available - it doesn't matter – just eat what looks good to you and try and have 12 – 16 hours between the dinner and breakfast and your body will just slip naturally back into fat-burning mode again.

You are likely to find that you feel wonderful eating real foods and burning primarily fat for fuel and want to keep on eating this way. The research supports the concept that, for most people, somewhere around 30% of your energy coming from GOOD carbs is a very health-promoting way to eat. The research also supports the idea that varying what you eat often is an important concept. Our ancestors didn't eat the same all the time – it varied not only from day to day but seasonally as well depending on what was plentiful at the time – be it bison or blueberries.

Because the science in this area is changing very rapidly, I encourage you to sign up to receive my blog posts where I am writing about new discoveries I have made. See – www.ITookCharge.nz/Blog, as I intend to make the information I share with you valid in the long-term.

If you have a friend whom you think might enjoy this book, please send them the link to visit www.ITookCharge.nz and read the "Look Inside" eBook, which includes the first chapter. You might well find yourself a buddy (or accountability partner) to do the 'Rapid Reset' with you. Having this kind of support from a buddy greatly increases your chances of success.

May this book help you find your own pathway to achieving your goals.

"The woman who follows the crowd will usually go no further than the crowd. The woman who walks alone is likely to find herself in places no one has ever been before."

Eda LeShan

CHAPTER 17

Take Charge of Your Sexiness

"Be the change you want to see in your relationship"

Me

17.1
Why Am I Writing This Chapter?

An essential element of our wellbeing is having successful relationships with others, and these relationships often challenge us to grow as a person. But let's face it, intimate relationships can be hard to maintain year after year after year, and one of the important glues that can help hold a relationship together is great sex.

If the sex is not great then you probably are little better than friends, so you might want to look at whether you're willing to settle for a long-term friendship or if YOU want to invest effort towards having an amazing, loving, and intimate long-term relationship.

Having an orgasm is a delicious experience, flooding your body with the feel-good hormones dopamine, oxytocin and endorphins, which counteract the negative effects of stress in an almost magical way. An orgasm will also give you a surge of HGH (don't make that an excuse not to exercise), and multiple studies have shown that women who orgasm regularly live longer, and on average, look seven years younger than their calendar age.

However, the benefits of great sex go far deeper than this by helping you to feel good about yourself, more connected to your partner, and more confident in your approach to life and just – sexy!

If you have skipped the rest of the book to get to the fun part, please go back to read and apply the rest of the book first. Otherwise you might be disappointed with the results.

Before you're ready to play, and to be your sexiest, juiciest and most playful self, you need to have your hormones in balance and to have detoxed your mind. This means you probably have had to make more than a few changes in your life. If you are stressed and your cortisol levels are high, you are not very likely to have an orgasm (maybe if you use a vibrator). Yes, I know that I said that multiple orgasms would give you pretty much a complete hormonal reset, but you probably have to get the basics right before this will work. Sorry!

The elephant in the room, which nobody really seems to talk about, is that surveys show that the majority of women (around 70% - 80%) never have an orgasm from vaginal intercourse.

Is this the way it needs to be? Absolutely not!

I think that many people's thinking on this subject is a bit confused and doesn't do anything to help you have a wonderful, juicy, and playful sex life.

For instance, I have heard a woman doctor, who lectures to other doctors on sexuality, suggest that they should redefine an orgasm as the whole of the sexual act after penetration. There is little doubt that penetrative sex, with the right person, is probably a delicious experience, but to pretend that this is an orgasm I don't think is giving anyone the right message. This doctor further suggested that vaginal contractions be called a climax, and be looked on as the cherry on top of your dessert!

It actually gets worse than this. I listened to a recent interview with John Gray, the author of 'Men Are From Mars, Women are from Venus', the biggest selling relationship book of all time. He said something along the lines of "orgasms are not as important for women as they are for men, as for women the feelings of closeness and intimacy of having sex is often enough" - which may be true. But to me, this is a huge copout for men. Would you rather have sex with closeness and intimacy and no orgasm, or amazing, heart-connected sex with multiple orgasms? Duh! Without tremendous feelings of closeness and intimacy you are unlikely to have an orgasm – let alone multiple orgasms.

This kind of thinking perpetuates the idea that it's okay for men to have an orgasm every time they have sex, while their partners often either don't have an orgasm or fake one to preserve the sense of having a mutual experience. With this kind of scenario, it is not entirely surprising that, after a while, many women might start to feel they can't be bothered with sex, and men might feel they don't get enough sex because women don't like it.

This can make your relationship really hard.

I also believe that sexual and relationship advice has focused for way too long on the erogenous zones of your body: "Just use this position and stimulate the clitoris (or the G spot or the deep spot) and you will have an orgasm". What such advice completely ignores is that the most important sexual organ that needs to be engaged in the process is a woman's mind.

If you think you CAN'T have multiple orgasms, then you WON'T have them. Your mind is VERY POWERFUL in this regard. Yet it's a routine part of the act for many stage hypnotists to bring a woman up on stage and give them multiple orgasms, purely by engaging their minds.

I know from my own experience that what looks like relatively minor changes in my approach to sex have made an enormous difference to me. Interestingly, all of the changes I have made have been, to my mind, in the way that I think about my partner, and who I am in our relationship, both in and out of the bedroom. What you do is way less important than who you are – how you feel about yourself and your emotional interactions with your partner.

I am not pretending to be a sex therapist that can solve all your problems. I'm just a guy doing my best to help you have as much fun as possible, as part of boosting your overall wellbeing. Also, based on my experience, once you start to get well, by using the tools I have given you, you will have so much energy and such a thirst for joy, that great sex will become an important desire for you.

I am seeking to nudge you in the direction of not accepting that the status quo is all there is so that you will do whatever it takes to achieve a joyful life, coming from a place of wellness.

17.2
But My Man Thinks Everything Is Fine!

What can you do to change the situation if your partner does not engage your mind and excite you in bed?

Unfortunately, I expect you will find that your partner might resist very strongly if you try and tell them what to do - for most men that pushes all the wrong buttons.

I will put my hand up and confess that I used to be part of this unconscious group until I was in a counselling session with my ex-wife when she said, "oh, the sex was okay, I guess". Ooooouch - that felt a lot like a kick in the balls. At that point in my life I had read multiple relationship and sex books (including 'Men Are from Mars, Women Are from Venus'), but I obviously hadn't got the right advice for me.

I decided that there must be something really important that I was missing, so I went on a mission to find it.

Fortunately, I found a very few amazing teachers out there who share their wonderful knowledge. Mainly about how to engage your partner's mind, share your emotions, build your confidence to share hot passionate sex, and build an amazing relationship that just keeps getting better. So life is very different for me now.

Alex Allman and David Deida were the key teachers for me, and they teach programs for women as well. On your behalf, I looked quite hard for women teaching the same sort of material and only found Jaiya teaching in a way that felt like a more universal approach to me. I think this may have something to do with sex being very different for individual women and, for women, sex seems to be far more complicated than it is for a man, so that teaching on this subject by women is often highly colored by how it is for them personally. If you want to change your experience it is going to require you to become very honest with yourself (and ideally also with your partner), about why the sex isn't working the way it should be (but don't ever confess to faking orgasms). It is also going to require you to become a bit proactive about creating the sex life you deserve.

You may think this is an impossible task because men and women want totally different things out of sex. However, recent research done by Alex Allman shows that this idea is wrong and that even though it's hidden by a completely different vocabulary around sex, both men and women want the same three things from sex:

1. We all love to give, so in sex that equates to our partner being a great receiver. In other words, they show that they really love what we do to them during sex.

2. We all want a partner who is comfortable and confident about his or her own sexuality. That means that if you are authentic and comfortable and confident in expressing your own desires around sex, this will help to give your partner the confidence to be authentic with you.

3. The last thing we all want is to be totally accepted for who we are. For instance, no matter what weird faces or noises we make when we are having an orgasm, there is no judgment; no matter what is said, there is no judgment.

According to Alex, if you are all of these three things then you are likely to be awesome in bed.

You need to realize that for a man, engaging his mind is also important- not quite as important as it is for you, granted, but still important. If you do a seductive strip in front of him, he will get an immediate erection, but if you tell him to "get hard right now, I want sex", of course, he won't. So if you lead by example and make some efforts to engage your partner's mind, you will be pleasantly surprised by how much better things will become.

You could also buy him the sequel to this book that I am going to write for men but, in the meantime, you could try some of the following ideas.

17.3
Find Your Feminine

David Deida teaches more of a spiritual approach to sex, and he likens the attraction between men and women to the two poles of a magnet. In practical terms, this means that if you want to bring out the masculine in your partner's sexuality, you need to offer the complementary element by being in your feminine. The more feminine you are in the way you behave, the more masculine he will become.

If, like many women you are a working mum, you likely get home stressed at the end of your working day only to have to deal with your children's demands and get a meal ready for your family, then get them sorted ready for tomorrow, then get the children off to bed. You almost certainly spend your evening in your stressed, 'tend and befriend' mode and you are not looking after yourself. Because if you are not dealing with your stress adequately, then your limbic system is telling you very subtly that you need to look after everyone else.

There are two potential barriers to you to being in your most feminine sexual polarity with this scenario:

Firstly, if you are working in a job where you have to be very decisive and in your masculine mode or your workplace is male-dominated, then you are likely to come home under that masculine influence and in your masculine mode – therefore little sexual polarity.

Secondly, because of the nudging from your stress hormones to 'tend', the probability is that you have also taken on doing some tasks for your partner that he is actually quite capable of doing for himself, and probably didn't ask you to do in the first place. Unfortunately, this means he starts to feel to you a bit like just another child you have to look after, which completely kills any sexual polarity between you.

If these scenarios are happening to you, then you need to bring these feelings to your awareness and use your insight to find a better way. Here are some suggestions on how to find your feminine to become the feminine pole that will create and attract the masculinity of your partner, so that sparks will fly and the juice will flow.

17.4

Feminine Meditation

De-stress yourself with a feminine meditation, which may take the form of a sacred dance - any form of dance or ritual movement done with the intention to connect with your divine feminine. Since the feminine tends to be about flow and movement and changes all the time, the masculine idea of sitting in stillness to meditate may not appeal to you at all, especially if you want to awaken your feminine.

One way in which you could do this is to turn on your favorite dance music and dance naked in front of a mirror, celebrating the bits you like and focusing on loving your wobbly bits as you dance. This will get your mind away from your day and get the energy moving in your body in a way that will enhance your femininity. The more you can love your body, the more your man will love your body – there is nothing more off-putting for a man than a woman denigrating her own body.

Feminine meditation can be a very empowering way to awaken your self-love, which is an important part of you being ready to truly love another.

17.5
Orgasmic Meditation

OM (Orgasmic Meditation), also known as DOing (Deliberate Orgasm), can be a very powerful way to involve your partner in a very intimate way, to help address a 'pleasure-deficit disorder'. Many women report that, even if they are having orgasms during sex, they have a deep hunger for something unknown, which OM can satisfy.

In OM, a partner uses the tip of their index finger (one of the most sensitive places on the body) to very gently stroke the most sensitive parts of a woman's clitoris (in the 1 o'clock position as the stroker is looking at it).

If having somebody stroke the tip of your clitoris for 15 minutes sounds a bit weird, many women report the experience can be deeply satisfying, in a way that they have not been able to achieve from anything else. It seems that there are a couple of potential reasons why this is likely:

1. The practice can completely decouple orgasm from sex so that the woman can focus on the pleasurable sensations she is getting. For this to happen it's important that both parties accept from the outset that this is not a precursor for sex. You should ideally agree to have a minimum of five 'no sex' sessions before you take things further.

Fun Fact

If you have 'a headache' then meditating will get rid of about 90% of headaches, so that's not really a viable excuse is it.

Even better, if you orgasm (doesn't matter how) this will stop the vast majority of migraine headaches in their tracks. It does this because all the endorphins, dopamine and oxytocin released during an orgasm expands the blood vessels in your brain.

And better – the rush of blood and oxygen to your brain makes your brain go wild.

And better – about a third of women report masturbating to give them a better sleep – and you know what that does to you, don't you.

2. The intense focus by both on a very small spot can induce a very intense energy exchange between the partners, to the extent that often the stroker can sort of feel some of the feelings of the woman being stroked.

It needs to be a completely goalless practice, with no expectations from either side on what might happen especially, as for first timers, your ego can really get in the way with feelings of skepticism or embarrassment.

It's a very powerful but relatively simple practice, and especially if you give a little feedback in the early stages to help your partner get it right for you, then this is probably all you need to know. However, if you want to know more go to my website, www.ITookCharge.nz/OM for links to where you can go for more detailed information.

17.6
All Day Foreplay

It's sad that most people talk about their 'sex life', as though it is something that is somehow separate from the rest of their life. Unfortunately, many men think of foreplay as that five minutes of stroking and touching 'you have to do before you get to the sex' – I wish, as a sex, we males were different, but there are things you can do to help change that.

I now understand that, as soon as you get to anything physical and naked, that's having sex, so what do I mean by all-day foreplay? It's all those little things you can do to show him that you're a sexual being, that you find him sexy, and that you are a woman and he is your man.

So this might look like:

Walking up behind him while he is making his breakfast and giving his ass a pat or a squeeze, while you kiss the back of his neck.

Sending him a text during the day saying how much you're looking forward to playing with him tonight. You can be as raunchy as you think he can handle - he is unlikely to be working late after a text like that!

Invite him to stay in bed and enjoy the show as you get dressed. Choose some of his favorite underwear and dress yourself very slowly and seductively in front of him. This is you setting the mood for the rest of the day so, now every time you send him a message; he will replay the show in his head.

Let him be your hero – when you have a jar of pickles to open, pass it to him saying "Honey can you open this for me". This will give him a wee surge of testosterone because he was able to do this for you, that he just wouldn't get if you opened it for yourself. Men want to be your hero because it helps him to feel like a man, which is exactly what you want him to feel. I'm sure you could get that lid off if you really tried, but don't – ever, when he is around.

Wait for him to open the door for you!

Give him a big smoochy kiss and a sensuous cuddle when he gets home to get his mind thinking about what might happen later in the evening - or right then if there are no children around.

17.7
The Power of Positive Reinforcement

You all know about the power of making positive comments, don't you? You know you can't go wrong saying how much you love his cock, don't you? However, did you know that ANY positive comment actually works for BOTH OF YOU, in a very special way?

For instance, let's say one of the things that attracted you to your partner in the first place was his broad, well-muscled shoulders.

Now, if you tell him that you love his sexy shoulders then he will think 'Wow she still thinks I'm sexy, especially my shoulders – Hmm, maybe I will actually go to the gym tomorrow and spend a bit of time with some weights to keep them looking great'.

So you have done two great things for him. You have made him feel sexy, and you have also motivated him to look after his body to keep it looking sexy for YOU.

The other less well-known and fun part of commenting on his sexy shoulders, is that ALL our brains are hard-wired to have beliefs that are congruent with what we say. So every time you say he has sexy shoulders, you are reinforcing in your own mind just how sexy you think his shoulders are.

This means that every time you check out the new guy that walks into the room, his shoulders will be more likely to compare unfavorably with your partner's, which does very nice things for your attraction to him and therefore your relationship.

17.8
It Works on You Too

If you have some body image issues you can also use your brain's need to have beliefs consistent with what you say to help you feel better about your body.

So, for instance, if there's something about your legs that you are not totally comfortable with then spend a few minutes occasionally being grateful for them. Next time you're sitting there rubbing some moisturizer on them, you could tell your legs out loud how strong they are or how wonderful they are at getting you around and allowing you to play with your children and dance with your partner, or how wonderful and stroke-able they feel and how much you love their curves, etc.

Once you have done this a few times you will be amazed at how differently you feel about your legs or whatever body part you have been having issues with.

17.9
Keeping It Hot Long-Term

Another time you can use your brain's need to have beliefs consistent with what you say is during the afterglow after sex when you are both very open and vulnerable.

If you've just had a lovely session when things went pretty well for both of you, then you could say, "It just keeps getting better, doesn't it." Again, this works for both of you in that you will really think it did just get better but, because he's also very open, he will likely think "Yes it does, doesn't it."

This is a very powerful way for both of you to think that what you've got is pretty special and that together you are a pretty hot item, which will do a lot to help reduce the need for either of you to look elsewhere for excitement.

Unfortunately, a man's limbic system is pre-programmed to look for sexual variety, as this enhances the chances of his genes surviving. However, a man is more than his limbic brain, so as long as you recognize the underlying programming and work with him to bring a variety of moods and stimulants into your sex life, then this doesn't have to be a problem. There is good evidence that this should not include watching porn together.

Be creative. Try grabbing a rug and leading him out onto the back lawn on a hot, full moon night. This can be a lot of fun – it's amazing how the spice of potentially being caught by the neighbors can fire things up.

Or maybe he's gone to bed before you, so you put on some sexy music and do a slow strip just out of reach. If he tries to grab, you say, "no touching allowed". You have just created a little fantasy, which likely stimulates both of your imaginations. Using a 'fantasy' in such a way has been shown to be a powerful glue for many couples.

It's really important for all your relationships that you learn to set boundaries and say "No", "Yes" or "Wait" and also to respect it when your partner uses these words. It's also important that you help to create an environment where either of you can feel 'safe' to express a desire to try something new – it may not turn out to be something you want to do long-term, but it can be a lot of fun trying.

Only by creating a 'safe' environment like this in your relationship can you deepen your understanding of each other's pleasure maps, to uncover new possibilities for pleasure and play, and thus become more effective and compassionate lovers.

17.10
Get Physical

You might want to re-read Chapter 14.1.5 Get an Oxytocin Fix at this point, because any form of touch, but particularly on your naked skin, starts to build your oxytocin levels towards an orgasm. Women seem to know this instinctively, but sometimes your partner may need a little encouragement.

Do you want him to hold your hand, stroke your arm, put his arm around you, smack your bum, and give you a full-body massage ... the works? The best way you can teach him that this is what you want, is to touch him in ways that you want to be touched – he will respond to the oxytocin fix as well. Just grab his hand while you are sitting together.

If your partner is not touching you where or in a way that's working for you, you may need to find a way to guide him in the right direction. Telling him "don't touch me there, touch me up here" is never going to work, as you will sound like a teacher, but there's usually another way to get the desired result.

For instance, you can guide his body with yours. So you could use your arm to guide his arm and hand to where you want him to touch you, and then use sounds and movement to encourage him when he gets it right.

You will be pleasantly surprised at how easy it can be to achieve the desired result and how much better things can be. It just requires you to be a bit proactive to move things to where you want them to be.

Many women prefer a really light touch, especially early on, and probably the only way to communicate this is by telling him. You may have some nervousness about expressing needs like this because of past experiences, but it important for your self-love that you become more confident about setting boundaries.

17.11
Flaunt Your Pheromones

One of the primal criteria preprogramed into men's brains, which used to be important in finding a mate who could successfully carry his genes, was 'did she smell healthy'. This is why we now have a huge perfume industry that tries to help you to smell good, and thus attractive to men.

This industry has also been searching (so far unsuccessfully) for the one elusive human pheromone that would make you attractive to all men. I personally suspect they are unlikely ever to find a single such wonder chemical.

Apparently, some men secrete significant amounts of androsterone (a precursor to testosterone) through their skin, which seems to give them sex appeal no matter what they look like. Women also secrete much smaller amounts of androsterone as well.

The only female equivalent found so far is a compound called copulin which is secreted, in vaginal fluids, particularly around ovulation. Copulin has been demonstrated to induce men to produce more testosterone. Copulin secretion also to tends to bring women who live together or frequently associate, into ovulating at the same time.

There is no doubt that you have a unique, personal scent that your baby and your partner will respond to. Moreover, there is some evidence that women will respond positively to someone who smells like their partner, but are these scents pheromones? Probably not.

Rather than waiting for that elusive magical pheromone, you can 'Take Charge' of the way you smell. You may recall in Chapter 9 Bugs Are Important, I talked about not using soap in the shower to allow your skin microbiome to stabilize into a healthy balance and thus allow your natural personal scent to come through.

If you want to take advantage of the impact of your natural personal scent or pheromones on your partner, there are now a couple of options. You could try rubbing a live natural yoghurt all over your body, as I did in Thailand. We are now starting to see the development of probiotics specifically designed for the skin.

The trend setter is called Mother Dirt, AO+ Mist, which is designed to rebalance your skin microbiome, even allowing you not to shower if you so choose (although why you would beats me). As well as allowing your natural personal scent to show through, because of a rebalanced skin microbiome, this product is claimed to improve skin appearance including sensitivity, blotchiness, oiliness, and dryness. Early research suggests that these are reasonable claims. I'm sure we will see many more products coming into this space in the future.

In the meantime, if the idea appeals to you, try one of these options yourself and maybe on your partner as well. I am confident you will enjoy their natural personal scent. In my experience, the scent of my partner changes throughout her cycle and can send some very delicious signals. Are these pheromones? Again, probably not. They may just be changes in her skin microbiome in response to her hormonal patterns but, what I do know, is that the way she smells is an important component of our erotic life.

17.12
Change Your Mind-set

You are worth it, so detox your mind. It's really important that you take active steps to clear any resentment you may have around him - see Chapter 14 Detoxing Your Mind, so that you can have a complete, adult relationship with him.

David Deida talks about the way relationships have changed since the time of sexual liberation towards the end of the last century. Before this, the archetypal relationship was between the 'submissive housewife' and the 'macho jerk', where most men did not attempt to get in touch with their feminine side and most women were too suppressed to be in touch with their masculine side.

Fortunately, relationships have evolved since then but, for a while, the pendulum swung rather too far the other way towards 'career woman' and 'sensitive new-age guy'. In this kind of relationship, women were striving to be independent of men, by having their own careers, but to some extent they lost touch with their femininity. Some men, in their attempts to be more supportive of their women and her career and to help look after their family, to some extent lost touch with their masculinity. The unfortunate side effect of this evolution of relationships was that people became less polarized sexually because of the emphasis on getting in touch with the duality of our natures, be it masculine or feminine.

The associated lack of 'magnetic' attraction obviously doesn't make for great sex.

Fortunately, we are in a time when relationships are evolving further. To move into the next stage of relationships you need to embrace the fact that if you want to have hot, passionate sex with your partner you need to let go of any need to be in control, totally embrace your feminine, and become the magnetic pole that attracts his masculine.

One of the most powerful things you can do to enhance your love life is to become present in the NOW. Forget tomorrows to do list and focus ALL your attention on your lover. Ideally you would allow yourself to become very vulnerable, and open your heart to him with love. You can do this as easily as saying it, either internally or out loud, i.e. " .... I open my heart to you with love". If you think it's appropriate, you can invite your partner to do the same.

And if you can bring yourself to do this with your lovemaking, then you have made wonderful steps with detoxing your mind so that very magical things will start to happen with your relationships, and magical things will start to happen for your overall wellbeing.

"The road will ALWAYS be rocky...

It might never be EASY...

But if you decide to have the necessary maturity, courage, and self-esteem, you can actually enjoy and grow and become very happy in your relationships with the opposite sex."

Alex Allman

Appendix A
Recommended Supplements

Most supplements get made in a chemical factory, so do not contain the important co-factors associated the nutrients in their biological form. My Waihi Bush Organic Farm (WBOF) products are entirely food based, meaning they are made only from foods, plants or herbs; substances your body is familiar with using. My team and I scour the world to find the highest quality ingredients (Certified Organic and Local, if possible). These products incorporate all the knowledge and experience I have gained over the last 27 years.

If you choose to use other products to support you on your journey to wellness, remember to choose supplements that are derived from food wherever possible.

I recommend the following products to support you through the 'Rapid Reset' phase and beyond.

A.1 Pancake #2 – Stress Hormones

Dr Wilson's Super Adrenal Stress Formula

The Dr Wilson's formula is designed to support your adrenal glands back to health and contains a superior balance of vitamins and minerals in a time-release caplet, which is why it is included in the 'Rapid Reset Pack'. The slow release feature means your blood levels stay relatively constant for about four hours and you don't pee them out to waste shortly after taking them.

Available online from www.waihibush.co.nz/products/other-products.

Do you need to keep on taking it after the 'Rapid Reset' phase? In theory not, because of the following:

1. You are doing your preferred method of 'Mind Detox' most days, thus reducing the load on your adrenal glands.

2. Your leaky gut has healed and your gut microbiome is in a healthier balance, so your bugs are producing many of your Vitamins for you.

3. You are taking your WBOF Daily Boost for Woman most days which supplies high levels of Minerals and useful amounts of many Vitamins.

However, the real answer is maybe because of the following:

1. If you had symptoms of low adrenal function, your adrenal glands could

still take a while to get back to full health.

2.   Everyone is different.

Ask yourself if your energy levels and libido are where you would like them to be, and wait for your body's response to that question – it will come, I promise you. If the answer is no, then I suggest you take them for another month and then ask yourself the same question.

A.2 Pancake #4 - Minerals

WBOF Daily Boost for Women

Unless you live close to a glacier or desert where the soils are geologically very young (or you keep your garden young by adding lots of seaweed), then your food does not provide all the minerals your body needs to be healthy. This means you need to supplement your minerals with a product like my Daily Boost for Women.

If you are looking to use another product bear in mind, that in nature, minerals are always bound to another compound, like an amino acid, so in high-quality products, minerals are bound, or "chelated," with an amino acid to allow them to be absorbed more effectively.

An alternative, could be Vital Earth Mineral Blend Fulvic-Humic, which are derived from ancient deposits and are highly bioavailable. I suggest you start with ¼ - ½ dose and work up gradually if you feel like more is needed. If you choose another source, you need to select a high-quality, chelated multimineral.

A.3 Pancake #5 – Hormone Balance

WBOF Daily Boost for Woman

The best way to balance your sex hormones is to use phytoestrogens (See Chapter 7.4.6). Daily Boost for Woman provides about 80mg per day of Lignans from flax flour.

As an alternative you could use Coumestans from a red clover extract, which provides about 40 mg per day.

A.4 Pancake #7 – Pro Biotics

WBOF Gut Support is a world-class synbiotic powder which includes probiotics, prebiotics and enzymes to dissolve gut plaque, and is designed to heal and rebalance the gut.

You should also include locally produced Organic fermented vegetables in your diet on a regular basis. The Urban Monk range is available in NZ, online from www.waihibush.co.nz/products/other-products.

As an alternative, look for locally produced Organic fermented vegetables.

A.5 Pancake #9 – Omega-3

Step 1 - WBOF Super Boost Omega-3 Blend - this unique organic flax seed oil blend provides both the primary and secondary Omega-3 and Omega-6 you need during the first two months (including the 'Rapid Reset' phase). Take 1-2 servings daily.

After about two months the genes for creating your own secondary Omega-3 and Omega-6 are likely to be up-regulated and working for you. You are then likely to be ready to try switching to:

Step 2 - WBOF Flax Original – this is pure flaxseed oil rich in Omega-3. Take 1-2 servings daily and be very aware of how your body responds to the change.

If, after somewhere between six months to six years you start to get symptoms like dry skin or hair, it's likely that your body has gone past the desired 1:1 balance. This will suggest that you are likely to be ready to switch to:

Step 3 - WBOF Flax Balance – this is a blend of flaxseed oil and safflower oil which provides a balance of Omega-3 and Omega-6. Take 1-2 serving daily and be very aware of how your body responds to the change. If this blend feels good to you, then take this for the rest of your life to provide the Omega-3 and Omega-6 your body needs to build the 500 million healthy new cells you make each day.

Getting a blood test to find out your body's Omega-6/Omega-3 ratio used to be an expensive option, but the cost is dropping with the recent introduction of testing a dried blood spot from a finger prick, so you might want to try getting a blood test to help you decide which blend is for you.

As an alternative to Step 1, look for a quality blend of Evening Primrose oil and blackcurrant or fish oil and take with a quality flax seed oil – remember that if it doesn't taste good, it's not good for you.

When you are ready for Step 2 you can stop taking the Evening Primrose oil and blackcurrant or fish oil blend.

When you are ready for Step 3 you will find that most manufacturers of quality flax seed oil also have a blend which supplies a balanced ratio of Omega-3 and Omega-6.

A.6 Pancake #10 – Body Detox

WBOF Gut Support

The MOST important thing you need to achieve to support your body to detox is to have a bowel movement 1-2 times daily. Take this supplement as often as you need to achieve such regularity – usually one serving per day.

It would also help if you did a two weekly bowel detox with this product at the beginning of spring and autumn for the rest of your life. If you love the flavor, it is safe to take on an ongoing basis.

I have been designing foods that support wellness for over 27 years and have put together a 'Rapid Reset Pack', which contains all the products you need for your 21-day 'Rapid Reset'. If you choose to, you can purchase the recommended products either as a bundle (including bone broth), by subscription or individually from www.ITookCharge.nz/RapidResetPantry for delivery worldwide.

Appendix B
Take Care of Your Mouth

As I discussed in Chapter 9 Bugs Are Important, your mouth is the first line of defense for anything entering your digestive system. Also that what is happening in your mouth can be a significant source of chronic inflammation. It's important you realize that everything that is happening in your mouth affects your entire immune system – you are all interconnected.

So, if you have some metal in your mouth like an amalgam filling, or a crown or a brace wire that may be challenging your immune system, then your immune system is being challenged continuously as long as that is in your mouth. This has the highly undesirable effect of reducing your immune system's ability to respond to any new challenge that arises.

Just as there is a rapidly growing number of Functional Medicine practitioners who look at the big picture of your health. There is also a rapidly growing number of Biological Dentists who are informed about the issues I am discussing briefly in this Appendix and will be willing to work with you to find a solution to help you to be well. So here is what I have learnt on my journey.

B.1 Cavities

Tooth decay is the most prevalent chronic disease, affecting more than half the world's population, and the WHO (World Health Organization) states that tooth decay shares common risk factors with the four leading chronic diseases - cardiovascular diseases, cancer, chronic respiratory diseases and diabetes.

This means that most people have some form of dental fillings, but usually did not discuss the materials used to fill the cavities with their dentist. Dental amalgam has been the go-to dental filling material for more than 150 years because it's affordable and durable. However about half the metallic content of the amalgam used is liquid mercury, a heavy metal known to be toxic, causing brain, heart, kidney, lung and immune system damage.

The safety of mercury in your teeth has been debated for many years, and the official position of some authorities, such as the NZ Dental Association and the US FDA, is that dental amalgam is safe for use in adults. However, the European Union has banned the use of amalgam fillings in 2018, for children under the age of 15 and for pregnant or nursing women.

A very recently published study of nearly 15,000 individuals in the USA showed that those with more than eight fillings had about 150% more mercury in their blood than those with no amalgam fillings. In the USA, 25% of the population has 11 or more fillings. The data from this survey suggests that a big chunk of the population is getting enough mercury to be adversely affecting their health. The research data further suggests that the gut microbiome is converting some of this mercury to a form called methylmercury that is substantially more toxic than metallic mercury.

While it is widely accepted that mercury is the most poisonous, nonradioactive, naturally occurring substance on a planet, the official position of most dental organizations is that the amount of mercury you are exposed to from amalgam fillings is acceptable. On the other hand, the WHO has stated that there is no 'safe' level of mercury exposure.

Given that it is not cheap to have all your mercury amalgam fillings removed, YOU need to assess how comfortable you are with the level of mercury in your mouth.

Another factor you may wish to consider in this debate is that there are now studies linking amalgam fillings and mercury toxicity to gut dysbiosis and the development of leaky gut. If you have serious health issues, such as an autoimmune condition, your body's ability to heal from this is likely to be enhanced by having your amalgam fillings removed. The less well you are, the more likely you are to benefit from having them safely removed.

About twenty years ago I watched a documentary discussing the safety of mercury fillings, and the chairman of the New Zealand Dental Association reassured everyone about the safety of mercury for use in dental fillings. However, during the interview, he let slip that all the amalgam waste not used in the fillings must be stored under liquid in the dental surgery while awaiting disposal, so I thought "it's not safe in the dental surgery, but it is safe in my mouth" - Hmmm. This was enough to convince me that I wanted my mouth full of mercury removed.

At my next dental visit, I told my dentist that I wanted all my amalgam fillings removed. He asked "Why? They are perfectly safe". So I asked him if it was correct that the amalgam waste not used in fillings had to be stored under liquid to prevent the off-gassing of mercury vapor into the surgery -"Yes it does". So I said, "you're telling me that amalgam is not safe in your surgery, but it is safe in my mouth". There was a very long pause, and then he said, "Okay, I'll do your white dentistry." Unfortunately, this was not his specialty, so he didn't take the required precautions to protect me (or himself and his staff) from the mercury released during the removal process, so I ended up with significant memory problems for several months while my body detoxed my mercury levels.

I hope you will take from this that you really don't want any amalgam fillings in your mouth because they will be continuously releasing mercury into your body, particularly when you have a hot drink, chew food, clean your teeth or grind your teeth while you're asleep.

Also, if you do choose to have them removed, it's important you find a biological dentist who specializes in white dentistry so that they are removed safely and replaced with safer alternatives – the latest recommendations on how to achieve this are called the Safe Mercury Amalgam Removal Technique (SMART).

B.2 Root Canals

"In my experience, up to 40% of the root canals done in the past have some level of bacterial infection that is visible on imaging."

Carey O'Rielly, DDS

The second most likely intervention in your mouth is called a root canal, which is the usual remedy when you have a painful infected tooth. The dentist goes in and kills the nerve, removes what they can of the dead material, sterilizes the pulp chamber where the nerve used to be and seals it up. They will then tell you that the tooth is now 'non-vital'; sterile and perfectly 'safe'.

The bit they don't tell you is that 'non-vital' means dead tissue which your immune system rejects, forming a protective barrier around the tooth that prevents access by antibiotics and the white blood cells of your immune system to the dead tooth.

The other bit they don't tell you is that each tooth has over 4,000 meters of very fine tubules in the dentin layer, which are designed to carry nutrients into your live tooth. Because it is physically impossible to sterilize all 4,000 meters of these tubules, they form a perfect environment for an explosion of anaerobic bacteria living in the dead tooth – over 80 different, potentially toxic species have been found in root canal tooth samples.

These factors combined mean that there is a low proportion of teeth which have root canals, that do not carry a silent infection.

Every time you bite down on this tooth some of these bacteria are forced out into your bloodstream, providing a huge on-going challenge to your immune system and promoting chronic inflammation in your body.

If you have existing root canals and background inflammation, your immune system is almost certainly being continuously compromised and you would be prudent to consult a biological dentist to discuss other treatment options. The success rate used to be quite low, but very new technologies are reducing the rate of visible infections, but you would be wise to check out the existence of silent infections.

B.3 Cavitations

Cavitations can form when you have a tooth extracted, particularly a wisdom tooth. Bacteria may invade the hole in the bone where the tooth came from, especially if the extraction site is not allowed to bleed and flush the area clean. Gum tissue can then grow over the hole, followed by bone, which can leave potentially highly toxic bacteria living happily in a cavity in your jaw bone, being fed by you and leaking toxins into your body, but not accessible to your immune system or antibiotics. It's a very similar scenario to what can happen with a root canal, but they can be very difficult to detect on an x-ray, potentially leaving you wondering why you have FLC syndrome.

Fortunately, about ten years ago, a major technological advance was achieved with the use of 3-dimensional scanners like the CT scan. This has led to an explosion of cavitation detections from what were previously unexplained infections and pain.

An informed dentist will not insist on packing the site of an extracted tooth with gauze to try and stop the bleeding as quickly as possible. Rather they will encourage bleeding to help flush the extraction site clean and allow it to heal cleanly. If you do end up with a cavitation in your jaw, a biological dentist can cut into the hole and clean it out so that it can heal and your immune system will heave a sigh of relief.

B.4 My Experience

I grew up in an age where the State paid for well-meaning dental nurses to look after children's teeth and they drilled and filled your teeth with amalgam with great enthusiasm, so I had a mouth full of mercury amalgams when I made the decision to have them removed.

As I have already mentioned, the removal did not go smoothly and in fact I found many years later that the dentist had left small pockets of amalgam in all my teeth - welcome to round two of amalgam removal, done much more safely this time.

All this seems to have contributed to me having ongoing issues with gingivitis, and after several years of doing all the right things suggested by my dentist and my dental hygienist, things were getting slowly but progressively worse. Because of the way I think, I decided that there must be a better way of doing this, so I started looking in the research literature for alternatives. I now use a four-pronged approach using new technologies:

Step 1 - was a battery operated, Ionic action toothbrush developed in Japan. It works because dental plaque is bonded to your teeth by positive ions. The tiny negative ion flow produced by the toothbrush when in use, breaks this plaque bonding mechanism. Several research studies have shown the result to be around 50% better plaque removal than ordinary tooth brushing. This was step one and eliminated my gum bleeding and has given me whiter teeth than anything my dentist could do for me (including the use of overnight whitener held on by a custom mold). The brand I use is called hyG.

Step 2 - was to start using a water flosser which uses rapidly pulsating high- pressure water to remove any food deposits from between the teeth and below the gum line while breaking up clumps of plaque. Research has shown that it is substantially more effective than dental floss for reducing gingivitis and gingival bleeding, and at removing plaque. It is particularly effective at penetrating below the gum line, which has been shown to reduce this hard- to-access plaque and contribute to a reduction in gum pocket depth.

You do have to be a bit careful not to jet too hard below the gum line as you could potentially damage the gum trying to heal back onto the tooth.

I find it a very effective and easy-to-use alternative to the unpleasant dental floss and bottlebrush approach recommended by my dental hygienist - I wish I had discovered it years ago. The brand I use is a Waterpik.

Step 3 - was to start using a prebiotic, nutritional formulation toothpaste designed to support a balanced oral microbiome and re-mineralize your teeth. This has given me a much fresher mouth in the morning and reduced tooth sensitivity, which are both effects of having a healthy microbiome.

The brand I use is called Revitin. I have not been able to find any similar products as all the potential alternatives contain essential oils as flavorings, which would distort your oral microbiome.

Step 4 - which I started at the same time as Step 3, was to use a probiotic lozenge that contains specific strains of the bacteria, Streptococcus salivarius M18.

Research has shown that when used with regular oral hygiene, this strain is effective in promoting a healthy, balanced microbiome in your mouth by inhibiting the growth of S. mutans, S. pyogenes and S. sobrinus which are the main species that contribute to tooth cavities. M18 is also capable of producing enzymes that have been shown to inhibit the accumulation and acidification of plaque.

The brand I use is called Blis M18.

B.5 My Results

Now all my gum bleeding has gone, and my gum pockets are decreasing in size and my teeth are a nice white color. Also, my dentist has finally stopped suggesting that I need to have my gums surgically pared away (root planing), so the tartar in the gum pockets can be cleaned up – well worth the changes to the way I do things, I reckon.

Further Reading Suggestions

Biobehavioral responses to stress in females: Tend-and-befriend, not fight-or-flight. Taylor, S. E., Klein, L. C., Lewis, B. P., Gruenewald, T. L., Gurung, R. A. R, & Updegraff, J. A. (2000). Psychological Review, 107, 441-429.

Creating A Bug Free Mind – The Secret to Progress. Andy Shaw, 2010

Eat Dirt - Why Leaky Gut May Be the Root Cause of Your Health Problems and 5 Surprising Steps to Cure It. Josh Axe. 2016

Eat Fat, Get Thin - Why the Fat We Eat Is the Key to Sustained Weight Loss and Vibrant Health. Mark Hyman, 2016

Fats that Heal Fats that Kill – The complete guide to fats, oils, cholesterol and human health. Udo Erasmus, 1993

Grain Brain - The Surprising Truth about Wheat, Carbs, and Sugar - Your Brain's Silent Killers. David Perlmutter, 2014

Iodine: Why you need it, Why you can't live without it. David Brownstein, 2014

My Stroke of Insight – A Brain Scientists Personal Journey. Jill Bolte Taylor, 2009

No Grain, No Pain – A 30-day Diet for Eliminating the Root Cause of Chronic Pain. Peter Osborne, 2016

Revolutionary Sex – The Secret To Mind-Blowing Sex & Intimacy. Alex Allman, 2006

Rushing Woman's Syndrome – The impact of a never ending to-do list on your health. Libby Weaver, 2011

SuperCharge Your Brain. David Jockers, 2013

The Autoimmune Solution - Prevent and Reverse the Full Spectrum of Inflammatory Symptoms and Diseases. Amy Myers 2017

The End of Alzheimer's - The First Program to Prevent and Reverse Cognitive Decline. Dale Bredesen, 2017

The Hormone Cure - Reclaim Balance, Sleep and Sex Drive; Lose Weight; Feel Focused, Vital, and Energized Naturally with the Gottfried Protocol. Sara Gottfried, 2014

The Hormone Fix – Burn Fat Naturally, Boost Energy, Sleep Better, and Stop Hot Flashes, the Keto-Green Way. Anna Cabeca, 2018

The Iodine Crisis: What You Don't Know About Iodine Can Wreck Your Life Lynne Farrow, 2013.

The Microbiome Diet- The Scientifically Proven Way to Restore Your Gut Health and Achieve Permanent Weight Loss. Raphael Kellman, 2015

The Omega Plan: the Medically Proven Diet That Gives You the Essential Nutrients You Need. Artemis Simopoulos & Jo Robinson, 1998

The Way of the Superior Man – A spiritual Guide to Mastering the Challenges of Women, Work and Sexual Desire. David Deida, 2011

What Your Doctor May Not Tell You About Menopause – The Breakthrough Book on Natural Progesterone. John Lee, 2004

DEDICATION

I dedicate this book to my partner Lara, who embodies what this book is about and to all those who are dealing with the Feel Like Crap syndrome.

May you find another way and a solution in this book.

ACKNOWLEDGMENTS

I first want to thank my parents for the loving upbringing they gave me, and particularly my father, who always encouraged me to ask Why.

To my partner Lara, you bring joy to my life, and I couldn't have written this book without you. Your wisdom and love have made me a better man and teacher.

To my editor, Alan Baddock, whose ability to find any weakness in my arguments, his insight and skills, have helped to make this book what it is.

To our Jack Russel dog, Pippin, for reminding me every morning that life is so full of love and joy and excitement.

To my wonderful family and staff, who have coped with me taking lots of time out to get this book written.

To my designer Les Stoddart, Copyfast who created the cover design and internal layout.

To my customers of the last 27 years, who have challenged me to find the information I need to answer their questions accurately.

To my beta test group of 13 women and two men who road-tested the book and the 'Rapid Reset' protocol and provided valuable tweaks to make it more understandable for all those who follow.

To the many, many researchers and authors who have made such huge advances in understanding how the human body works. This is my best attempt to translate your work into an actionable plan to improve women's wellness.

ABOUT THE AUTHOR

David Musgrave first started producing flaxseed oil with health in mind in 1992. This was prompted by the rapid results seen when he gave some imported oil to his youngest son Oliver, who had had major eczema for two and a half years after his measles immunization.

Before this, David spent 20 years as a research scientist in agriculture. For the last 27 years, he has actively researched the role of nutrition, mind and body toxicity in optimizing health and seen major benefits in the health of himself, family and customers.

This knowledge has been used to both develop innovative products and to write this book for you.

Lightning Source UK Ltd.
Milton Keynes UK
UKHW021133250222
399234UK00007B/1211